Non-Epileptic Seizures

Non-Epileptic Seizures

Second Edition

Edited by

John R. Gates, M.D.
Clinical Professor of Neurology, University of Minnesota Medical School, Minneapolis; Director, Adult Services, Minnesota Epilepsy Group, P.A., United Hospital and Children's Clinics and Hospitals, St. Paul

A. James Rowan, M.D.
Professor of Neurology, Mount Sinai School of Medicine of the City University of New York, New York; Chief of Neurology Service, Bronx Veterans Affairs Medical Center, Bronx, New York

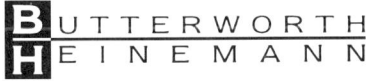

Boston   Oxford   Auckland   Johannesburg   Melbourne   New Delhi

Copyright © 2000 by Butterworth–Heinemann

 A member of the Reed Elsevier group

All rights reserved.

No part of this publication may be reproduced, stored in a retrieval system, or transmitted in any form or by any means, electronic, mechanical, photocopying, recording, or otherwise, without the prior written permission of the publisher.

Every effort has been made to ensure that the drug dosage schedules within this text are accurate and conform to standards accepted at time of publication. However, as treatment recommendations vary in the light of continuing research and clinical experience, the reader is advised to verify drug dosage schedules herein with information found on product information sheets. This is especially true in cases of new or infrequently used drugs.

∞ Recognizing the importance of preserving what has been written, Butterworth–Heinemann prints its books on acid-free paper whenever possible.

 Butterworth–Heinemann supports the efforts of American Forests and the Global ReLeaf program in its campaign for the betterment of trees, forests, and our environment.

Library of Congress Cataloging-in-Publication Data
ISBN 0-7506-7026-6

British Library Cataloguing-in-Publication Data
A catalogue record for this book is available from the British Library.

The publisher offers special discounts on bulk orders of this book.
For information, please contact:

Manager of Special Sales
Butterworth–Heinemann
225 Wildwood Avenue
Woburn, MA 01801-2041
Tel: 781-904-2500
Fax: 781-904-2620

For information on all Butterworth–Heinemann publications available, contact our World Wide Web home page at: http://www.bh.com

10 9 8 7 6 5 4 3 2 1

Printed in the United States of America

This book is dedicated to the memory of Fritz E. Dreifuss, M.B., F.R.C.P., F.R.A.C.P., and Ronald L. Martin, M.D.

These two men were giants in their respective fields, and it is only appropriate to dedicate a multidisciplinary book that captures the extraordinary spirit of collaborative cooperation and consensus building that characterized them both.

Contents

Contributing Authors   xi
Preface   xvii

I. NEUROLOGIC ASPECTS OF NON-EPILEPTIC SEIZURES IN THE ADULT AND PEDIATRIC PATIENT

1. Epidemiology and Classification of Non-Epileptic Events   3
   John R. Gates

2. Diagnosis of Non-Epileptic Seizures   15
   A. James Rowan

3. Unusual Epileptic Events and Non-Epileptic Seizures: Differential Diagnosis and Coexistence   31
   Orrin Devinsky and Joel O. Paraiso

4. Non-Epileptic Paroxysmal Neurologic Events   51
   Frederick Andermann

5. Parasomnia Purgatory: Epileptic/Non-Epileptic Parasomnia Interface   71
   Mark W. Mahowald and Carlos H. Schenck

6. Non-Epileptic Seizures in Children   95
   Frank J. Ritter and Prakash Kotagal

7. Part Summary: Neurologic Aspects of Non-Epileptic Seizures in the Adult and Pediatric Patient   111
   John R. Gates

II. PSYCHOLOGICAL AND NEUROPSYCHOLOGICAL EVALUATION OF THE PATIENT WITH NON-EPILEPTIC SEIZURES

8. Use of Neuropsychological Testing to Differentiate Neurologic from Non-Neurologic Disorders   115
   John A. Walker

9. Cognitive and Psychological Functioning in Patients with Non-Epileptic Seizures   123
   Sara J. Swanson, Jane A. Springer, Selim R. Benbadis, and George L. Morris III

10. Neuropsychological Performance and Cognitive Complaints in Epileptic and Non-Epileptic Seizure Patients   139
Gail L. Risse, Sharon L. Mason, and D. Kent Mercer

11. Depression and Anxiety in Patients with Non-Epileptic versus Epileptic Seizures   151
Nancy Donofrio, Kenneth Perrine, Kenneth R. Alper, and Orrin Devinsky

12. Relationship between Quality of Life Variables and Personality Factors in Patients with Epilepsy and Non-Epileptic Seizures   159
David W. Loring, Kimford J. Meador, Don W. King, and Bruce P. Hermann

13. Part Summary: Psychological and Neuropsychological Evaluation of the Patient with Non-Epileptic Seizures   169
Carl B. Dodrill and Mark D. Holmes

III. COGNITIVE AND PSYCHOLOGICAL FUNCTIONING AND TREATMENT OF THE PEDIATRIC PATIENT WITH NON-EPILEPTIC SEIZURES

14. Cognitive Features and Predisposing Factors in Children with Psychogenic Seizures   185
Ann Hempel

15. Characteristics of Pediatric Non-Epileptic Seizure Patients: A Retrospective Study   197
Jane Williams and Mitzie L. Grant

16. Psychological Assessment and Treatment of Non-Epileptic Seizures and Related Symptoms in Children and Adolescents   207
Audrey M. W. Ho, Marilyn J. Ransby, Kevin Farrell, Mary Connolly, and Nancy Thornton

17. Adolescents' and Parents' Perception of Non-Epileptic Seizures: A Retrospective and Qualitative Glance   227
Lucyna M. Lach and Louis Peltz

18. Munchausen Syndrome by Proxy and Svengali Syndrome   237
Fritz E. Dreifuss and John R. Gates

19. Part Summary: Cognitive and Psychological Functioning and Treatment of the Pediatric Patient with Non-Epileptic Seizures   245
Ann Hempel

IV. PSYCHIATRIC ASPECTS OF THE PATIENT WITH NON-EPILEPTIC SEIZURES

20. Nosology, Classification, and Differential Diagnosis
    of Non-Epileptic Seizures: An Alternative Proposal 253
    Ronald L. Martin and John R. Gates

21. Relationship of Remote and Recent Life Events to the Onset
    and Course of Non-Epileptic Seizures 269
    Elizabeth S. Bowman

22. Non-Epileptic Seizures as a Paradigm for Research
    on Historical Theories of Conversion 285
    Kenneth R. Alper

23. Use of Hypnosis to Differentiate Epileptic from
    Non-Epileptic Events 295
    John J. Barry and Orit Atzmon

24. On the Psychobiology of Non-Epileptic Seizures 305
    Dietrich Blumer

25. Treatment of the Adult Patient with Non-Epileptic
    Seizures 311
    Venkat Ramani

    Index 317

Contributing Authors

Kenneth R. Alper, M.D.
Assistant Professor of Psychiatry and Neurology, New York University School of Medicine, New York; Attending Neuropsychiatrist, New York University Comprehensive Epilepsy Center, New York

Frederick Andermann, M.D., F.R.C.P.C.
Professor of Neurology and Pediatrics, McGill University Faculty of Medicine, Montreal, Quebec; Director of Epilepsy Service, Montreal Neurological Hospital and Institute

Orit Atzmon, Ph.D.
Researcher, Department of Psychiatry and Behavioral Science, Stanford University Medical Center, Stanford, California

John J. Barry, M.D.
Assistant Professor of Psychiatry, Stanford University Medical Center, Stanford, California

Selim R. Benbadis, M.D.
Associate Professor of Neurology, Director of Comprehensive Epilepsy Center, University of South Florida College of Medicine, Tampa

Dietrich Blumer, M.D.
Professor of Psychiatry, University of Tennessee, Memphis, College of Medicine, Memphis

Elizabeth S. Bowman, M.D.
Associate Professor of Psychiatry, Indiana University School of Medicine, Indianapolis

Mary Connolly, M.B., F.R.C.P.C.
Clinical Assistant Professor of Pediatrics, University of British Columbia Faculty of Medicine, Vancouver; Pediatric Neurologist, British Columbia Children's and Women's Hospital, Vancouver

Orrin Devinsky, M.D.
Professor of Neurology, New York University School of Medicine, New York; Director, New York University Comprehensive Epilepsy Center, New York; Chief of Neurology, Hospital for Joint Diseases, New York

Carl B. Dodrill, Ph.D.
Professor of Neurology and Neurological Surgery, University of Washington School of Medicine, Seattle; Associate Director of Regional Epilepsy Center, Harborview Medical Center, Seattle

Nancy Donofrio, M.A.
Graduate Student in Clinical and Health Psychology, Allegheny University of the Health Sciences, Philadelphia; Neuropsychology Intern, Brown University Clinical Psychology Internship Consortium, Providence, Rhode Island

Fritz E. Dreifuss, M.B., F.R.C.P., F.R.A.C.P.
Former Professor of Neurology and Director, F. E. Dreifuss Comprehensive Epilepsy Program, University of Virginia School of Medicine, Charlottesville; Neurologist, University of Virginia Hospital, Charlottesville

Kevin Farrell, M.B., Ch.B., F.R.C.P.C., F.R.C.P.E.
Professor of Pediatrics, University of British Columbia Faculty of Medicine, Vancouver; Director of Epilepsy Service, British Columbia Children's and Women's Hospital, Vancouver

John R. Gates, M.D.
Clinical Professor of Neurology, University of Minnesota Medical School, Minneapolis; Director, Adult Services, Minnesota Epilepsy Group, P.A., United Hospital and Children's Clinics and Hospitals, St. Paul

Mitzie L. Grant, Ph.D.
Assistant Professor of Psychiatry, Allegheny University of the Health Sciences, Philadelphia; Clinical Neuropsychologist, St. Christopher's Hospital for Children, Philadelphia

Ann Hempel, Ph.D.
Pediatric Neuropsychologist, Minnesota Epilepsy Group, P.A., St. Paul

Bruce P. Hermann, Ph.D.
Professor of Neurology, University of Wisconsin Medical School, Madison

Audrey M. W. Ho, Ph.D.
Adjunct Professor of Clinical Psychology, University of British Columbia Faculty of Medicine, Vancouver; Clinical Psychologist, British Columbia Children's and Women's Hospital, Vancouver

Mark D. Holmes, M.D.
Department of Neurology, University of Washington School of Medicine, Seattle; Director of EEG and Clinical Neurophysiology Laboratory, Harborview Medical Center, Seattle

Don W. King, M.D.
Professor of Neurology, Medical College of Georgia School of Medicine, Augusta; Medical Director, Adult Epilepsy Monitoring Unit, Medical College of Georgia Hospitals and Clinics, Augusta

Prakash Kotagal, M.D.
Section of Pediatric Epilepsy, Cleveland Clinic Foundation, Cleveland

Lucyna M. Lach, B.A., M.S.W., C.S.W.
Project Director, Brain and Behaviour Program, Hospital for Sick Children Research Institute, Toronto, Ontario; Social Worker, Neurology Program, Hospital for Sick Children, Toronto; Ph.D. Candidate, Faculty of Social Work, University of Toronto Faculty of Medicine, Toronto

David W. Loring, Ph.D.
Professor and Director of Adult Neuropsychology Service, Medical College of Georgia School of Medicine, Augusta

Mark W. Mahowald, M.D.
Professor of Neurology, University of Minnesota Medical School, Minneapolis; Director of Minnesota Regional Sleep Disorders Center, Hennepin County Medical Center, Minneapolis

Ronald L. Martin, M.D.
Former Professor and Chair of Psychiatry and Behavioral Sciences, University of Kansas School of Medicine, Wichita

Sharon L. Mason, M.A., L.P.
Psychologist, United Hospital, St. Paul, Minnesota

Kimford J. Meador, M.D.
Professor and Director, Section of Behavioral Neurology, Medical College of Georgia School of Medicine, Augusta

D. Kent Mercer, Psy.D.
Clinical Director of Neuropsychology Services, Larry Pollock, Ph.D., and Associates, Houston

George L. Morris III, M.D.
Associate Professor of Neurology, Medical College of Wisconsin, Milwaukee

Joel O. Paraiso, M.D.
Neurologist, Amsterdam, New York

Louis Peltz, M.D., M.Sc., F.R.C.P.
Lecturer, Department of Psychiatry, University of Toronto Faculty of Medicine, Toronto, Ontario; Staff Psychiatrist, Department of Psychiatry, Hospital for Sick Children, Toronto; Clinical Director, Child and Family Services, Credit Valley Hospital, Mississauga, Ontario

Kenneth Perrine, Ph.D.
Clinical Assistant Professor of Neurology, New York University School of Medicine, New York; Chief of Neuropsychology, Department of Neurology, Hospital for Joint Diseases, New York

Venkat Ramani, M.D.
Professor of Neurology, Albany Medical College, Albany, New York; Attending Neurologist, Albany Medical Center Hospital, Albany

Marilyn J. Ransby, Ph.D., R.Psych.
Graduate Student in Educational Psychology, University of British Columbia Faculty of Medicine, Vancouver; Psychology Intern Graduate, British Columbia Children's Hospital, Vancouver

Gail L. Risse, Ph.D.
Director of Psychological Services, Minnesota Epilepsy Group, P.A., St. Paul; Clinical Neuropsychologist, Epilepsy Group, United Hospital, St. Paul

Frank J. Ritter, M.D.
Clinical Assistant Professor of Neurology, University of Minnesota Medical School, Minneapolis; Director, Pediatric Services, Minnesota Epilepsy Group, P.A., St. Paul; Director, Pediatric Services, United and Children's Clinics and Hospitals, St. Paul

A. James Rowan, M.D.
Professor of Neurology, Mount Sinai School of Medicine of the City University of New York, New York; Chief of Neurology Service, Bronx Veterans Affairs Medical Center, Bronx, New York

Carlos H. Schenck, M.D.
Associate Professor of Psychiatry, University of Minnesota Medical School, Minneapolis; Senior Staff Psychiatrist and Staff Physician, Minnesota Regional Sleep Disorders Center, Hennepin County Medical Center, Minneapolis

Jane A. Springer, Ph.D.
Consulting Neuropsychologist, University of Iowa Hospitals and Clinics, Iowa City; Neuropsychologist, Covenant Medical Center, Waterloo, Iowa

Sara J. Swanson, Ph.D.
Assistant Professor of Neurology, Medical College of Wisconsin, Milwaukee

Nancy Thornton, R.N., M.Sc.N., C.N.N(C)
Research Study Nurse, Department of Neurology, British Columbia Children's and Women's Hospital, Vancouver

John A. Walker, Ph.D.
Assistant Professor of Neurology, University of California, San Francisco, School of Medicine, San Francisco

Jane Williams, Ph.D.
Associate Professor of Pediatrics, University of Arkansas for Medical Sciences College of Medicine, Little Rock; Staff, Arkansas Children's Hospital, Little Rock

Preface

This book is the result of the continued outgrowth of two important conferences. The first conference was titled "The Dilemma of Non-Epileptic (Pseudo-Epileptic) Seizures" and was held in March 1990, in Fort Lauderdale, Florida. The second conference was titled "Non-Epileptic Seizures: A Consensus Conference on Diagnosis and Treatment" and was held in April 1996, in Bethesda, Maryland. These two conferences brought together experts from the multiple disciplines of neurology, psychiatry, and neuropsychology for both adult and pediatric patients to exchange views and to develop a consensus perspective on this group of complex disorders.

Since the late 1970s, an explosion has taken place in our knowledge about non-epileptic seizures, initially owing to the growth and widespread application of intensive video-electroencephalographic monitoring, a critical element that increases diagnostic capability. It soon became apparent that non-epileptic seizures are far more common and varied than originally suspected. At the same time, interest in the problem has grown among neuropsychologists and psychiatrists who have attempted to define the personality characteristics for concomitant *DSM-IV* disorders that characterize this spectrum of paroxysmal disturbances.

As a result of these events and the unique interaction among the disciplines of neurology, psychiatry, and neuropsychology, a synthesis of current knowledge about non-epileptic seizures is available. The chapters in this edition represent updated material by the foremost experts in their respective fields. The editors hope that both readers and patients benefit from the insights offered and that the direction of research is further clarified.

Finally, the editors would like to express their thanks to Ann Hempel, who co-edited Part III, Cognitive and Psychological Functioning and Treatment of the Pediatric Patient with Non-Epileptic Seizures.

JOHN R. GATES
A. JAMES ROWAN

PART I

Neurologic Aspects of Non-Epileptic Seizures in the Adult and Pediatric Patient

CHAPTER 1

Epidemiology and Classification of Non-Epileptic Events

John R. Gates

History

The distinction between non-epileptic seizures (NES) and epilepsy has been known since ancient times. Even the Greeks were aware of a paroxysmal disturbance distinct from epilepsy. As reviewed by Trimble,[1] epilepsy and hysteria have often been intertwined and have been of strong interest to medical historians. At times, both disorders have been confused with possession, demonology, or divinity. Hippocrates, in his *Diseases of Women*,[2] described the clinical presentation of NES that he clearly separated from epilepsy and named the *sacred disease*. Aerates also classified epilepsy into two varieties: the ordinary and the hysterical.[3] The latter disorder, following the ideas of the time, was thought to be due to the wanderings of the uterus. Both early Greek writers emphasized abdominal geneses of seizures, especially uterine, forever creating a feminine attribute to hysteria, and the idea that the paroxysms reminiscent of epilepsy form part of the clinical pattern of the disorder.

In 1684, Willis moved the origin of hysteria from the abdomen to the brain but again emphasized the association with epilepsy and speculated on an epileptic and a non-epileptic pathophysiology that had a similar basis.[4]

As reviewed by Trimble,[1] the association between hysteria and epilepsy "reached its zenith in the eighteenth and nineteenth centuries, particularly in France." The French introduced the term *hysteroepilepsy*, implying a clear association between the two disorders. Apparently most authors accepted the concept of *accés distincts*, in which it was clear that the same patients were having both epileptic and hysterical seizures. Others claimed the existence of *accés complexes*, in which there was a combination of the two disorders in the same patient. Briquet, and later Charco,[1] believed that a hysteroepilepsy with mixed attacks was, in reality, a form of hysteria, but others continued to raise questions concerning the existence of some intermediate condition. Briquet's classic association of epilepsy and nondominant hemiparesis is still a common presentation.

Gowers also emphasized the difference between the seizures of epilepsy and those of hysteria by discussing the two disorders in his classic 1881 monograph.[5] As pointed out by Trimble,[1]

> In practice, most authors have attempted to emphasize differences between the seizures of epilepsy and those of hysteria, many drawing up tables for differential diagnosis of the condition. In clinical practice, this has been enhanced by the fact that the treatment of epilepsy has gradually fallen almost entirely into the province of neurology and the treatment of hysteria into that of psychiatry, the reverse of the position of 100 years ago. However, the potential lack of experience of psychiatrists in the diagnosis and management of epilepsy, and in neurologists the diagnosis of hysteria, has led to many practical difficulties. One of these is that the assessment of many of these difficult cases evolves at the borderline between the two specialties.

Epidemiology

The incidence of NES is probably significantly higher than most clinicians realize. Only one true epidemiologic study has been performed. This was a small series published by Sigurdardottir and Olafsson.[6] Not surprisingly, however, this study did conclude that NES appears to equal approximately 5% of the incidence of epilepsy, a number that had previously been identified by Scott as a rough estimate.[7]

Sigurdardottir and Olafssonn,[6] realizing the unique epidemiologic resource of their remarkably stable population of Iceland, as well as the availability of a single comprehensive neurophysiologic laboratory from which all data were obtained, identified 14 patients aged 16–54 (mean 27.6 years), 11 of whom (78.6%) were women. The average population of Iceland during the study period for persons older than 15 years was 200,000, with an average annual incidence of NES of 1.4 per 100,000, compared with 35 per 100,000 for epilepsy in persons younger than 15 years old.

A remarkable additional observation was that seven of the patients (50%) also had epilepsy. Seizure types included generalized tonic-clonic seizures (N = 3), generalized tonic-clonic and myoclonic seizures (N = 2), tonic seizures (N = 1), and absence seizures (N = 1). Two of the seven patients had juvenile myoclonic epilepsy. All patients received long-term video-electroencephalographic (EEG) monitoring to confirm the diagnostic characterization, with 19.5 hours as the mean number of long-term video monitoring hours needed and a range of 6–146 hours.

Previous studies have suggested that the incidence of NES is 5–20% in an outpatient epilepsy population, with a higher incidence of 10–40% for inpatients studied at epilepsy centers.[8] Certainly one of the more controversial areas is the coexistence of epileptic seizures and NES. In the Icelandic study, the coincidence was 50%. In previous studies from Minnesota, Gates[9] found the coincidence to be approximately 58% in a highly referred epilepsy population.

Nonetheless, in a paper by Wilkus and Dodrill[10] from the University of Washington, Seattle, only 23 patients, 3.6% of a total sample of 643, had both epileptic seizures and NES recorded during their monitoring. This group was meticulous in identifying patients as having epileptic seizures, only including those with video-EEG–recorded seizures. They excluded patients with interictal epileptiform abnormalities. However, as noted by the authors, their average length of stay for monitoring was only 5.7 days, compared with the Gates et al. study, which averaged a length of stay of more than 21 days, identifying a 27% coincidence of clearly recorded epileptic and non-epileptic events (NEE), with the additional 31% of mixed patients consequently identified by history and active interictal discharges. Methodologic issues likely explain the difference in these two populations. Nonetheless, as identified from the Icelandic study,[6] it is very likely that considerably more than a mere 3.6% have both epilepsy and NEE, thereby making the diagnostic dilemma even more challenging.

Terminology

Clearly, one of the most confusing aspects of paroxysmal events that are not of epileptic origin is the remarkable diversity of terminology that exists in the literature for describing them. As discussed in the historical section, epilepsy and hysteria have often been closely intertwined and have been of strong interest to medical historians. At times, both disorders have been confused with possession, demonology, and divinity. In recent times, the most popular term promoted in the literature has been *pseudoseizure*. Other terms used have been *hysterical pseudoseizures*, *pseudoepileptic seizures*, *hysteroepileptic psychogenic seizures*, and *non-epileptic seizures*.

Those who use the term *pseudoseizure* presumably adopted it from the more neutral-meaning resource of medical terminology (i.e., the term *pseudocyst*). On the other hand, a term such as *pseudo* (i.e., relating to a pretended intellectual state) is clearly pejorative, carrying the connotation of false or deceptive. Inasmuch as people with seizures that are non-epileptic in origin do have a true illness, the term *pseudoseizure* is therefore best avoided. Obviously, the term *hysterical epilepsy*, or any

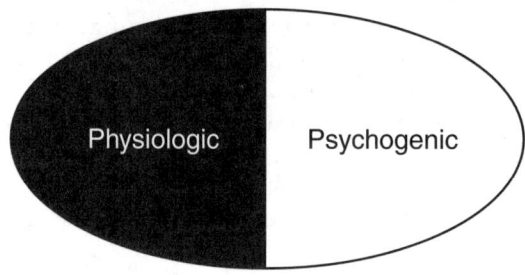

FIGURE 1.1. Division of non-epileptic events into physiologic and psychogenic.

combination thereof in which "hysterical" is included, also implies a pejorative overtone that is unacceptable to most professionals. Although originally a specific psychiatric term, in popular language *hysteria* has significantly connotative negativity. The descriptive word *hysterical* implies a specific psychiatric diagnosis of conversion. Consequently, it would appear prudent to develop a consistent terminology that is denotatively acceptable and connotatively as neutral as possible. For this purpose, the term *non-epileptic seizure* is suggested. Figure 1.1 represents the subcategorization of NEE into those of physiologic and psychogenic origin.

Physiologic Non-Epileptic Events

It is essential to understand and remember that there is a significant subgroup of patients who have a physiologic explanation for their paroxysmal events other than that of epilepsy. Figure 1.2 is a diagram of the subdivision of physiologic NEE. These include syncope, paroxysmal toxic phenomena, nontoxic organic hallucinosis, non-epileptic myoclonus, the spectrum of a parasomniac sleep disorder, paroxysmal movement disorder, paroxysmal endocrine disturbances, paroxysms of acute neurologic insults, and transient ischemic cerebrovascular phenomena.

Syncope is probably the disorder most commonly confused with epilepsy in the non-epileptic physiologic category. It is not uncommon for patients to have isolated myoclonic jerks that can often be unilateral. Syncope may be triggered by significant psychogenic stimulation that suggests an NES of potential psychogenic origin. Use of a 24-hour cardiac monitor is not infrequently normal in patients who experience syncopal episodes of cardiac origin, and 72-hour or longer recordings are sometimes required.

Paroxysmal toxic phenomena, such as acute effects of cocaine overdose or other nontoxic organic hallucinosis, for example, during acute encephalitis, may also be confused with epilepsy and require appropriate definitive evaluation. In addition, if the patient has a family history of mild myoclonic disorders, including benign essential myoclonus, nontoxic

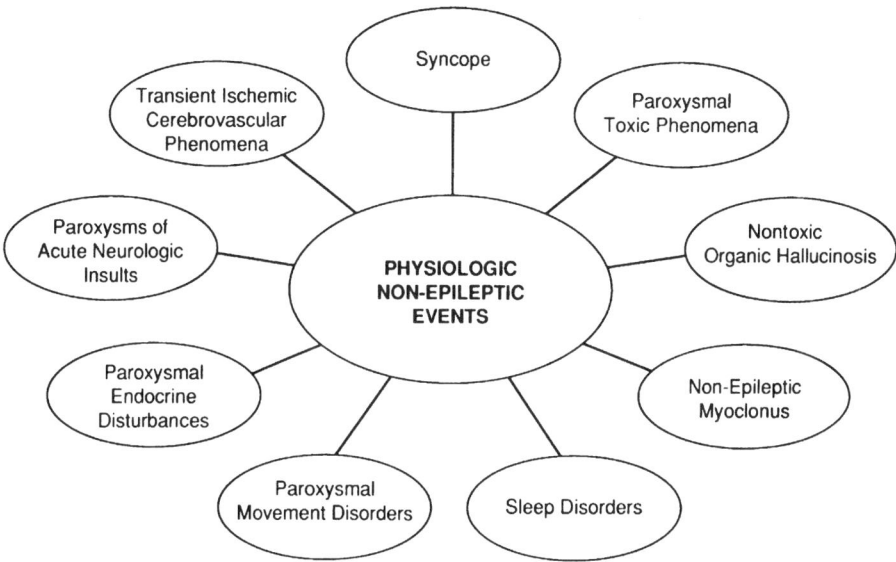

FIGURE 1.2. Physiologic non-epileptic events. Alternative diagnoses.

myoclonus, and spinal myoclonus (an exaggerated startle disease), these must be appropriately identified and distinguished from epilepsy.

The family of movement disorders can include paroxysmal kinesigenic choreoathetosis, paroxysmal dystonia, and paroxysmal ataxia. These disorders must be distinguished from epilepsy and not be inappropriately managed with anticonvulsants. The paroxysmal endocrine disorders such as carcinoid syndrome and pheochromocytoma must also be recognized. In addition to acute encephalitis, there are other acute neurologic insults that may be misinterpreted as epilepsy. Decerebrate attacks with extensive bihemispheric cortical damage or spinal release phenomena resulting from higher cortical compromise are often confused with epilepsy in patients who are in intensive care unit settings requiring appropriate clinical acumen to distinguish those symptoms from those of epilepsy.

Transient ischemic cerebrovascular phenomena include not only classic atherosclerotic attacks but also the full spectrum of disorders associated with migraine. With approximately 18% of the adult female population and 9% of the adult male population having migraine, the differentiation between a classic migraine attack and simple partial sensory seizure can be difficult in some patients, especially if it is a migraine equivalent with little or no accompanying headache.

These physiologic events are elucidated in greater detail in Chapters 4, 5, and 6.

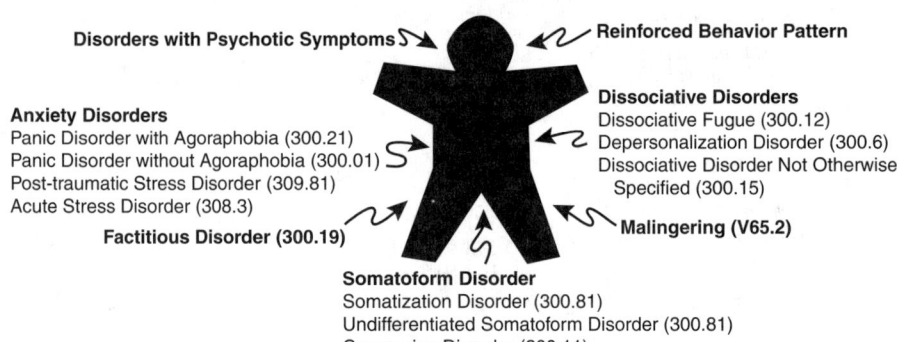

FIGURE 1.3. General diagnostic categories that may be observed in patients with non-epileptic events. See the *Diagnostic and Statistical Manual of Mental Disorders*, Fourth Edition (Washington, DC: American Psychiatric Association, 1994), for the meaning of numbers in parentheses.

Psychogenic Non-Epileptic Disorders

Since the publication of the *DSM-IV* (*Diagnostic and Statistical Manual of Mental Disorders*, Fourth Edition)[11] classification scheme, a more detailed description of psychiatric disorders in diagnostic categories in which to classify patients with NES has become available (Figure 1.3; see Chapter 20).

Somatoform Disorders

The one feature common to all somatoform disorders is the presence of physical symptoms that are suggestive of a medical condition but are not the result of a medical condition, the direct effects of a substance, or another mental disorder (for example, panic disorder or schizophrenia).[17] The physical symptoms are not believed to be under voluntary control. They must cause significant distress or impairment in social, occupational, or other areas of functioning. By far the largest group of patients with psychogenic NEE present with the somatoform disorder referred to as *conversion disorder*. As discussed elsewhere, the classic Briquet patient who presents with nondominant hemiparesis and psychogenic tonic-clonic seizures still thrives within our society. Of course, the essential feature of this disorder is the presence of symptoms that affect voluntary motor or sensory function, suggesting a neurologic or other general medical conditions. Furthermore, the initiation or exacerbation of the symptom complex is preceded by psychological conflicts or other stressors. There is no evidence that these symptoms are intentionally produced, and symptoms are not explainable by a neurologic or other general medical condition, the effects of substances, or the result of culturally sanctioned behaviors or experiences. The difficulties presented must be clinically significant, as is evident from marked distress, impairment in a basic area of functioning (for example, social or occupational), or the fact that it warrants medical evaluation.

According to the *DSM-IV*, approximately one-fourth to one-half of persons initially diagnosed with conversion disorders in early studies gave evidence of general medical causes. Furthermore, as many as one-third of individuals with conversion disorder symptoms have a current or prior coexisting neurologic condition, as is the case with regard to the sizable number of patients who present with both epileptic seizures and NEE. Behavioral features that may be associated with conversion disorders include the classic sign, *la belle indifférence*, dramatic or histrionic (hysterical) behavior, and/or extreme suggestibility. Symptoms of conversion disorder clearly occur more frequently in females than in males, with reported ratios varying from 2 to 1 to 10 to 1.[11] The *DSM-IV* identifies four conversion disorder subtypes: (1) with motor symptom or deficit, (2) with sensory symptom or deficit, (3) with seizures or convulsions, and (4) with mixed presentation. Clearly, symptoms that conform to these subtypes may mimic a variety of seizure classifications. In our experience, the presentation of conversion disorder as NEE tends to occur in younger to middle-aged women. Often a sexual abuse precipitant is discovered, although this is not exclusively the case.[12] The temporal association between the precipitant and the ultimate medically refractory paroxysmal event is highly variable, often spanning many years. More proximate stressors, such as the death of a loved one or another major life trauma, may serve as the trigger for a conversion disorder. It is critical that clinicians recognize the overdetermined, multifactorial nature of NEE.

The diagnoses of somatization disorder, undifferentiated somatoform disorder, and somatoform disorder not otherwise specified also fall under the *DSM-IV* rubric of somatoform disorders. The diagnostic criteria for somatization disorder require that the patient present with a variety of physical complaints that began before the age of 30 years. These symptoms must have resulted in treatment being sought or significant impairment in social, occupational, or other important areas of functioning. Specific physical complaints must include pain symptoms, gastrointestinal symptoms, sexual symptoms, and pseudoneurologic symptoms (i.e., seizure-like events, dissociative symptoms, and diminished level of consciousness). The symptoms must not be explained by a general medical condition, or the symptoms must be clearly in excess of any known general medical condition. Finally, symptoms are clearly not intentionally produced or feigned.

The criteria for undifferentiated somatoform disorder are less rigorous, requiring only one or more physical complaints that cannot be fully explained by a known medical condition or that are clearly in excess of a known medical condition. The symptoms that cause clinically significant distress are of at least 6 months' duration, cannot be accounted for by another mental disorder, and are not intentionally produced. Individuals with these disorders may present with histrionic behavioral pictures, significant symptoms of depression or anxiety, and deeply ingrained characterologic difficulties. Issues of substance abuse and secondary gain should be carefully evaluated, as in any of these conditions.

The diagnosis of somatoform disorder not otherwise specified is appropriate when physical symptoms are of less than 6 months' duration and are not due to a known medical or another mental disorder. Obviously, patients presenting with these disorders who evidence NES require exhaustive step-by-step diagnostic evaluations to evaluate the reported medical concerns clearly and definitively. These patients are often difficult to treat and may reject any recommendations for psychiatric or psychological follow-up.

We have observed a number of non-epileptic patients who are ultimately diagnosed as having hypochondriasis. These individuals have irrational fears of having a serious disease. Their concerns are often based on a misinterpretation of bodily symptoms. Although this belief is not of delusional intensity, it persists despite appropriate and sufficient medical evaluation and reassurance. The disturbance lasts for at least 6 months and causes clinically significant distress in at least one major area of functioning. Depression, anxiety, and obsessive-compulsive features are frequently present, and psychosocial distress clearly exacerbates the disorder.

Dissociative Disorders

A number of patients who present with NES meet the diagnostic criteria for one of several dissociative disorders. The critical feature of the dissociative disorder is "a disruption in the usually integrated functions of consciousness, memory, identity, or perception of the environment. The disturbance may be sudden or gradual, transient or chronic."[11] Our experience at the Minnesota Epilepsy Group has suggested that NEE may be observed in at least three separate dissociative disorders: dissociative fugue, depersonalization disorder, and dissociative disorder not otherwise specified.

The critical feature of dissociative fugue is sudden and unexpected travel away from one's home or customary place of daily activities with subsequent inability to recall some or all of one's past.[11] The travel may range from brief wanderings involving only hours to more lengthy time periods involving weeks or months. Such activity is typically accompanied by confusion about personal identity and is not explained by direct physiologic effects of a substance or a general medical condition.

The symptoms must cause clinically significant distress or impairment in a major area of functioning. Associated features include depression, dysphoria, grief, shame, guilt, psychological distress, and occasionally suicidal and aggressive impulses. The onset of dissociative fugue is typically related to severely traumatic or overwhelming life events. Recovery is typically rapid, although refractory dissociative amnesia may persist in some cases.

The critical features of depersonalization disorder involve persistent or recurrent episodes of depersonalization characterized by feelings of detachment or estrangement from oneself. The phenomenology of such events involves persons feeling as though they are an automaton or an outside observer of their own mental processes, body, or life. It is important to note that various types of sensory anesthesia as well as subjective feelings of loss of control of one's actions (including speech) are often present. Although reality testing remains intact, the experience causes clinically significant distress or impairment in a major area of functioning. Such depersonalization experiences might be misinterpreted as an aura or simple partial seizure by the patient who is familiar with seizure disorders or the physician before long-term video-EEG monitoring.

Dissociative disorders not otherwise specified represent a category designed for those disorders in which the predominant feature is a dissociative symptom (disruption in integrative ego functions) that does not meet the criteria for a specific dissociative disorder. In the context of NEE, this might include derealization (alteration in perception or experience of the external world so that it seems strange or unreal) without depersonalization or dissociative trance disorders, which involve "narrowing of awareness of immediate surroundings or stereotyped behaviors or movements that are experienced as being beyond one's control."[12] Dissociative trances that involve ideas of possession are often associated with stereotyped "involuntary" movements of amnesia and may have a clear cultural reference. A number of culture-bound syndromes are noted in *DSM-IV*. These include *amok* (Indonesia), *latah* (Malaysia), *piplokto* (the Arctic), and *ataque de nervious* (Latin America). For NES or depersonalization disorder not otherwise specified to be correctly diagnosed, the dissociative or trance disorder must be judged not to be a normal part of a broadly accepted cultural or religious practice.

Anxiety Disorders

Patients presenting with NES who evidence significant anxiety symptoms may ultimately be diagnosed with one of four anxiety disorders: (1) panic disorder without agoraphobia, (2) panic disorder with agoraphobia, (3) posttraumatic stress disorder, or (4) acute stress disorder. The principal features of panic disorder (both with and without agoraphobia) involve symptoms of a panic attack, concern about additional panic attacks, worry about the implications of the attack or its consequences, or a significant change in behavior resulting from the attacks.[11] Symptoms of a panic attack include cardiac irregularities (palpitations, pounding heart, accelerated heart rate), sweating, trembling or shaking, shortness of breath, chest pain, nausea, dizziness, derealization or depersonalization, paresthesia, and unreasonable fears of losing control or dying. Clearly, many of these symptoms might be misinterpreted by an individual familiar with seizure disorders as an aura or simple partial seizure. The more dissociative symptoms (depersonalization and derealization) often mimic symptoms of a complex partial seizure.

Whereas the features of panic disorder principally involve panic attacks, the principal features of post-traumatic stress disorder and acute stress disorder involve more generalized anxiety symptoms and more prominent dissociative symptoms. The main difference in the two disorders is that post-traumatic stress disorder is of greater than 1 month's duration, whereas acute stress disorder lasts for a minimum of 2 days and a maximum of 4 weeks and occurs within 4 weeks of the traumatic event. Should the symptoms emerge more than 4 weeks after the period, the event is classified as a post-traumatic stress disorder. The diagnostic criteria for both post-traumatic stress disorder and acute stress disorder require that the patient has experienced or witnessed or was confronted with an event that involved actual or threatened death or serious injury or a threat to the physical integrity of others. Furthermore, the person's response involved a strong sense of fear, helplessness, or horror. It should be made clear that the events referred to in the *DSM-IV* are *severe* stressors, outside the realm of normal experience. These patients persistently re-experience the traumatic event despite avoidance of stimuli associated with the event and dissociative defenses, resulting in a numbing of general responsiveness. These patients also evidence persistent symptoms of increased arousal (sleep difficulties, anger management difficulties, hypervigilance). The principal features of these disorders that present as NES involve dissociative symptoms. These result in a subjective sense of numbing, diminished emotional responsiveness, reduced awareness of surroundings, and periods of derealization and depersonalization.

Disorders with Psychotic Symptoms

We have observed a number of patients whose seizure-like events are ultimately found to be the result of psychotic symptomatology. Schizophrenia and other psychotic disorders (schizophreniform disorder, schizoaffective disorder, delusional disorder, brief psychotic disorder, and psychotic disorders not otherwise specified) may present a variety of behavioral and affective symptoms that mimic seizures. In addition, symptoms of individuals with severe mood disorders (depressive disorders and bipolar disorders) that include psychotic manifestations may be misinterpreted as paroxysmal seizure activity.

Factitious Disorder and Malingering

Factitious disorder and malingering are similar in that each involves intentionally produced or feigned symptoms. The critical difference in the two diagnostic entities involves the individual's motivation in producing the symptom picture. In factitious disorder, the patient produces symptoms to assume the sick role. Such individuals are preoccupied with being admitted to the hospital. They usually do not restrict their symptomatology to the nervous system. They may present their "medical history" in a dramatic fashion but become vague and at times self-contradictory when they are questioned in detail. They are often intelligent and have more than a casual knowledge of the illness in question. Individuals with factitious disorder who present symptoms of epilepsy often complain of other physical difficulties once the non-epileptic diagnosis is made. Diagnosis of factitious disorder not otherwise specified may be given in cases of Munchausen disease by proxy. This is most commonly seen in children[4] and is particularly distress related in that the young patient is often experiencing anxiety from being separated from the offending caretaker.

Although malingering also involves the intentional production of feigning of symptoms, the malingerer is motivated by secondary gain. External incentives such as avoiding responsibilities, obtaining financial compensation, and attempting to present mitigating circumstances in criminal procedures are related to the onset and maintenance of the symptoms. It is important that the clinician recognize the need to evaluate such secondary gain issues, not only in the NES patient but in all patients. In addition to secondary gain of sympathy and emotional support, many patients receive significant financial benefits from their apparent seizure difficulties. It is incumbent on the clinician to evaluate such secondary gain issues carefully and to clarify whether there is any pending litigation or other potential financial gain.

Addressing issues of secondary gain in patients who present with NES can be difficult. In patients who have a lengthy history (e.g., more than 2 years) of a lifestyle that involves significant secondary gain, effective treatment tends to be particularly difficult.

Reinforced Behavior Patterns

A final patient group that has once again eluded *DSM-IV* classification is made up of cognitively impaired patients in whom NES has developed as a result of reinforced behavior patterns. Such patients have essentially been operantly conditioned to produce paroxysmal events, typically by direct modeling or shaping by successive approximations. Such events tend to produce reinforcing changes in their environment.

References

1. Trimble MR. Pseudoseizures. Neurol Clin 1986;4:531–548.
2. Tempkin O. The Falling Sickness. Baltimore: Johns Hopkins, 1945.
3. Massey EW. History of Epilepsy and Hysteria. In T Riley, A Roy (eds), Pseudoseizures. Baltimore: Williams & Wilkins, 1982;1–20.
4. Gates JR. Nonepileptic Events. New York: Churchill Livingstone, 1995.

5. Alper K. Nonepileptic seizures. Neurol Clin 1994;1:153–173.
6. Sigurdardottir KR, Olafsson E. Incidence of psychogenic seizures in adults: a population-based study in Iceland. Epilepsia 1998;39:749–752.
7. Gates JR. Diagnosis and Treatment of Nonepileptic Seizures. In HW McConnell, PJ Snyder (eds), Psychiatric Comorbidity in Epilepsy. Washington, DC: American Psychiatric Press, 1998;187–204..
8. Gates JR, Luciano D, Devinski O. The Classification and Treatment of Nonepileptic Events. In O Devinski, WA Theodore (eds), Epilepsy and Behavior. New York: Wiley-Liss, 1991;251–263.
9. Gates JR, Ramani V, Whalens SM. Ictal characteristics of pseudoseizures. Arch Neurol 1985;42:1183–1187.
10. Wilkus RJ, Dodrill CB. Factors affecting the outcome of MMPI and neuropsychological assessments of psychogenic and epileptic seizure patients. Epilepsia 1989;30:339–347.
11. American Psychiatric Association. Diagnostic and Statistical Manual of Mental Disorders (4th ed). Washington, DC: American Psychiatric Association, 1994.
12. Goodwin JM. Childhood Sexual Abuse and Non-Epileptic Seizures. In AJ Rowan, JR Gates (eds), Non-Epileptic Seizures. Boston: Butterworth–Heinemann, 1993;181–192.

CHAPTER 2

Diagnosis of Non-Epileptic Seizures

A. James Rowan

The differential diagnosis of non-epileptic seizures (NES) includes a wide variety of psychiatric and physiologic conditions in addition to epilepsy itself.[1] Many of these conditions may be suspected on historical grounds alone, provided that accurate information is available. Unfortunately, it is often difficult to obtain critical historical evidence. How often has a neurologist been confronted with a patient in whom the chief complaint is unobserved loss of consciousness or episodic loss of memory? This chapter discusses epileptic versus psychogenic NES, physiologic non-epileptic events that resemble epileptic seizures, psychogenic conditions that resemble epileptic seizures, and diagnostic protocol for treatment of epileptic versus non-epileptic seizures.

The classification of psychogenic NES, a subject still under review, is discussed in depth in Chapter 1. There are a number of classification schemes, some of limited utility. It is likely that subsequent research will result in a multiaxial classification system, similar to that used in the *DSM-IV* (*Diagnostic and Statistical Manual of Mental Disorders*, Fourth Edition). This chapter reviews psychogenic NES based on the observed phenomenology and its resemblance to epileptic seizures. Although believed by some to be of limited utility, this approach constitutes a starting point and indeed may provide clues to the underlying psychiatric condition and its (presumed) associated cerebral dysfunction.

Historical Features That Suggest a Diagnosis of Psychogenic Non-Epileptic Seizures

In the consultation room, patients with psychogenic NES may appear no different from their epileptic counterparts. They frequently have had seizures for years, have been seen by several neurologists, and have not responded satisfactorily to multiple anti-epileptic drug regimens.[1,2]

High Seizure Frequency, Often with Multiple Daily Events

Flurries of multiple seizures or daily seizures can be seen in intractable epilepsy, rendering this criterion nondiagnostic in itself.[3] However, in patients with epilepsy, a continuing pattern of high seizure frequency in spite of adequate treatment is unusual. Increased or increasing seizure frequency in epileptic patients often is associated with some intercurrent event such as illness or anti-epileptic drug (AED) noncompliance, whereas patients with psychogenic NES may give no such history. Even though this criterion is flawed, it should prompt the clinician to reconsider the patient's diagnosis.

Little or No Response to Anti-Epileptic Drugs

Patients with epilepsy usually respond to AED therapy, either completely or partially. The response may be long lasting or temporary and may be related to the specific drug or drugs selected. Patients with psychogenic NES likewise may respond to AEDs, but the response, if present, is likely to be temporary. It is not unusual to obtain a history of lack of response to all AEDs in patients with psychogenic NES, prompting the clinician to re-evaluate the clinical problem.[1,2]

Paradoxical Response to Anti-Epileptic Drugs

It is unusual for patients with epilepsy to experience increased seizure frequency after receiving AED therapy. There is controversy regarding a paradoxical response to certain AEDs (e.g., phenytoin) when serum levels reach the toxic range. However, some patients with psychogenic NES show a surprising intolerance for AEDs, ascribing multiple symptoms to AED side effects, and indicate that their seizures actually increase when AED levels rise. AED intolerance and an inverse relationship between seizure frequency and AED levels should arouse suspicion of NES.[1]

Events Occur Only in the Presence of Others or Only When Alone

Although it is possible that events occur only in the presence of others or only when patients with epilepsy are alone, this should raise questions regarding the true diagnosis. Many patients with psychogenic NES report seizures that never have been observed by others. The clinician must, therefore, rely solely on self-reports. This is always an uncomfortable situation, but the patient may escape definitive diagnosis if suspicion is allayed because of convincing reports in conjunction with an abnormal electroencephalogram (EEG). Other patients with psychogenic NES have seizures only in the presence of others, for example, family members, in which case secondary gain may be a critical element.

Lack of Concern or Excessive Emotional Response to Seizures

Many patients with NES display a surprising lack of concern for their seizures, akin to the classic *la belle indifférence,* even in the face of high seizure frequency. Such a presentation is very unusual in patients with true epilepsy. Excessive emotional reaction to seizure occurrence may be seen in both conditions, although weeping or exaggerated emotions may point to the possibility of NES.[1,2]

History of Sexual Abuse

Evidence suggests that a history of sexual abuse, especially in childhood but also in adult life, is common in patients with psychogenic NES. The differential incidence of sexual abuse among epileptic patients, those with NES, and the general population is not known. Such information may not be offered spontaneously and must be specifically elicited.[2]

Experience with Epilepsy

Many patients with psychogenic NES have had some experience with epilepsy. It may take the form of a personal history of epilepsy, epilepsy in the family, or experience as a professional (e.g., a hospital worker). Such experience may provide a template for the clinical expression of NES.[1]

Repeated Hospitalizations or Emergency Department Visits

Some patients with NES have repeated flurries of seizures or even pseudo–status epilepticus, leading to multiple hospitalizations or emergency department visits. Such a history may also be found in patients with epilepsy, although this is uncommon. Patients with pseudostatus epilepticus have been described who have been treated with large doses of intravenous drugs and even general anesthesia. Clearly, accurate diagnosis can prevent potentially life-threatening iatrogenic complications.[4]

No History of Injury as a Result of Seizures

Injuries of various sorts, including tongue biting, fractures, and lacerations, are common in epilepsy but infrequent in psychogenic NES. Injuries in NES do occur, however, and may be an indicator of the severity of the underlying psychiatric disorder.[4,5]

Associated Psychiatric Disorders

Psychiatric problems may be associated with epilepsy but are always present in patients with psychogenic NES. Depression, for example, is common in both NES and epilepsy. Patients with NES, however, often have more than one psychiatric diagnosis. The presence of a psychiatric disorder should suggest the possibility of NES but must be considered in concert with other indicators.[1,2]

Clinical Signs Associated with Psychogenic Non-Epileptic Seizures[4,5]

No clinical signs are specific to psychogenic NES; all features associated with NES may be observed in patients with epileptic seizures. Nonetheless, a combination of suggestive clinical features can support a diagnosis of NES, which must be confirmed by specific studies (see below). Although not complete, the following items are commonly associated with psychogenic NES.

Emotional Trigger

Sometimes an obvious emotional precipitant of NES is apparent—for example, a personal loss, an altercation, or frustration. Many patients with epilepsy report stress as an important precipitating factor in their seizures, although this is difficult to confirm in most cases.

Gradual Onset and Gradual Cessation

Epileptic seizures are characterized by an abrupt onset, and some NES are similarly abrupt. On the other hand, many NES are characterized by a slow, gradual beginning, becoming increasingly vigorous as the seizure progresses. In such cases, seizure cessation may likewise be gradual, unlike the sudden termination of most epileptic events.

Nonphysiologic Progression

Epileptic seizures usually have a specific progression and a recognizable pattern based on anatomic and physiologic principles. Obvious examples are the jacksonian march and the generalized tonic-clonic convulsion. In contrast, psychogenic NES, particularly those with motor manifestations, often do not appear to follow the "rules." Thus, generalized motor activity may precede loss of consciousness; progressive involvement of body parts may not follow a known anatomic pattern. Unfortunately, even seizures of apparently bizarre appearance may be epileptic in origin—for example, those of frontal lobe origin (see Epileptic Seizures, later).

Out-of-Phase Motor Activity

Out-of-phase motor activity has long been considered a hallmark of psychogenic NES due to its bizarre nature and apparent lack of adherence to logical anatomic or physiologic foundation. It is now clear, however, that this motor pattern is observed in patients with frontal lobe seizures and cannot be considered specific for NES.

Intermittent Motor Activity

A frequent characteristic of psychogenic NES is waxing and waning motor activity over the course of the seizure. Repetitive movements may stop completely, only to start again with renewed vigor. In addition, clonic activity frequently can be modified by grasping the involved limb or changing the patient's position.

Dystonic Posturing

Dystonic posturing is not uncommon in psychogenic NES, ranging from flexion and inversion of the feet to full-blown opisthotonus. Twisting movements of the limbs and trunk are also seen. As is the case with other motor manifestations, such movements are suggestive but not diagnostic of NES.

Ability of Examiner to Modify Motor Activity

The amplitude, persistence, or type of motor activity in psychogenic NES often can be modified or even eliminated temporarily by grasping a limb, moving a limb, or changing the patient's position. Such modification is difficult, if not impossible, in true seizures, in particular tonic-clonic convulsions.

Pelvic Movements

Pelvic movements, in particular forward pelvic thrusting (as contrasted with retrothrusting), certainly are encountered in psychogenic NES and have long been considered highly suggestive, if not diagnostic, of the condition. Intensive video-EEG monitoring has revealed that such movements may be encountered in complex partial seizures (CPS), either of frontal or temporal origin.

Crying

Crying during an event is a distinctly unusual symptom in epileptic seizures but is not an infrequent occurrence in NES. We have encountered crying before, during, and after documented psychogenic NES. In many cases, the crying is highly emotionally charged, either interrupting ongoing motor activity or concurrent with it.

Avoidance Behavior during an Event

Avoidance behavior during an event is an inconstant sign, but when present it is suggestive of NES. For example, if the patient's arm is held aloft over the face, the limb may fall to the side. Blinking or averting the face to threat is another suggestive sign.

Typical Event Can Be Provoked by Suggestion

Provoking an event typical of the patient's spontaneous seizures by using techniques of suggestion is one of the most reliable signs of NES. Several techniques have been tried with success, including intravenous saline and placement of alcohol pads over the carotid arteries. The particular method used is of less importance than the experience and the ability of the examiner to effectively deliver the suggestion that a seizure may occur. The ethics of using this technique are controversial.

Differential Diagnosis of Non-Epileptic Seizures

The differential diagnosis of NES includes epilepsy itself; physiologic events, which are non-epileptic; and psychogenic episodes.

Epileptic Seizures

Psychogenic NES may mimic any type of epileptic seizure, and the differentiation may be difficult, if not impossible, on purely clinical grounds. In particular, seizures that originate in the frontal lobe, including the supplemental motor cortex, pose great difficulty. Until relatively recently, frontal seizures were no doubt frequently diagnosed as NES because of their often bizarre manifestations. For example, to-and-fro movements of the arms, bicycling movements of the legs, bizarre vocalizations such as barking, sudden jerking movements of the body, and wild flailing movements may be observed.[6] Motor activity may be discontinuous, and the patient may appear to be awake and responsive. Thus, many of the suggestive signs of NES are incorporated into the phenomenology of frontal seizures.

Supplementary motor seizures (SMS) comprise a subdivision of frontal seizures and have been studied with special reference to their differentiation from NES. Typically, SMS arise from sleep with sudden awakening. Tonic posturing of the upper extremities follows, with or without tonic extension of the legs. This phase is relatively brief, and vigorous thrashing movements ensue. Consciousness is apparently preserved throughout. The thrashing comes to an abrupt end, and the patient experiences little postictal confusion.[6]

In comparison with NES, SMS are shorter in duration. An ictal cry with SMS tends to be monotonous, in contrast to the emotionally laden cry of NES. The tonic abduction seen in SMS is not associated with NES. Thrashing movements are seen in both and do not provide differential information. SMS may involve the legs only but not the head only. The opposite is the case with NES.

CPS of temporal lobe origin usually follow a recognizable pattern and are highly stereotyped. However, many of the manifestations of true CPS may be incorporated into NES resembling CPS, including simple automatisms, staring, more complex motor activities, apparent confusional state, and lack of memory for the event.[7]

Convulsive NES are those events that bear a resemblance to generalized convulsions—tonic-clonic, tonic, clonic, clonic-tonic-clonic—with or without other associated motor phenomena. In some cases, the resemblance may be surprisingly close, whereas in others it is only superficial. A number of studies of convulsive NES have yielded information that aids the clinical differentiation from true seizures, although no single feature can be said to be diagnostic.

NES resembling absence seizures or petit mal are encountered from time to time. We have seen a number of such cases, including a young woman with multiple daily attacks who was treated for true absence seizures. Differentiation on clinical grounds is impossible inasmuch as the only signs are staring and unresponsiveness.[7]

NES resembling simple partial or focal seizures present a difficult problem. Focal NES with objective manifestations such as tonic posturing or repetitive motor activity may appear identical to true focal seizures. The problem is further complicated by the fact that the EEG in focal seizures is often normal, even during the ictal event. Diagnosis in such cases must rest on associated factors such as lack of stereotypy, precipitation by suggestion, and alteration of motor activity by the examiner. In cases of simple partial NES with subjective symptoms such as a cephalic or epigastric sensation, differentiation from a true "aura" may be impossible.

Physiologic Non-Epileptic Seizures

Attacks of physiologic origin often resemble epilepsy or psychogenic NES. Differentiation is usually possible on clinical grounds with the aid of ancillary studies. Such events, however, are frequently misdiagnosed because of lack of accurate historical information or the inability of the examiner to observe an attack. What follows is a partial listing of physiologic events that have been mistaken for epileptic attacks or NES of psychogenic origin.

Syncope

Syncopal attacks, whether of vasovagal or cardiac origin, are frequently mistaken for epilepsy. This is particularly true in the case of convulsive syncope. Typical premonitory symptoms such as lightheadedness, gradual loss of consciousness, brief duration, and lack of postictal confusion usually point to the diagnosis. In convulsive syncope, the syncopal attack is followed by motor activity, usually clonic in type, which is of brief duration. A tonic event may also be observed. Again, the typical postictal confusion of a generalized convulsion is absent. Convulsive syncope may occur in circumstances in which the individual does not fall or collapse to a horizontal position, thus further compromising cerebral blood flow.

Paroxysmal Movement Disorders

Paroxysmal movement disorders—for example, paroxysmal kinesigenic choreoathetosis and paroxysmal dystonia—may be misdiagnosed by the inexperienced or by those who have not witnessed the attacks. The typical clinical picture of paroxysmal basal ganglia dysfunction without altered awareness in a young person is usually sufficient to differentiate such attacks from epilepsy.

Migraine

The diagnosis of migraine is usually not difficult when a typical stereotyped headache is present, with or without neurologic signs and symptoms. Difficulty arises when the headache is minor or absent. In such cases, the patient may present with paroxysmal hemiparesis, discoordination, somatosensory symptoms, language difficulty, or visual symptoms (positive or negative). One helpful feature is the rarity of so-called negative symptoms, such as hemiparesis, as a manifestation of epilepsy. If one is fortunate enough to be able to record the EEG during or shortly after the attack, localized slowing without epileptiform features supports the diagnosis of migraine. In the case of positive visual symptoms (e.g., flashing lights), differentiation from epilepsy may not be possible without EEG confirmation. We recorded several attacks of "flashbulbs" from a child who was thought to have a migraine equivalent. During periods when he was symptomatic (and fully alert), the EEG demonstrated electrographic seizure activity originating in the right occipital lobe.

Sleep Disorders

As is more completely discussed in Chapter 5, there are many parasomnias that masquerade as epileptic or psychogenic disorders.[8] The growth of sleep medicine and documentation by polysomnography have been instrumental in increasing our understanding of these often bizarre symptoms.

Narcolepsy is a well-known example, wherein repeated episodes of sleep may be mistaken for attacks of loss of consciousness. Further, attacks of cataplexy may be thought to represent massive myoclonus. Demonstration of sleep onset with a typical rapid eye movement (REM) period during polysomnography or a multiple sleep latency test should confirm the diagnosis.

Night Terrors

Night terrors (or sleep terrors) occur mainly in young children and are thought to represent a psychiatric problem or possible CPS. These events arise out of slow-wave sleep; the child suddenly bolts up with a look of abject fear, screaming and crying inconsolably. Attempts to calm the child are fruitless, and he or she appears to be unresponsive. Recovery is accompanied by a confusional state, and the child has little or no memory of the event.[8]

Enuresis

Nocturnal enuresis occurs in slow-wave sleep and sometimes raises the question of an unrecognized seizure. Several studies failed to provide such evidence. Thus, nocturnal enuresis in the absence of other evidence should not be considered a sign of a seizure disorder.[8]

Sleepwalking

Sleepwalking is considered a disorder of arousal with intrusion of the waking state on REM sleep. The condition is relatively common in children (up to 17%) and is characterized by complex behaviors that may resemble CPS. The individual may appear to be awake but cannot react appropriately to the environment. No memory of the event is retained. Careful observation and appropriate laboratory testing, including EEG recording during the event, can usually clarify the diagnosis.[8]

Rapid Eye Movement Behavior Disorder

REM behavior disorder, a recently described parasomnia, was previously thought to be a psychiatric or epileptic disorder, due mainly to its bizarre manifestations. It is thought to be due to a failure of the motor inhibitory centers of the brain stem during REM sleep. Thus, patients may "act out" their dreams, which may be of violent content. Thus, patients may cry out, bolt out of bed, and run, seeking to escape an enemy or a frightening circumstance. Injuries have occurred such as falling or striking a wall or piece of furniture. Sleeping partners have reported being struck or kicked. In fact, some patients have gone to elaborate lengths to remove potentially dangerous objects from the bedroom, and their partners often resort to separate sleeping arrangements. The diagnosis may be suspected on purely clinical grounds and confirmed by polysomnography. Treatment with tricyclic antidepressants may afford relief.

Cardiac Events

Intermittent arrhythmias, such as ventricular tachycardia or Stokes-Adams attacks, can result in episodic loss of consciousness and even convulsive movements, raising the question of epilepsy. The diagnosis may be suspected by the history and confirmed by appropriate cardiac studies such as Holter monitoring.

Transient Ischemic Attacks

Transient ischemic attacks usually present no problem in diagnosis because of the fact that intermittent hemiparesis, dysphasia, and vision loss are unusual manifestations of epilepsy. If a transient ischemic attack is manifested mainly by sensory symptoms, differentiation from a focal sensory seizure may be more difficult. Usually the duration of the attack, presence of known cerebrovascular disease, and absence of epileptiform activity on the EEG suggest the correct diagnosis.

Transient Global Amnesia

Transient global amnesia may present diagnostic difficulties, usually because the physician does not have an opportunity to observe the patient's attack. If the history as given by observers suggests a confusional state, a diagnosis of CPS can be considered. Careful questioning reveals typical features, such as repeated questioning, bewilderment, some apparent confusion, ability to carry out complex actions, and complete lack of memory for the event, and therefore should suggest the diagnosis. The EEG is normal.

Psychiatric Conditions: Fugue States and Psychogenic Amnesia

Fugue states and psychogenic amnesia are psychiatric conditions that are encountered uncommonly. Fugue is differentiated from psychogenic amnesia mainly by definition; that is, fugue involves travel, whereas psychogenic amnesia does not. The individual is amnesic for all actions, which may be carried out flawlessly. Differentiation from CPS, in particular the postictal state, may be difficult. The long duration of the attacks mitigates against a diagnosis of epilepsy. Evidence of a psychiatric disorder usually exists, and EEG studies are normal.[9]

Malingering

Malingering may be the basis of apparent confusional or amnesic states. Such individuals may have pending legal action or other primary gains to account for their actions. In the end, the diagnosis may be suspected but not provable.

Diagnostic Procedures for Non-Epileptic Seizures

Diagnostic procedures for NES and epilepsy are similar, although it must be emphasized that definitive diagnosis may be more difficult in patients with suspected NES. An adequate series of EEG studies is critical, including routine and activation EEGs. An EEG after sleep deprivation is important, especially if a routine study is normal. All patients should have an imaging study, in particular magnetic resonance imaging, which is more sensitive than computed tomography in detailing deep temporal structures. A standard laboratory battery should include anti-epileptic drug levels if applicable. If cardiac or cerebrovascular disease is suspected, Holter monitoring or noninvasive carotid studies should be carried out.

Although the above studies provide important data in evaluating patients for possible NES, the generally agreed-on standard for diagnosis is the recording of a typical event during intensive video-EEG monitoring. Ideally, more than one event should be recorded to determine their similarity, and the event must be typical of those experienced spontaneously. The event must then be reviewed with family members or others who have witnessed the patient's seizures to ensure that it is indeed typical. If seizure frequency is relatively high, at least three events a week, daytime intensive monitoring for 6 to 8 hours may be sufficient. With relatively low seizure frequencies, prolonged monitoring may be required. In general, the use of ambulatory cassette EEG is not recommended as a definitive diagnostic procedure. If multiple seizure types are reported, each type of event should be recorded to exclude coexisting epilepsy (approximately 20% of patients).

During intensive video-EEG monitoring, an opportunity is provided for the examiner to gain important information regarding NES by direct intervention. The presence or absence of responsiveness may be determined, and the character of any observed motor activity may be ascertained. The examiner should attempt to alter repetitive, tonic, or dystonic manifestations, and avoidance testing should be carried out. Pupillary reactivity can be determined and plantar responses evaluated.

If no spontaneous event occurs, some centers make an attempt to precipitate a typical seizure by applying suggestion.[9] This may take the form of intravenous saline, application of alcohol pads over the carotid arteries, or application of a tuning fork to the head. Patients should be told that the procedure is likely to evoke their typical seizures and that recording such an event is important in understanding the problem and arriving at appropriate treatment. The interaction between patient and examiner is a critical determinant of success, regardless of the method used.

Electroencephalographic Findings

Ictal

Before the onset of an event, there should be no depression or ongoing background activity, and a premonitory epileptiform discharge must be absent. During the event, the EEG often is obscured to a great extent by muscle and movement artifact. Due to the intermittence of motor activity, however, artifact-free intervals are frequently observed. During these times, there should be no electrographic seizure activity and no generalized or localized slowing. Indeed, alpha activity may be observed intermittently, which supports the diagnosis of NES. After the event, an alpha rhythm without evidence of postictal slowing should be immediately re-established.

Interictal

It is important to note that the interictal EEG in patients with NES may be normal or abnormal. In fact, it may well contain epileptiform discharges, especially if NES and epilepsy coexist. Conversely, a normal EEG is not infrequent in patients with epilepsy. Thus, caution is advised when considering the significance of interictal EEG findings.

Prolactin

Considerable literature exists on the changes in serum prolactin after the occurrence of various seizure types.[10,11] Of several hormone studies, including cortisol, only prolactin has shown relatively consistent results. Generalized tonic-clonic convulsions result in a marked increase in prolactin levels (at least twofold, often more) in 90–100% of patients, with peak levels occurring 15–30 minutes after the event. This has been the case in studies of patients undergoing electroconvulsive therapy as well as those with spontaneous convulsions. Prolactin elevations after CPS are less consistent (43–100%). Simple partial seizures infrequently elevate prolactin levels (10%), and no change in prolactin has resulted from absence attacks. Finally, prolactin usually does not rise after NES. Thus, the lack of a prolactin response may provide support for a diagnosis of NES but cannot be considered definitive, especially in patients with apparent partial or absence seizures or in females in whom any breast stimulation is part of their ictus; in these patients, a false evaluation of prolactin can occur in NES.

Neuropsychological Testing

Neuropsychological testing may provide supportive data for an NES diagnosis.[12,13] In particular, the Minnesota Multiphasic Personality Inventory (MMPI) has been administered to patients with epilepsy and compared with those who have NES. Patients with NES may demonstrate higher scores on the hypochondriasis, hysteria, schizophrenia, and psychopathic deviate scales than patients with epilepsy. Wilkus et al. (1984)[12] were able to classify correctly 80% of patients with NES and 88% of epileptic patients using their configural rules. Wilkus and Dodrill later reported that patients who have a major change in affect but minor motor activity during NES have a more disturbed MMPI pattern than patients with partial seizures. Conversely, patients with minimal change in affect and major motor features during NES were not distinguishable from patients with generalized convulsions. Other authors have found more variable results in distinguishing NES from epilepsy using the MMPI. Thus, the MMPI may provide supportive data for an NES diagnosis but, at this time, as with other measures of NES, they cannot be considered definitive.

Until recently, patients with a diagnosis of psychogenic NES "fell between the cracks." Neurologists were reluctant to manage such patients after the diagnosis was made, and many were referred to psychiatrists. Psychiatrists, in turn, had little experience dealing with NES patients. Furthermore, many patients with NES have a somatoform disorder, considered by many to be difficult to treat with conventional psychotherapy. Epilepsy centers using intensive video-EEG monitoring realized that NES was relatively common and that such patients should enjoy the benefits of comprehensive care, as did those with epilepsy. Thus, the concept of a multidisciplinary approach to management of patients with NES gained currency.

Approaches to Outpatient Treatment of Non-Epileptic Seizures

The Minnesota Epilepsy Group pioneered inpatient management of NES patients, and their results indicate the success of the concept of multidisciplinary management. Their approach requires a relatively intensive and prolonged hospitalization. An alternative approach, multidisciplinary outpatient management of NES in a specialized clinic (the NES Clinic), has been used successfully at Mount Sinai Medical Center in New York.

Patients referred to the NES Clinic must have a confirmed diagnosis of NES. Clinical evaluation includes the features described in the section on diagnostic procedures, the most important of which is daytime intensive monitoring. At least one seizure must be recorded on EEG and videotape that is typical of the patient's usual events. A conference is held with the patient, the patient's family, and an epileptologist during which the patient's history is reviewed and the results of the daytime intensive monitoring study are discussed. The videotape is reviewed with the family, sometimes separately and sometimes with the patient in attendance. The presence of the patient in the videotape review may be a delicate matter, and the decision is based on the desires of the patient and clinical judgment. After confirmation that the event is typical, the diagnosis is presented to the patient. This is a critical moment, and the presentation must be made with compassion and sensitivity. A positive, optimistic attitude indicates to the patient that a definitive diagnosis has been made. The patient is assured that the seizures are real but are not epileptic and cannot be treated with anti-epileptic medicines. Acknowledgment is made that the seizures have been a great burden, with significant disruption of the patient's life. It is then pointed out that many people experience this type of seizure, and many have been helped. The concept of a specialized clinic is introduced; in such a clinic, the patient is seen and followed by a team of experts including his or her neurologist. Emphasis is given to the success that the clinic has enjoyed. It has been found that patients respond to a caring attitude and are nearly always willing to participate in the program.

The NES Clinic team consists of two neurologists, the epilepsy fellow, a psychiatrist, and a social worker. The team meets once a month, during which new patients are introduced and a management plan is devised. In addition, the progress of past patients is reviewed, with confirmation or revision of the therapeutic plans. During the team meeting, appointments with the social worker and psychiatrist are made for the new patient. During the initial visits with the social worker, a detailed social history is taken, including living and vocational circumstances, family constellation, educational background, possible environmental stressors, and the like. The initial psychiatric evaluation relies heavily on administration of the Structured Clinical Interview (SCI) for the *DSM-IV*. The SCI allows objective diagnoses from the *DSM-IV*. In addition, a psychiatric interview elicits information not covered by the SCI—for example, a history of sexual abuse and possible models in the patient's background for NES. After the evaluation process is completed, the patient returns to the NES Clinic, where the team discusses the evaluation results and formulates a treatment plan. Sometimes, for geographic or personal reasons (e.g., the patient may already be seeing a psychiatrist with whom he or she has a therapeutic relationship), the patient is not followed in the NES Clinic. In these circumstances, the team's recommendations are forwarded to the local practitioner, and interval follow-up visits at the team meetings are scheduled to evaluate the patient's progress.

For patients who remain in the NES Clinic, weekly visits with the social worker are scheduled, as are visits with the psychiatrist as required. In addition, a weekly group psychotherapy session is held. Each month, the team reviews the patient's progress. The method of therapeutic intervention depends on the specific diagnosis or diagnoses that result from the evaluation process. Some patients are treated with psychotropic drugs, for example, those with significant depression or panic disorder. Some receive no medication and, instead, participate in individual or group psychotherapy. Still others require only supportive therapy. In such cases, a main goal is to convince the patient not to "doctor shop" for solutions that are not available.

Outcomes from Outpatient Cancer

Three of the first 10 patients evaluated had epileptiform abnormalities on EEG, and one was known to have epilepsy. Five patients were taking anti-epileptic drugs at the time they were first seen, and all 10 had been treated at some time with AEDs. One patient had had a craniotomy for posterior fossa meningioma, and another had previous resection of cerebellopontine angle meningiomas. One had a documented learning disability, and one was of borderline intelligence.

By definition, all NES patients (with the exception of malingerers) have a psychiatric disorder. Seven of the first 10 patients received psychiatric treatment in the past, and six reported some form of sexual abuse. Eight qualified for a diagnosis other than somatoform disorder, and many of these carried multiple diagnoses. Five had current or previous mood disorders and, surprisingly, eight had anxiety disorders, more specifically, panic disorder with agoraphobia. In none was panic or phobias part of the initial presentation.[14–16]

It should be noted that two patients were involved in litigation at the time of evaluation. For one, settlement of the case resulted in amelioration of the patient's symptoms. The other patient's litigation continues, as do the NES symptoms. The presence of litigation appears to complicate therapy, which may be ineffective until settlement is reached.

References

1. Rowan M, Gates JR (eds). Non-Epileptic Seizures. Boston: Butterworth–Heinemann, 1993.
2. Scott DR. Recognition and Diagnostic Aspects of Nonepileptic Seizures. In MA Riley, A Roy (eds), Pseudoseizures. Baltimore: Williams & Wilkins, 1982;21–34.
3. Reynolds JR. Epilepsy: Its Symptoms, Treatment, and Relation to Other Chronic Diseases. London: John-Churchill, 1861;286–288; facsimile edition, Abbott Laboratories, 1991.
4. Leis AA, Ross MA, Summers AK. Psychogenic seizures: ictal characteristics and diagnostic pitfalls. Neurology 1992;42:95.
5. Gulick TA, Spinks IP, King DW. Pseudoseizures: ictal phenomena. Neurology 1982;32:3440.
6. Kanner AM, Morris HH, Lüders H, et al. Supplementary motor seizures mimicking pseudoseizures: some clinical differences. Neurology 1990;40:1404.

7. Rowan M, Rosenbaum DH. Ictal Amnesia and Fugue States. In DB Smith, DM Treiman, MR Thimble (eds), Advances in Neurology, vol 55. Neurobehavioral Problems in Epilepsy. New York: Raven, 1991;357–368.
8. Mahowald MW, Schenck CH. REM Sleep Behavior Disorder. In MH Kryger, T Roth, WC Dement (eds), Principles and Practice of Sleep Medicine. Philadelphia: Saunders, 1989;389–401.
9. French JA, Kaner AM, Rosenbaum DH, Rowan AS. Do techniques of suggestion aid the differential diagnosis of epileptic vs. psychogenic seizures? Epilepsia 1987;28:612.
10. Trimble M. Serum prolactin in epilepsy and hysteria. BMJ 1978;2:1682.
11. Sperling MR, Pritchard PB, Engel E, et al. Prolactin in partial epilepsy: an indicator of limbic seizures. Ann Neurol 1986;17:7, 727.
12. Wilkus RJ, Dodrill CB. Factors affecting the outcome of MMPI and neuropsychological assessments of psychogenic and epileptic seizure patients. Epilepsia 1989;30:339.
13. Sackellares JC, Giordani B, Berent S, et al. Patients with pseudoseizures: intellectual and cognitive performance. Neurology 1985;35:116.
14. French JA, Rosenbaum DH, Rowan M. Outcome in 55 patients with documented psychogenic seizures: clinical and EEG correlates. Epilepsia 1938;29:653.
15. Gatfield PD, Gold SB. Prognosis and differential diagnosis of conversion reactions: a follow-up study. Dis Nerv Syst 1963;23:623.
16. Williams DT, Gold AP, Shrout P, et al. The impact of psychiatric intervention on patients with uncontrolled seizures. J Nerv Ment Dis 1979;167:626–631.

CHAPTER 3

Unusual Epileptic Events and Non-Epileptic Seizures: Differential Diagnosis and Coexistence

Orrin Devinsky and Joel O. Paraiso

Epileptic seizures (ES) are spontaneous, paroxysmal episodes of altered behavior caused by excessive neuronal discharges. The spectrum of altered behavior is broad and may include weird and indescribable feelings; hallucinations and illusions involving any sensory modality; psychic phenomena such as *déjà vu*, forced thinking, and out-of-body experiences; affective and autonomic symptoms (fear, vomiting); impaired consciousness; and involuntary movements ranging from a momentary jerk (myoclonus), which is considered a shiver, to intense and prolonged convulsions.

Paroxysmal altered behaviors may result from a diverse group of non-neurologic disorders. Various medical as well as psychiatric conditions can present with paroxysmal behavioral changes that can be misinterpreted as epilepsy (Table 3.1). These non-epileptic paroxysmal disorders are common and can mimic many epileptic seizure types.

Correct diagnosis of paroxysmal behavior is essential. Failure to recognize seizures can prevent prompt diagnosis and treatment of curable etiologies. Alternatively, incorrectly diagnosing epilepsy can cause permanent loss of self-esteem and employment and, in many cases, obscure the recognition and treatment of the true underlying disorder.

TABLE 3.1
Non-Epileptic Paroxysmal Disorders

I. Cardiovascular
   A. Syncope
      1. Reflex (vasovagal, carotid sinus, glossopharyngeal)
      2. Respiratory (cough, Valsalva)
      3. Decreased cardiac output
         a. Decreased left ventricular filling
            i. Hypovolemia/dehydration (orthostatic)
            ii. Pulmonary embolism
         b. Arrhythmias
         c. Aortic stenosis
      4. Decreased systemic venous resistance—autonomic dysfunction
         a. Neurogenic
         b. Medication effect
   B. Breath-holding spells
      1. Cyanotic
      2. Noncyanotic
   C. Mitral valve prolapse
II. Cerebrovascular
    Transient ischemic attacks
III. Migraine
IV. Movement disorders
    A. Tics, Tourette's syndrome
    B. Myoclonus
    C. Startle attacks (hyperexplexia)
    D. Chorea and paroxysmal choreoathetosis
    E. Shuddering attacks
    F. Spasmus nutans
V. Sleep disorders
   A. Narcolepsy
   B. Night terrors (*pavor nocturnus*)
   C. Somnambulism
   D. Rapid eye movement sleep disorder
   E. Benign sleep jerks
   F. Periodic leg movements (nocturnal myoclonus)
VI. Metabolic-toxic
    A. Endocrine
       1. Hypo- or hyperglycemia
       2. Cushing's syndrome
    B. Drug ingestion
       1. Toxicity from prescription drugs
       2. Illegal drugs (e.g., heroin, cocaine)
VII. Gastrointestinal disorders
VIII. Psychiatric disorders
      A. Panic disorder
      B. Somatization disorder
      C. Dissociative disorder
      D. Intermittent explosive disorder (episodic dyscontrol)
      E. Psychogenic seizures (conversion disorder)
IX. Malingering

The clinical presentations of non-epileptic seizures (NES) are varied. Generalized convulsive, nonconvulsive, focal motor, and subjective symptoms (i.e., amnesia and various episodic sensations involving any sensory modality) occur. The clinical diagnosis of non-epileptic psychogenic seizures is difficult and has traditionally relied on identification of bizarre or atypical paroxysmal behavioral changes, especially in patients with known psychological or psychiatric disorders. Our concepts regarding the behavioral spectrum of epileptic and non-epileptic seizures have been radically transformed by the information obtained from video-electroencephalographic (EEG) monitoring.

Historical features traditionally associated with NES, such as a histrionic (hysterical) personality style, *la belle indifférence* (unconcern for deficits or problems), depression, anxiety disorder, and a history of physical or sexual abuse, are neither exclusive for nor typical of NES patients. These historical features, although they may be important to identify and have an impact on treatment, cannot reliably distinguish NES from ES. Further, although one or more of these features may raise suspicion of NES, the common coexistence of NES and ES in one particular patient decreases their diagnostic value.[1-3] Primary or secondary gain issues are often identified in NES patients[4,5] but can be absent in NES and present in ES patients. When spells are triggered by emotional factors, NES are often considered. However, in our experience it is more common that patients with ES report that emotional stress provokes seizures than do patients with NES. Uncontrolled seizure activity in spite of high or multiple antiepileptic drugs (AEDs) and frequent emergency room visits or hospitalizations should suggest possible NES but is consistent with medically refractory seizures. Atypical emotional reaction to the seizure (i.e., unconcern after a "convulsive episode" or excessive crying) can suggest NES but is nonspecific. Some patients with tonic-clonic seizures state that they are not particularly bothered by the seizures, especially if they occur during sleep and are not associated with tongue biting. Absence of physical injuries (e.g., tongue biting, abrasion) during convulsive attacks also is traditionally associated with NES but is quite nonspecific. Many tonic-clonic seizures do not cause any physical trauma, and NES can be associated with self-inflicted or accidental injuries.[6,7] A history of physical or emotional abuse or psychiatric disease is common among patients with NES. NES patients also have an increased frequency of a personal history and probably a family or friend's history of epilepsy. Attacks that occur during sleep have been considered ES or a sleep disorder; however, NES can also occur during apparent sleep.[8]

The clinical features of NES vary.[1,4,9,10] Clinical observations suggesting NES are summarized in Table 3.2. Differentiating ES from NES based on visual inspection can be notoriously difficult. Epileptologists often show videotapes of unusual ES and NES that most physicians and many experts incorrectly diagnose without knowledge of the simultaneous EEG.

TABLE 3.2
Clinical Characteristics of Convulsive Non-Epileptic Seizures

Onset
  Gradual
Duration
  Varied/prolonged
Clinical presentation
  Discontinuous activity
  Erratic progression
  Discoordinated motor activity
  Dystonic posturing
  Pelvic thrusting
  Noninvolvement of facial musculature during a generalized event
  Crying during or after event
  Lack of gradual cessation of clonic activity
  Disorientation to person after the event
Provocation test
  Usually positive
Electroencephalography
  Ictal
    Usually unchanged from baseline except for prominent muscle and movement artifact
  Postictal
    Usually unchanged from baseline

However, the vast majority of ES and NES can be clinically distinguished with experience. No single clinical feature distinguishes NES from ES; one must rely on a cluster of features. Absence, atypical absence, tonic, myoclonic, simple partial, complex partial, and tonic-clonic seizures have distinct clinical pictures. There is considerable variability, but usually within a defined range. In adults, for example, most tonic-clonic seizures last for 40–200 seconds. The duration, gradual slowing in the frequency of clonic jerks at offset, and unnatural facial contractions usually allow reliable differentiation from "convulsive NES." Frontal lobe complex partial seizures (see Frontal Lobe Seizures, later) represent perhaps the most common ES type to be confused with NES. The combination of sudden onset of complex movements (often beginning in the trunk), nocturnal occurrence, and brief but highly stereotypic duration (e.g., always within a range of 10–14 seconds) should always make one very suspicious of frontal lobe complex partial seizures.

With NES, the onset is usually gradual and disjointed.[11] Unlike ES, the duration of NES often varies and is commonly prolonged (>5 minutes of ictal activity).[6,9,11] The "ictal event" itself may present with discontinuous, uncoordinated activity with erratic progression. Stopping and starting of ictal motor activity is much more common in ES than in NES, but complex partial status can mimic this pattern. In NES, however, there is often vigorous motor activity for a brief period, and the patient seems to "take a rest" before resuming another round of NES. Pelvic thrusting, thrashing or flailing movements, out-of-phase clonic or jerking movements (this is a nonspecific feature in which one arm flexes while the other extends), tremors, and lack of facial muscle involvement during a generalized event are more common in NES than ES.[1,4,9,11,12] The lack of gradual slowing in the rate of clonic activity near the end of a convulsive spell is very helpful, because NES rarely come close to accurately imitating the ending of a convulsion (i.e., most of the time rapid shaking ends abruptly).[1]

Convulsive NES are common.[1,4,6,11–13] These apparent convulsions can be associated with opisthotonic posturing, out-of-sequence movements, or other features that suggest but cannot be used in isolation to diagnose non-epileptic convulsions. Vocalizations (e.g., moaning, crying, gasping, choking, and groaning) can occur at the onset of a convulsive NES[4,9,11] and often differ significantly in quality from the intense and unnatural vocalization of force expiration against the contracted laryngeal musculature that occurs near the onset of many tonic-clonic seizures. Urinary incontinence is more common with convulsive ES than with NES but does not distinguish these events because patients with ES often have no incontinence and, uncommonly, patients with NES can have incontinence.[9,6,11]

Subjective symptoms suggesting auras (e.g., lightheadedness, dizziness, headache, nausea, and focal or generalized numbness) are common in patients who have convulsive NES.[1,6,11] Some patients are well informed about the historical features of epilepsy and provide remarkably "good" stories of their auras (e.g., rising abdominal sensation and a bad smell).

Diagnostic Tests Help to Distinguish Epileptic and Non-Epileptic Seizures

Routine Electroencephalography

Although most patients with NES do not have epilepsy, the two disorders can coexist in 10–40% of patients. Thus, the finding of interictal epileptiform activity can support the diagnosis of epilepsy in a patient but does not establish that current events are epileptic. One or more normal interictal EEGs can never exclude the diagnosis of epilepsy.

Video-Electroencephalographic Monitoring

Correlating the EEG and clinical changes during a paroxysmal behavioral event with video-EEG remains the most reliable method to differentiate NES from ES.[4] NES are not associated with EEG changes during the ictal or postictal periods.[1,4,6] In contrast, complex partial and tonic-clonic seizures are almost always associated with characteristic ictal patterns and postictal slowing. However, frontal lobe complex partial and simple partial seizures from any region may not be associated with ictal EEG changes. Prominent movement and muscle artifact often compromise the recording during NES. Interictal EEGs of NES patients may be abnormal, revealing either slowing or, occasionally, epileptiform activity. Because 10–40% of patients with NES can have both ES and NES, epileptic seizures with characteristic ictal patterns are occasionally documented in NES patients.[6,14]

Prolactin Levels

Significantly elevated serum prolactin levels occur after tonic-clonic seizures and temporal lobe epilepsy (TLE) and to a lesser degree among those with extratemporal lobe epilepsy.[15–17] Complex partial seizures are more likely to elevate prolactin levels than are simple partial seizures. Unfortunately, frontal lobe complex partial seizures, which are often difficult to distinguish from NES, are not consistently associated with elevated prolactin. To further confound diagnostic specificity, we have observed four- to fivefold increases in prolactin levels after convulsive syncope. With convulsive NES, mild elevations of prolactin levels may be found, but marked (>2.0–2.5 times) baseline levels do not occur.[18,19] Prolactin levels are most helpful when obtained within 15 minutes after a tonic-clonic or complex partial seizure, because levels begin to fall after this period, obscuring the difference between ES and NES.

Epileptic Seizures Misdiagnosed as Non-Epileptic

Most studies and reviews distinguishing NES from ES focus on features of NES. However, certain ES are misdiagnosed as psychogenic, especially when the clinical manifestations are bizarre or do not conform to expected patterns. Because physicians usually do not have the opportunity to witness stereotypic paroxysmal behaviors, misdiagnosis is common. Although NES are more commonly misdiagnosed as ES, the converse probably occurs with greater regularity than might be suspected.

The most common reasons for misdiagnosis of ES are summarized in Table 3.3. In many cases, normal laboratory studies such as EEGs or coexistence of behavioral disorders lead physicians to discount the possibility of epilepsy. However, physicians should be cautious about making this diagnosis on such results alone. An important caveat in diagnosing NES can be invoked to explain many cases in which ES are misdiagnosed as NES: *Never rely on a single clinical feature.* One must make the diagnosis of ES or NES based on the combination of many features. When the clinical and laboratory features suggest both ES and NES, one must approach

TABLE 3.3
Factors That Lead to Misdiagnosis of Epileptic Seizures as Non-Epileptic Seizures

Feature	Comment
Clinical	
Bizarre subjective features (e.g., out-of-body-experience, forced thinking)	Occur with frontal and temporal partial seizures.
Bizarre automatism (e.g., pelvic thrusting, masturbation, rocking)	Occurs with frontal and less often with extrafrontal complex partial seizures.
Ictal or postictal emotional display	Ictal laughing is more common than ictal crying (rare); postictal crying is usually functional.
Prolonged duration	Can occur with all seizure types; witness or patient combines ictal and postictal phases.
Lack of physical injury with "convulsion"	Common with tonic-clonic and other seizure types.
Preserved consciousness with bilateral motor activity	Common with supplementary motor area seizures.
Preserved consciousness during automatism or fluent ictal speech that is not recalled	Occur with right temporal and less often with left extratemporal or extratemporal seizures.
Lack of stereotypic seizures (i.e., clinical features change)	Clinical features of seizures can fluctuate a fair amount (e.g., presence or absence of aura, variable aura; variable duration); however, certain patterns are often stereotypic.
Prominent anxiety, depression, or histrionic behavioral traits	Occurs in patients with epileptic seizures (ES).
History of physical or sexual abuse	Occurs in patients with ES.
Psychological or psychiatric disorders	Common in patients with ES.
Failure to fully respond to multiple anti-epileptic drugs	Defines refractory epilepsy.
Electroencephalography (EEG)	
One or multiple normal interictal EEGs	Occur with frontal lobe and less often extrafrontal seizure foci.
Normal EEG during a simple partial seizure	Common.
Normal EEG during a complex partial seizure	Occurs with frontal and less often extrafrontal complex partial seizures.
Only muscle and movement artifact during a "convulsion"	Can occur; look for evidence of postictal slowing compared to preictal baseline.
Other laboratory studies	
Lack of elevated prolactin level after an "ictal event"	Occurs with extratemporal complex partial and all simple partial seizures; if blood, take >15 mins after a seizure.
Normal neuroimaging studies	Common with partial and the rule in generalized epilepsies.

diagnosis with great humility. Both disorders may be present but, in most cases, some of the data are misleading or inaccurate. Table 3.4 summarizes the seizure types that are most commonly misdiagnosed as psychogenic.

Frontal Lobe Seizures

Frontal lobe seizures are most often misdiagnosed as NES because many features have been used by epileptologists to help define NES. These features include (1) bizarre automatisms that may include sexual (e.g., pelvic thrusting, genital manipulation) or vocal (e.g., grunts, screams, curses) components, (2) lack of interictal or ictal EEG changes, (3) failure to respond to AEDs, (4) interictal personality and behavioral disorders, (5) preserved consciousness during bilateral motor seizures (most often with supplementary motor foci), and (6) lack of postictal phase (i.e., no confusion, lethargy). Table 3.4 summarizes the clinical features of frontal lobe seizures.

Seizures that arise from primary motor or adjacent premotor cortex usually produce stereotypic motor seizures, often with a characteristic spread, the jacksonian march, reflecting the sequential activation of the motor cortex. Because of the robust interconnections with the primary sensory cortex, many of these seizures cause sensory phenomena or the "sensation of movement." Although simple partial motor seizures are more likely to have ictal EEG changes than are nonmotor simple partial seizures,[20] many lack EEG changes. Furthermore, neuroimaging studies may also be normal. Occasionally, superior or mesial foci in the motor cortex cause bizarre, gross movements involving proximal muscles that appear functional. In some cases, the patient uses the contralateral arm to hold down the "wild limb," further supporting an apparent theatrical performance to some onlookers.

Supplementary motor area (SMA) seizures may be misdiagnosed as NES because of their unusual behavioral features and often subtle or absent EEG changes (see Table 3.3). Onset is often abrupt with violent motor activity, usually without warning. However, some patients experience sensory auras, such as numbness, tingling, pulling, or nonspecific head sensations.[21-23] The classic fencer's posture of unilateral head or eye deviation with arm abduction and elbow flexion is not the most common motor pattern.[24] Rather, various combinations of tonic posturing and clonic movements involving contralateral or bilateral upper extremities or all four extremities are observed. Twisting movements of the truncal muscles can occur, and tonic, dystonic, and clonic movements are common. Seizure may manifest as brief attacks.[25] Speech arrest is common, but loud vocalizations such as grunts can occur. Preserved consciousness is typical unless the seizure becomes secondarily generalized. Patient or witness reports of preserved awareness and recall, despite bilateral motor activity,

TABLE 3.4
Epileptic Seizures Misdiagnosed as Psychogenic

Frontal lobe complex partial seizures
- Frequent stereotype seizures, often in clusters
- Brief duration (<1 min)
- Minimal postictal confusion and lethargy
- Complex motor automatisms
- Kicking, rocking, thrashing, rubbing, scratching, genital manipulation, head nodding, vocalization (hum, squeals, shouting obscenities)
- Urinary incontinence
- Frequent episodes of complex partial status epilepticus

Supplementary motor area seizures
- Unilateral head and/or eye deviation, arm abduction, elbow flexion (head looks at the hand—fencer's posture)
- Bilateral upper and/or lower extremity tonic or clonic activity with preserved consciousness
- Vocalization (grunts, hum)
- Speech arrest

Temporal lobe simple partial seizures
- Forced thinking
- Autoscopy (out-of-body experiences, seeing one's double)
- Depersonalization (alteration in one's sense of personal reality and experience of self)
- Derealization (alteration in one's sense of external reality)
- Fear, panic
- Depression
- Complex visual or auditory hallucinations

Temporal lobe complex partial seizures
- Laughing; rarely, crying
- Vocalization
  - Repetition of a word or phrase, either side
  - Fluent speech (right temporal seizures)
  - Walking
- Continuation of ongoing behavior

Reflex epilepsies
- Light—flickering, sudden intensity changes, television/video
- Language—reading, writing, speaking
- Cognition
- Startle
- Somatosensory-proprioceptive
- Auditory
- Eating
- Vestibular
- Hot-water immersion
- Self-induced

Myoclonic jerks

Hypothalamic hamartomas and seizures
- Laughing
- Precocious puberty
- Interictal aggressive behavior

suggest a "conversion convulsion" to many physicians. Preserved consciousness during NES mimicking tonic-clonic seizures distinguishes these from tonic-clonic seizures but not from SMA seizures. SMA seizures can be frequent, often occurring in clusters, mainly during sleep.[26,27] Interictal and ictal EEG changes vary from prominent epileptiform activity over the ipsilateral or contralateral superior frontal region to normal patterns.

Complex partial seizures from prefrontal, cingulate, or orbitofrontal areas are also commonly misdiagnosed as NES due to their unusual features and commonly normal ictal and interictal recordings.[28,29] Complex motor automatisms, including kicking, rocking, thrashing, rubbing, scratching, and head nodding, can occur.[23,28,30–33] Sexual automatisms, such as pelvic thrusting, masturbatory activity, and exhibitionism, also may occur.[34,35] Vocalizations, including shouting obscenities, have been associated with frontal lobe CPS. The seizures, which occur frequently (at least 10 per day), are brief in duration, lasting an average of less than 1 minute.[28] Clustering of seizures and complex partial status epilepticus are common.[28] Seizures often occur at night. Scalp EEG recordings may be normal or falsely localizing, reflecting patterns of spread rather than onset.[28,31] Subdural and depth electrode recordings are typically required during surgical evaluation to define the ictal focus.[28]

Temporal Lobe Seizures

The temporal lobe is the most common site of simple partial seizure focus.[36] Autonomic phenomena, such as piloerection, vomiting, increased heart rate or blood pressure, pallor, and sweating, are common during temporal lobe seizures.[37–41] Subjective symptoms associated with temporal lobe foci are extremely diverse, manifesting as paroxysmal alteration in autonomic, cognitive, speech, emotional, and special sensory functioning, with illusions, hallucinations, increased sensitivity, or defective sensation in olfaction, taste, hearing, and higher-order visual processing (see Table 3.4). Episodes usually are brief, lasting between 30 and 180 seconds, and are generally not associated with changes on the scalp EEG recordings.[20] Visceral or indescribable body or head sensations are common. Forced thinking and alterations in the speed of mental processes or time perception can occur during temporal lobe seizures.[37] *Déjà vu* (feeling of familiarity) and *jamais vu* (feeling of unfamiliarity) usually occur with right temporal seizures.[42,43] *Déjà vu* or *jamais entendu*, similar events in the auditory realm, also occur with TLE. Forced recollections of past memories occur as simple partial seizures originating from mesial or lateral temporal regions.[24,37] Depersonalization, an alteration or loss of the sense of self, and derealization, altered perception of the external world (e.g., dreamy state), can occur.[44] Autoscopy, a phenomenon in which one experiences a sense of having an external double or an out-of-body experience with the perception of seeing oneself from the outside, occurs with temporal and extratemporal seizure foci.[45] Ictal emotions, such as unprovoked fear, anxiety, anger, hate, depression, embarrassment, joy, love, religious ecstasy, and sexual feelings, can occur.[37,46,47] Visual illusions and hallucinations are common, occurring in approximately 20% of TLE patients.[24,48,49] Visual illusion can involve distortions in size, shape, color, luminescence, motion, and distance.[37,49-51] Visual hallucinations are typically complex, including visual scenes or people. Complex visual hallucinations and hallucinations that involve several sensory modalities (e.g., seeing a person who talks) often arise from the right temporal cortex. Complex auditory hallucinations such as music and voices are common among TLE patients.[24,49] Simple auditory hallucinations (e.g., buzzing, ambulance sound, or clicking) are common and suggest posterosuperior temporal involvement.[24,38,49,52]

Complex partial seizures comprise 55% of all adult seizures, and most arise from the temporal lobe.[36,53] Temporal lobe complex partial seizures are characterized by impaired consciousness, usually accompanied by oral or upper extremity automatisms,[29,48,54] and are followed by mild confusion and lethargy. Seizures typically last between 1 and 2 minutes.[37,38] However, the postictal phase of confusion may be prolonged, leading witnesses to estimate that the seizure lasted 20 minutes, and possibly contributing to confusion with NES. Automatisms in TLE may consist of de novo activity or preservation of an already existing behavior.[42,55] Oral-alimentary are the most common automatisms, consisting of lip smacking, swallowing, sucking, puckering, chewing, and other movements.[38,56] Manual (upper extremity, hand) automatisms are common and consist of simple repetitive behaviors such as fumbling or picking that may progress to more complex forms of stereotypic behavior. Unilateral upper extremity automatisms are associated with ictal discharges in the ipsilateral temporal lobe.[56] In contrast, dystonic movements are associated with ictal discharges in the contralateral temporal lobe. Gestural automatisms overlap with manual automatisms. Gestural automatisms consist of stereotypic semipurposeful motor activity, such as nose, neck, or chest rubbing; smiling; and grimacing.[56] Other motor changes such as walking or continuation or cessation of ongoing motor activity (e.g., pouring a glass of water, driving a car, walking) can occur during temporal lobe seizures. Occasionally, patients run or try to "escape" their environment during a complex partial seizure. Emotional automatisms such as laughing or crying[57] occur during temporal and frontal seizures.[58-61] Automatisms may extend into the postictal period, at which time they are more reactive to the environment.[38] Ictal automatisms with preserved responsiveness and CPS with fluent speech usually occur with nondominant temporal lobe foci.[62] With rapid spread from temporal to frontal areas, automatisms characteristic of frontal lobe CPS may occur with temporal foci. After temporal lobe CPS, patients usually are lethargic and confused for seconds to minutes. Recovery often is gradual, and patients generally have amnesia for the event, although intermediate levels of awareness and memory are possible. Many patients report that they are "half here and half there" or "removed but yet present." Patients may subsequently report that they can hear what people are saying but cannot respond to them. In many such cases, recall for events during the seizure is incomplete.

Reflex Epilepsy

Five percent to 6% of patients with epilepsy have seizures that can be activated by specific stimuli—that is, a reflex.[63] The reflex epilepsies can be provoked by diverse stimuli and cause either partial or generalized seizures. Diagnosis of reflex epilepsy often provides clues to the epilepsy syndrome and treatment. Because of the unusual nature of some provocative factors such as cognition or emotion, physicians may incorrectly diagnose NES.

Light Stimuli

Photosensitive epilepsy is the most common form of reflex epilepsy, occurring most often in 10- to 15-year-olds, with a female predominance. Genetic factors often are present. The EEG signature of photosensitive epilepsy is a photoconvulsive response (generalized spike or polyspike and wave discharges) during intermittent light stimulation. Among patients with a photoparoxysmal response, 70% have seizures evoked by a light stimulus. Approximately 40% of patients with photosensitive epilepsy only have light stimulus–induced seizures. Common environmental triggers include sunlight passing through trees in a moving vehicle, sudden bright or reflected lights, and strobes. Occasionally, patients have seizures induced by visual patterns, usually vertical or horizontal lines (e.g., venetian blinds, striped or plaid patterns). Video games can provoke seizures. Photosensitive epilepsies usually remit by the third decade. Treatment includes identification and avoidance of environmental triggers. Dark (especially blue sunglasses) or polarized glasses and viewing televisions from greater than 7 feet can help.[63] Valproate is effective in most patients, as are benzodiazepines and ethosuximide.

Reading, Speaking, and Writing

Myoclonic jerks of the jaw and laryngeal muscles can be evoked by reading and less often by speaking or writing.[64] These seizures are most often associated with left perisylvian foci, but generalized spike and slow-wave discharges also occur.[63] Ethosuximide, valproate, and benzodiazepines are often effective in reading epilepsy.

Cognition

A variety of mental activities, including playing chess or card games, making a decision, and performing mathematics or visuospatial tasks, can evoke myoclonic seizures. In many patients, more than one specific trigger exists. The seizures usually are bilateral and maximally involve proximal upper extremities. Interictal and ictal EEGs reveal generalized spike and polyspike and slow-wave discharges.[65] Many of these patients have juvenile myoclonic epilepsy.[66] Valproate and benzodiazepines often are effective.

Startle

Sudden and unexpected auditory, tactile (e.g., stumbling) or, rarely, visual stimuli can evoke unilateral or bilateral tonic seizures, often with adversive eye and head deviation. Most patients have spastic or tetraplegic cerebral palsy and mental retardation; many have genetic or metabolic disorders, with the initial cerebral insult before age 2 years in children with perirolandic encephalomalacia. Startle seizures usually begin between ages 2 and 8 years and are often preceded by spontaneous seizures.

Somatosensory and Proprioceptive Stimuli

Tactile stimuli can evoke seizures without startle, that is, somatosensory reflex epilepsy. Seizures usually are tonic and generally involve the stimulated hand or face. Parietal lobe seizure foci are typical, often associated with structural lesions. Proprioceptive changes can rarely evoke seizures. Most "movement-induced" seizures probably result from positional changes, not movement. The disorder most often complicates nonketotic hyperglycemia in elderly patients with unilateral sensory or motor deficits, but can occur sporadically.

Complex Auditory Stimuli

Seizures induced by music, voices, or other complex auditory stimuli are rare and usually occur in patients with partial epilepsy. In musicogenic epilepsy, specific songs or types of music evoke partial or secondary generalized seizures that arise from either hemisphere. Nonmusical stimuli such as a frequency-band of church bells or a person's voice can also provoke seizures.

Other Stimuli

Eating, vestibular stimulation, and hot-water immersion can occasionally evoke seizures.

Self-Induced Seizures

Visual self-stimulation is the most common form of self-induced seizures, which can be induced by proprioception and other stimuli. Patients may be compulsively attracted to sunlight, wave their hand with open fingers in front of a light source to cause intermittent photic stimulation, or adjust the vertical hold on a television to provoke seizures. Self-induced seizures are often difficult to control with AEDs. Antipsychotic and anticompulsive drugs may help.

Myoclonic Jerks

Myoclonic seizures are the most characteristic feature of juvenile myoclonic epilepsy and may occasionally be the only seizure type. When myoclonic jerks occur in isolation, they may be misidentified as tremors due to anxiety or movement disorders. Benign nocturnal myoclonus (hypnic jerks) must be distinguished from epileptic myoclonus. Although epileptic myoclonus often occurs during the transition into or during the early stages of sleep, benign nocturnal myoclonus is restricted to this period. If EEG recordings are made, hypnic jerks are not associated with epileptiform discharges, in contrast to myoclonic seizures. Also, nocturnal epileptic myoclonus is more likely to occur as a cluster of jerks, in contrast to the usual single benign hypnic jerks. Only episodes of myoclonus during wakefulness clearly support the diagnosis of juvenile myoclonic epilepsy unless nocturnal events are associated with epileptiform discharges. However, most of the patients we surveyed or their family members reported frequent, moderate-intensity myoclonic jerks shortly after falling asleep. In eliciting the history of myoclonic seizures, it is helpful to describe specific types of myoclonic jerks that are commonly reported, such as the shoulders and proximal upper extremities, neck, and facial and jaw muscles. In some cases, it was only when the physician imitated the jerk that the patient recognized the phenomenon as a common event. Myoclonic jerks usually were mild and only rarely caused the patient to fall. However, many patients reported dropping objects in association with myoclonic jerks. All seizure types occur most frequently during the first several hours after awakening or shortly before awakening. However, many patients report seizures occurring throughout the day without any peak period.

Hypothalamic Hamartomas and Gelastic Epilepsy

Gelastic seizures (ictal laughter) are a characteristic but nonspecific seizure type associated with hypothalamic hamartomas.[67-71] Gelastic seizures also occur with frontal and temporal seizure foci and probably result from spread to the cingulate gyrus.[72] Gelastic seizures resulting from hypothalamic hamartomas usually begin in infancy or childhood and are associated with cognitive delays, precocious puberty, and behavioral problems such as interictal aggression. The behavioral problems in these patients can be the most disabling feature of the disorder, because patients may assault family members and strangers. We have seen one patient with coexisting ES and NES. Complex partial, atypical absence, and tonic-clonic seizures often develop in later childhood or early adulthood. Diagnosis is based on magnetic resonance imaging studies demonstrating a hypothalamus; computed tomographic scans are usually normal. Response to AED is generally disappointing.[68,69] Temporal lobectomy is usually unsuccessful, but resection of the hypothalamic lesion can improve behavior, hormonal abnormalities, and seizure control,[70] although postresection morbidity can be significant.

Coexistence of Epileptic and Non-Epileptic Seizures

Coexistence of ES in a patient with NES ranges from 10% to 40% in most studies but more than 50% in some reports.[1,2,73-76] Just like ES, NES can be very stereotypic, with almost identical clinical features and durations from one event to the next. NES are usually clinically atypical of ES but can mimic any common seizure type. Because descriptions provided by family members or coworkers often are the basis of the diagnosis, care must be taken in assessing these histories. These descriptions may not be accurate in either their details of what happened (e.g., to which side did the head turn, which hand was held in a dystonic posture) or duration (i.e., there is a strong tendency to overestimate the duration). Witness and patient accounts can also be obscured by inaccurate and loose use of terms such as tonic-clonic (grand mal) seizures ("and I've seen 'em before!"), upward rolling of the eyeballs, and others.

Placebo activation of seizures can help diagnose NES.[60,61,77] Rarely, suggestive techniques with placebo can induce an ES, probably by evoking emotionally triggered seizures or coincidentally (the test is often done on inpatients in whom AEDs have been withdrawn). One must verify that a provoked seizure is typical of the patient's spontaneous activity by reviewing the videotape with witnesses.[78] History of a prolonged febrile seizure, significant head trauma, abnormalities on neurologic examination or neuroimaging studies that correlate with the ictal description, and abnormal interictal EEG strongly support the diagnosis of ES. However, ES coexist with NES, and historical findings cannot exclude possible NES. NES patients have a coexisting psychiatric diagnosis, depression being the most commonly associated condition. Many other psychopathologies have been observed.

We studied 20 patients with coexisting ES and NES (ES/NES) from a group of 99 consecutive NES patients.[1] We excluded 12 patients with a probable history of ES in the past due to lack of definite diagnostic data. We compared the 20 patients with ES and NES to control groups with only ES or only NES. All 20 ES/NES developed NES after ES. Clinical features of NES clearly differed from ES in 18 of 20 cases. The two patients with NES closely mimicking ES had "convulsive NES." In patients with ES/NES, their ES were similar to seizures in patients with only ES, and their NES were similar to spells in patients with only NES. ES/NES patients were similar to ES in electrodiagnostic and neuroimaging studies and similar to NES in psychiatric interviews and inventories.

The diagnosis and treatment of NES are facilitated by a multidisciplinary approach, including assessment by a neurologist (with video-EEG monitoring, provocative testing, etc.), a neuropsychiatrist (using psychiatric interview to explore primary and secondary gain), psychiatric inventories to identify depressive and anxiety disorders, a psychologist to explore psychological factors and neuropsychological functioning, and a social worker to explore family, work, and personal dynamics. In some cases, the diagnosis remains uncertain. Treatment and management are often challenging. Many patients with NES do not respond well to behavioral or psychiatric approaches despite vigorous attempts at psychotherapy to unravel the underlying psychopathology. However, just as failure to respond to numerous AEDs with documented therapeutic levels should raise a "red flag" for possible NES, failure to respond to vigorous behavioral and psychiatric therapies should prompt consideration that some, or all, episodes are epileptic.

References

1. Devinsky O, Sanchez-Villasenor F, Vazquez B, et al. Clinical profile of patients with epileptic and nonepileptic seizures. Neurology 1996;46: 530–533.
2. Ozkara C, Dreifuss FE. Differential diagnosis in pseudoepileptic seizures. Epilepsia 1993;34:294.
3. McDade G, Brown SW. Non-epileptic seizures: management and predictive factors of outcome. Seizure 1992;1:7.
4. Desai BT, Porter RJ, Penry JK. Psychogenic seizures: a study of 42 attacks in six patients, with intensive monitoring. Arch Neurol 1982;39:202.
5. Lesser RP. Psychogenic Seizures. In TA Pedley, BS Meidrum (eds), Recent Advances in Epilepsy. Edinburgh: Churchill Livingstone, 1985;273–296.
6. Luther JS, McNamara JO, Carwile S, et al. Pseudoepileptic seizures: methods and video analysis to aid diagnosis. Ann Neurol 1982;12:458.
7. Scott DF. Recognition and Diagnostic Aspects of Nonepileptic Seizures. In TL Riley, A Roy (eds), Pseudoseizures. Baltimore: Williams & Wilkins, 1982;21–33.
8. Thacker K, Devinsky O, Perrine K, et al. Nonepileptic seizures during apparent sleep. Ann Neurol 1993;33:414.
9. Gates JR, Ramani V, Whalen S, et al. Ictal characteristics of pseudoseizures. Arch Neurol 1985;42:1183.
10. Riley TL, Brannan WL. Recognition of pseudoseizures. J Fam Pract 1980; 10:213.

11. Gulick TA, Spinks RP, King DW. Pseudoseizures: ictal phenomena. Neurology 1982;32:24.
12. Cohen RJ, Suter C. Hysterical seizures: suggestion as a provocative EEG test. Ann Neurol 1982;11:391.
13. Holme GL, Sackellares JC, McKiernan J, et al. Evaluation of childhood pseudoseizures using EEG telemetry and video tape monitoring. J Pediatr 1980; 97:554.
14. King DW, Gallagher BB, Murvin AJ, et al. Pseudoseizures: diagnostic evaluation. Neurology 1982;32:18.
15. Trimble MR. Serum prolactin in epilepsy and hysteria. BMJ 1978;2:1682.
16. Collins WCJ, Lanigan O, Callaghan N. Plasma prolactin concentrations following epileptic and pseudoseizures. J Neurol Neurosurg Psychiatry 1983; 46:505.
17. Wroe SJ, Henley R, John R, et al. The clinical value of serum prolactin measurement in the differential diagnosis of complex partial seizures. Epilepsy Res 1989;3:248.
18. Laxer KD, Mullooly JP, Howell B. Prolactin changes after seizures classified by EEG monitoring. Neurology 1985;35:31.
19. Yerby MS, Van Belle G, Friel PN, et al. Serum prolactins in the diagnosis of epilepsy: sensitivity, specificity, and predictive value. Neurology 1987; 37:1224.
20. Devinsky O, Kelley K, Porter RJ, Theodore WH. Clinical and electroencephalographic features of simple partial seizures. Neurology 1988;38:1347.
21. Morris HH III, Dinner DS, Lüders H, et al. Supplementary motor seizures: clinical and electroencephalographic findings. Neurology 1988;38:1075.
22. Rasmussen T. Characteristics of a pure culture of frontal lobe epilepsy. Epilepsia 1983;24:482.
23. Salanova V, Morris HH, Van Ness P, et al. Frontal lobe seizures: electroclinical syndromes. Epilepsia 1995;36:16.
24. Penfield W, Jasper H. Epilepsy and the Functional Anatomy of the Human Brain. Boston: Little, Brown, 1954.
25. Benbadis SR, Kotagal P, Rothner AD. Supplementary motor area seizures presenting as stumbling episodes. Seizure 1995;4:241.
26. Fusco L, Iani C, Faedda MT, et al. Mesial frontal lobe epilepsy: a clinical entity not sufficiently described. J Epilepsy 1990;3:123.
27. Tinuper P, Cerullo A, Cirignotta F, et al. Nocturnal paroxysmal dystonia with short-lasting attacks: three cases with evidence for an epileptic frontal lobe origin of seizures. Epilepsia 1990;31:549.
28. Williamson PD, Spencer DD, Spencer SS, et al. Complex partial seizures of frontal lobe origin. Ann Neurol 1985;18:497.
29. Williamson PD, Spencer SS. Clinical and EEG features of complex partial seizures of extratemporal origin. Epilepsia 1986;27(Suppl 2): S46.
30. Laskowitz DT, Sperling MR, French JA, O'Connor MJ. The syndrome of frontal lobe epilepsy. Neurology 1995;45:780.

31. Geier S, Bancaud J, Talairach J, et al. Automatisms during frontal lobe epileptic seizures. Brain 1976;99:447.
32. Geier S, Bancaud J, Talairach J, et al. The seizures of frontal lobe epilepsy: a study of clinical manifestations. Neurology 1977;27:951.
33. Tharp BR. Orbital frontal seizures: a unique electroencephalographic and clinical syndrome. Epilepsia 1972;13:627.
34. Spencer SS, Spencer DD, Williamson PD, et al. Sexual automatisms in complex partial seizures. Neurology 1983;33:527.
35. Boone KB, Miller BL, Rosenberg L, et al. Neuropsychological and behavioral abnormalities in an adolescent with frontal lobe seizures. Neurology 1988;38:583.
36. Cahan LD, Sutherling W, McCulloough MA, et al. Review of the 20-year UCLA experience with surgery for epilepsy. Cleve Clin Q 1984;51:313.
37. Daly D. Ictal clinical manifestations of complex partial seizures. Adv Neurol 1975;11:57.
38. Williamson PD, Weiser HG, Delgado-Escueta AV. Clinical Characteristics of Partial Seizures. In J Engel (ed), Surgical Treatment of the Epilepsies. New York: Raven, 1987;101–120.
39. Devinsky O, Price BH, Cohen SI. Cardiac manifestations of complex partial seizures. Am J Med 1986;80:195.
40. Kotagal P. Seizure Symptomatology of Temporal Lobe Epilepsy. In H Lüders (ed), Epilepsy Surgery. New York: Raven, 1991;143–156.
41. Van Buren JM, Ajmone-Marsan C. A correlation of autonomic and EEG components in temporal lobe epilepsy. Arch Neurol 1960;3:683.
42. Gastaut H, Broughton R. Epileptic Seizures. Springfield, IL: Thomas, 1972.
43. Bancaud J, Brunet-Bourgin F, Chauvel P, Halgren E. Anatomical origin of *deja vu* and vivid "memories" in human temporal lobe epilepsy. Brain 1994;117:71.
44. Jackson JH. On right- or left-sided spasm at the onset of epileptic paroxysms, and on crude sensation warnings and elaborate mental states. Brain 1880;3:192–200.
45. Devinsky O, Feldmann E, Burrows K, et al. Autoscopic phenomena with seizures. Arch Neurol 1989;46:1080.
46. Williams D. The structure of emotions reflecting in epileptic seizures. Brain 1956;79:29.
47. Daly D. Ictal affect. Am J Psychiatry 1958;115:97.
48. King DW, Ajmone-Marsan C. Clinical features and ictal patterns in epileptic patients with EEG temporal lobe foci. Ann Neurol 1977;2:138.
49. Penfield W, Perot P. The brain's record of auditory and visual experience. Brain 1963;86:595.
50. Baldwin M. Hallucinations in Neurologic Syndromes. In LJ West (ed), Hallucinations. New York: Grune & Stratton, 1962;77–86.
51. Russell WR, Whitty CWM. Studies in traumatic epilepsy. 3: Visual fits. J Neurol Neurosurg Psychiatry 1955;18:79.

52. Weiser HG. Electroclinical Features of the Psychomotor Seizure. New York: Butterworth, 1983.
53. Jackson JH. On a particular variety of epilepsy ("intellectual aura"): one case with symptoms of organic brain disease. Brain 1988;11:179.
54. Delgado-Escueta AV, Swartz B, Chauvel P, et al. Clinical and CCTV-EFG evaluation in presurgical work-up of temporal and frontal lobe epilepsies. Epilepsy Res 1992;5(Suppl):37.
55. Penry JK, Dreifuss FE. Automatisms associated with the absence of petit mal epilepsy. Arch Neurol 1969;21:142.
56. Quesney LF. Clinical and EEG features of complex partial seizures of temporal lobe origin. Epilepsia 1986;27(Suppl 2):527.
57. Luciano D, Devinsky O, Perrine K. Crying seizures. Neurology 1993;43: 2113–2117.
58. Sackeim HA, Greenberg MS, Weiman AL, et al. Hemispheric asymmetry in the expression of positive and negative emotions. Neurologic evidence. Arch Neurol 1982;39:210.
59. Sethi PK, Rao TS. Gelastic, quiritarian, and cursive epilepsy. J Neurol Neurosurg Psychiatry 1976;39:823.
60. Guberman A. Psychogenic pseudoseizures in non-epileptic patients. Can J Psychiatry 1982;27:401.
61. Luther SJ, McNamara JO, Carwile S, et al. Pseudoepileptic seizures: methods and video analysis to aid diagnosis. Ann Neurol 1982;12:458.
62. Ebner A, Dinner DS, Noachtar S, Lüders H. Automatisms with preserved responsiveness. Neurology 1995;45:61.
63. Ritaccio AL. Reflex seizures. Neurol Clin 1994;12:57.
64. Geschwind N, Sherwin I. Language-induced epilepsy. Arch Neurol 1967;16:25.
65. Goossens LA, Andermann F, Andermann E, et al. Reflex seizures induced by calculation, card or board games, and spatial tasks: a review of 25 patients and delineation of the epileptic syndrome. Neurology 1990;40:1171.
66. Matsuoka H. A clinical and electroencephalographic study of juvenile myoclonic epilepsy: pathophysiological considerations based on the findings obtained from neuropsychological EEG activations. Seishin Shinkeigaku Zashi 1989;91:318.
67. Cascino GD, Andermann F, Berkovic SF, et al. Gelastic seizures and hypothalamic hamartomas: evaluation of patients undergoing chronic intracranial EEG monitoring and outcome of surgical treatment. Neurology 1993;43:747.
68. List CF, Dowman CE, Bagchi BK, Bebin J. Posterior hypothalamic hamartomas and gangliogliomas causing precocious puberty. Neurology 1958;8:164.
69. Matustik MC, Eisenberg HM, Meyer WJ. Gelastic (laughing) seizures and precocious puberty. Am J Dis Child 1981;135:837.
70. Berkovic SF, Andermann F, Melanson D, et al. Hypothalamic hamartomas and ictal laughter: evolution of a characteristic epileptic syndrome and diagnostic value of magnetic resonance imaging. Ann Neurol 1988;23:429.
71. Sato M, Ushio Y, Arita N, Mogami H. Hypothalamic hamartoma: report of two cases. Neurosurgery 1985;16:198.

72. Sammaritano MR, Adam C, Giard N, Saint-Hillaire JM. Frontal lobe origin of gelastic seizures with SEEG [Abstract]. Epilepsia 1993;34(Suppl 6):132.
73. Krumholz A, Niedermeyer E. Psychogenic seizures: a clinical study with follow-up data. Neurology 1983;33:498.
74. Ramani V. Intensive Monitoring of Psychogenic Seizures, Aggression, and Dyscontrol Syndromes. In RJ Gumnit (ed), Advances in Neurology, vol 46. Intensive Neurodiagnostic Monitoring. New York: Raven, 1986:203–217.
75. Lempert T, Schinidt D. Natural history and outcome of psychogenic seizures: a clinical study in 50 patients. J Neurol 1990;237:35.
76. Lesser RP. Psychogenic seizures. Psychosomatics 1986;27:823.
77. Lesser RP, Lüders H, Dinner DS. Evidence for epilepsy is rare in patients with psychogenic seizures. Neurology 1983;33:502.
78. Gumnit JR. Behavior disorders related to epilepsy. EEG Clin Neurophysiol 1985;37:313.

CHAPTER 4

Non-Epileptic Paroxysmal Neurologic Events

Frederick Andermann

A wide range of patients are referred for investigation of uncontrolled attacks that are considered to be potentially epileptic in nature. Because these episodes usually do not respond to anti-epileptic medication, lack of response should alert the observer to the possibility of their non-epileptic nature. Awareness of the various alternative diagnoses is important and should prevent unfounded treatment with anti-epileptic medication. Gowers[1] recognized that the problem with the diagnosis of epilepsy includes (1) the recognition of the occurrence of attacks, (2) the distinction of the attacks from other paroxysmal affections with which they may be confounded, and (3) the distinction of hysteroid from epileptic attacks. Clearly, the main problem in making a diagnosis of epilepsy or an epileptic seizure is that the event or events in question are short lived and sporadic and can occur too infrequently to be directly studied by the physician except in special circumstances. Furthermore, no test has been developed that is sufficiently sensitive or specific to reliably document the underlying epileptic abnormality in the interictal state.

Nonetheless, some conditions permit us to make a convincing diagnosis of epilepsy. A patient has *documented* epilepsy when seizures have been recorded on electroencephalography (EEG) with simultaneous visual observation either by trained observers or by camera. The diagnosis of epilepsy can be said to be *confirmed* when a clear description by a witness to the attack is supplemented by an epileptiform EEG abnormality and an abnormal imaging test that is consistent with the nature of the attack. However, the diagnosis of epilepsy should never be made on the basis of a test result alone because epileptiform abnormalities occur in approximately 2% of healthy subjects,[2] and lesions can be incidental and cause symptoms by other mechanisms.

Description of the attack, especially by an experienced observer, is very important because the subjective recollection of events by the patient is likely to be incomplete. An account of the aura at the onset of a seizure can only be obtained from the patient; however, patients commonly underestimate the extent of impairment of consciousness in their partial seizures and may claim full awareness of their seizures until an accident supervenes from a seizure while they are driving or performing some other sustained vigilance task in which interruption of attention can have significant consequences. The quality of the witnessed accounts depends on the frequency of observations, whether the observer was present at the very beginning, and the experience of the witness. Even a physician, unless specifically trained and familiar with seizure observation, can make an incorrect diagnosis. When the description of one witnessed account is unsatisfactory, more should be sought. In this era of rapid communication, a telephone call to a witness while the patient is in the office can be very valuable. Thus, in the diagnosis of epilepsy, the clinician is like a detective. The facts as related may or may not be reliable. Scattered clues must be pieced together, and the ability to make a correct diagnosis of a condition other than epilepsy is helped by awareness of the wide range of conditions with which it may be confused.

The causes for a mistaken diagnosis of epilepsy are legion. Unfortunately, they are more commonly the result of an error of comission than one of omission on the part of members of the medical community. As reviewed by Engel,[3] misinterpretation of benign or nonspecific EEG abnormalities is a frequent cause of misdiagnosis. Further, because syncope is common, not surprisingly it is often confused with epilepsy. Patients who initially present with non-epileptic psychogenic seizures do not usually voice their concern that they may be developing epilepsy but readily accept the diagnosis of epilepsy afterward. They complain of spells, strange turns, blackouts, falls, and shaking episodes. By contrast, patients with epileptic seizures often minimize their troubles until an undeniable tonic-clonic seizure occurs. Excessive parental concern is sometimes a cause for the misdiagnosis of epilepsy in young children. Exposure to information resources on epilepsy can contribute to the overinterpretation of symptoms and transform those of benign or non-epileptic phenomena to the very picture of epilepsy itself.

Alertness to the possible presence of paroxysmal disorders other than epilepsy should be present not only at the initial diagnostic encounter but also after the patient has been under treatment, especially if there is a lack of clear response to medication. Re-evaluation should be sought to confirm the diagnosis and exclude others in several situations. A sudden unanticipated change in the pattern of attacks or recurrence of attacks that had previously been controlled requires further investigation. Drug-seeking behavior, dramatic presentations with multiple attacks in public, and repeated visits to the emergency room also should invite healthy skepticism. New paroxysmal symptoms in a patient with epilepsy should not be automatically assumed to be due to the epilepsy. Common disorders such as those described in the following sections, including syncope, migraine, panic attacks, and sleep apnea, can develop in addition to epilepsy. Tables 4.1 to 4.4 provide a differential diagnosis by category of the predominantly presenting symptom: paroxysmal attacks, episodic abnormal movements, episodic abnormal sensations, and episodic abnormal mental state. These disorders are discussed categorically in the following text.

Syncope

The mechanisms and EEG findings of syncope and anoxic convulsions have been well described by Gastaut and Fisher-Williams[4] and by Aminoff et al.[5]

Patients who faint and are maintained in an upright or sitting position tend to have more prolonged impairment of consciousness and more prominent myoclonic jerks and may have an anoxic convulsion. Syncope may also be accompanied by incontinence, although this is exceptional.

Syncope may occur while sitting or even while lying down, which can lead to some difficulty in diagnosis. Possible psychogenic or other triggers should be thoroughly looked for in this situation because this type of syncope is not common.

Some patients, fortunately few, have a tendency toward serial syncope, which may be associated with asystole. One such man had bouts of attacks recurring during a single day on several occasions and, to the consternation of the cardiologist, asystole developed while the electrocardiogram was being taken. A diagnosis of cardiac epilepsy was suspected. This man had a strong family history of syncope involving his mother and his two sons, and the bouts of syncope were precipitated by tension and anxiety.

Deliberate stretching leading to syncope is sometimes seen in adolescents, who cannot adequately explain why they do this.[6] The mechanism is similar to the better-known cough or micturition syncope. Such episodes also have been described in the cognitively impaired.

Usually, the detailed history of the event enables a specific diagnosis. When no description is available, it may be wise to interpret the situation to the patient and the family with instructions to carefully observe any subsequent event and to have them return. This may clarify the diagnosis.

Intermittent ventricular tachyarrhythmia,[7] or the Romano-Ward syndrome,[8] can also lead to loss of consciousness and anoxic convulsion. Reflex cardiac arrest and Stokes-Adams syndrome must be considered as well.[9]

Acute manifestations of asthma can lead to anoxic events, which can result in an anoxic encephalopathy or death. Recurrent and fairly frequent

TABLE 4.1
Non-Epileptic Paroxysmal Disorders

Syncope
    Vasovagal syncope
    Convulsive syncope
    Syncope in specific situations: micturition syncope, tussive syncope, carotid sinus hypersensitivity, glossopharyngeal neuralgia
    Cardiac syncope: Stokes-Adams attack, tachyarrhythmias, prolonged QT syndrome, aortic stenosis, hypertrophic cardiomyopathy
    Orthostatic syncope: idiopathic orthostatic hypotension, Shy-Drager syndrome, autonomic neuropathy
    Deliberate syncope (or "fainting lark")
Movement disorders
    Habit spasm
    Tic
    Paroxysmal kinesigenic choreoathetosis
    Paroxysmal dystonia
    Paroxysmal ataxia
    Tremor
    Chorea
    Segmental dystonia
Non-epileptic myoclonus
    Hypnic jerks
    Spinal myoclonus
    Reticular myoclonus
    Palatal myoclonus
    Essential myoclonus
    Myoclonus and asterixis in toxic-metabolic states
Startle
    Startle reaction
    Startle disease: hyperexplexia
    Jumping Frenchmen, Malay *latah*, etc.
Migraine and head pains
    Classic migraine (with aura)
    Basilar artery migraine
    Cluster headache
    Chronic paroxysmal hemicrania
    Ice-pick headache
    Trigeminal neuralgia
Disorders in infants and children
    Jitteriness
    Shuddering
    Esophageal reflux (Sandifer's syndrome)
    Breath-holding attacks
    Alternating hemiplegia
Cerebrovascular disease
    Carotid territory transient ischemic attack (TIA): limb-shaking attack
    Vertebrobasilar TIA

Moyamoya disease
   Specific strokes: paramedian thalamic nuclei, fusiform gyrus, right parietal lobe
Sleep disorders
   Pavor nocturnus
   Jactatio capitis nocturna
   Confusional arousals
   Somnambulism
   Periodic leg movements of sleep or nocturnal myoclonus
   Sleep apnea syndrome
   Narcolepsy (including cataplexy)
   Other hypersomnias
   Rapid eye movement behavior disorder
Toxic-metabolic or infectious states
   Alcoholic blackouts
   Hallucinogens (LSD [lysergic acid diethylamide], mescaline)
   Strychnine and camphor poisoning
   Tetanus
   Rabies
   Hypoglycemia
   Porphyria
   Pheochromocytoma
   Carcinoid syndrome
   Mastocytosis
Diencephalic and brain stem disorders
   Decorticate and decerebrate posturing
   Diencephalic attacks
   Peduncular hallucinosis
   Kleine-Levin syndrome
Miscellaneous disorders
   Idiopathic drop attacks of the elderly
   Transient global amnesia
   Flumazenil-responsive recurring stupor
   Paroxysmal attacks in multiple sclerosis
Psychiatric disorders
   Psychogenic seizures
   Depersonalization
   Psychogenic amnesia
   Psychogenic fugue
   Panic attacks
   Hyperventilation anxiety attacks
   Intermittent explosive disorder (episodic dyscontrol)
   Schizophrenia

TABLE 4.2
Non-Epileptic Causes of Episodic Abnormal Movements

Bilateral motor activity
    Psychogenic seizure*
    Convulsive syncope
    Startle disorders
    Non-epileptic myoclonus
    Paroxysmal dyskinesias
    Other movement disorders
    Decorticate and decerebrate rigidity
    Parasomnias
    Rapid eye movement behavior disorder
    Rabies
    Tetanus
    Strychnine and camphor poisoning
Focal or segmental twitches, jerks, shakes, and postures
    Non-epileptic myoclonus
    Movement disorders
    Periodic leg movements of sleep (nocturnal myoclonus)
    Tonic spasms in multiple sclerosis
    Limb-shaking transient ischemic attack
    Esophageal reflux (Sandifer's syndrome) in children
Drop attacks
    Idiopathic drop attack of the elderly
    Syncope
    Cataplexy
    Vertebrobasilar transient ischemic attacks
Paralysis
    Transient ischemic attacks
    Hemiplegic migraine
    Alternating hemiplegia

*Can occur under any category in Tables 4.2, 4.3, and 4.4.

tonic attacks may occur without interictal epileptogenic discharge.[10] The mechanism is that of anoxic convulsions, which are uncommon in adults. Some asymmetry in the attacks of such patients may be related to an associated localized cerebral disturbance. Treatment should be directed to the asthma, the underlying cause. In considering this type of attack, it must also be kept in mind that children with asthma have an increased risk of seizures. Aminophylline may lower the seizure threshold, and this may be of more practical significance than is generally accepted.

Migraine

Migraine and epilepsy are distinct in their pathogenesis and in their genetic basis.[11,12] The two conditions may coexist or may interrelate in a number of

TABLE 4.3
Non-Epileptic Causes of Episodic Abnormal Sensations

Elementary visual hallucination
    Ocular disorders
    Disorders of optic pathway (phosphenes and photopsias)
    Classic migraine (with aura)
    Occipital lobe lesions
    Drugs
    Hypnagogic hallucinations
    Schizophrenia
Elementary auditory hallucinations
    Ear disorders (including Ménière's disease)
    Cranial bruits
    Palatal myoclonus
    Drugs
Vertigo
    Vestibular disorders (including Ménière's disease)
    Basilar artery migraine
    Brain stem disorders
Paresthesia and somatic sensations
    Transient ischemic attacks
    Multiple sclerosis
    Peripheral neuropathy
    Restless legs syndrome
    Hyperventilation anxiety attacks
    Hypnagogic hallucinations
    Schizophrenia
Abdominal sensation
    Migraine
    Drugs: side effects
    Gastrointestinal disorders
Autonomic flushing, pallor, sweating, palpitations
    Panic attacks
    Presyncope
    Hypoglycemia
    Pheochromocytoma
    Carcinoid syndrome
    Mastocytosis

ways. Since the days of Jackson and Gowers, it has been known that distinction between the two is occasionally difficult. A major difficulty in clarifying migraine-epilepsy relationships is the uncertainty of the frequency of migraine in the general population; estimates range from 1% to 60%. Migraine is extremely variable and, when diagnosed according to the criteria of the International Commission for the Study of Headache of the World Federation of Neurology, it is extremely common.[11,12] Unfortunately, definite clinical markers exist only in classic or complicated migraine.

TABLE 4.4
Non-Epileptic Causes of Episodic Abnormal Mental State

Blackout
  Syncope
  Concussion
  Sleep attack
Amnesia
  Transient global amnesias
  Daydreaming
  Sleep attack
  Alcoholic blackout
  Drugs
  Psychogenic amnesia
  Psychogenic fugue
Confusion
  Drugs and poisons
  Alcohol
  Hypoglycemia
  Porphyria
  Other toxic-metabolic states
  Hypersomnia (sleep drunkenness)
  Parasomnias
  Basilar artery migraine
  Flumazenine-responsive recurring stupor
  Strokes
Complex hallucinations
  Drugs and hallucinogens
  Delirium tremens
  Toxic encephalopathies
  Peduncular hallucinosis
  Vision or hearing loss
  Hypnagogic hallucinations
  Schizophrenia and other psychoses
Fear and rage
  Panic attacks
  Hyperventilation anxiety attacks
  Intermittent explosive disorder (episodic dyscontrol)
  Rapid eye movement behavior disorder

Patients with a classic migraine aura may at times progress to have clear epileptic manifestations, usually during or after the aura. These patients are unlikely to have seizures outside of classic migraine attacks, and anti-epileptic medication may not be necessary if the migraine can be controlled by preventive medications.

Occasionally, in patients who have seizures only at the time of a classic migraine attack, epilepsy, particularly temporal lobe epilepsy, may eventually develop. The early history may be forgotten by the patient and the family, and the frequency of events can only be shown by review of neurologic observations made over the years.

Migraine is a risk factor in occipital epilepsy, certainly in children and probably in adults as well. Like other epilepsies, occipital epilepsy is multifactorial in cause, and migraine with its known predilection for involvement of the posterior cerebral territory seems to be an important component.

Benign occipital epilepsy of childhood is often difficult to distinguish from migraine. The incidence of migrainous or vascular headache in patients with benign occipital epilepsy is very high in our experience and that of Gastaut and Zifkin.[13]

Benign rolandic epilepsy is also a migraine-related condition.[14] A positive family history of migraine is almost always present.

Epileptogenic EEG abnormalities are common in children with vascular headache and are similar to those found in the benign epilepsies of childhood.[15,16] Unless these children also have seizures, anti-epileptic medication is not required. When the headache requires treatment, one should remember that anti-epileptic drugs such as phenytoin have in the past been shown to be effective in treating migraine, at least in children, although these agents may not be the treatment of choice.

Basilar migraine, like classic migraine or confusional migraine, can lead to epileptic seizures.[17] The electrographic abnormalities may be impressive but, despite this, the prognosis of the epilepsy is usually benign.[18,19]

The interference with consciousness described in basilar migraine consists of stupor or drowsiness, but these patients can always be aroused. This feature should enable distinction from unconsciousness due to epilepsy.

The slow march of the migrainous aura is an important factor in differential diagnosis because the course of the migrainous auras is much longer than what is found in epileptic seizures.

Finally, migraine attacks may be induced by or follow a partial complex seizure.[20] Seizures can also result from a fixed lesion, usually caused by vascular occlusion related to migraine.

Acephalgic migraine may be mistaken for epilepsy, and it is sometimes the eventual onset of symptoms on the contralateral side that leads to the diagnosis. The slow migrainous march is again the clue to the nature of the attacks.

The term *abdominal epilepsy* is fortunately rarely used now. Abdominal pain with dizziness or vertigo and intense autonomic dysfunction in children is most often a migrainous manifestation. Only occasionally is abdominal pain without other obvious clinical manifestations indicative of temporal lobe epilepsy. The presence of "epileptogenic" EEG abnormalities in children with migraine has probably led to diagnostic difficulties in the past. One also no longer refers to *epileptic equivalents*, a term that arose out of diagnostic uncertainty and that has been rendered obsolete by lessons learned from electroclinical correlations.

Paroxysmal Dyskinesias

Paroxysmal kinesigenic choreoathetosis is a well-known, dominantly inherited disorder that responds to anti-epileptic medication such as carbamazepine or phenytoin.[21] Interestingly enough, such medications are often prescribed because an original diagnosis of epilepsy is made. The severity and frequency of the attacks tend to vary within the family. In addition to initiation of movement, emotion is an important trigger. On his way to work, one patient used to pass a yard where a big German shepherd lived. The dog would usually try to attack him through the fence. Once, to his consternation, he found that the gate was open and the dog had access to him. This led to his first attack of paroxysmal choreoathetosis.

Paroxysmal dystonia has been well described by Lance.[22] It is also dominantly inherited; the attacks are usually longer than those of paroxysmal kinesigenic choreoathetosis and do not respond to anti-epileptic medication.

Episodes of paroxysmal ataxia may be misinterpreted as representing cerebral seizures.[23] These usually occur in patients with ataxic or other fixed diffuse neurologic deficits, generally due to a perinatal encephalopathy. The attacks may last minutes or hours and do not respond to anti-epileptic medication. The person may be aware of some lateralized or localized increase in tone, and a dyskinetic component may be present. The major manifestations consist of ataxia and tremor. This disorder must also be distinguished from the two forms of familial paroxysmal ataxia: that in patients who respond to acetazolamide and that in those who do not.[24]

Valproic acid tends to bring out an underlying essential tremor that may be very pronounced and resemble asterixis. This tremor must be distinguished from myoclonus, which may be present as well. It is important to explain to the patient and family the role of these different mechanisms and the fact that valproic acid–induced tremor can be relieved if necessary by the additional use of beta-adrenergic blockers.

Focal stereotyped painful dystonic attacks may be activated or virtually only encountered during pregnancy. It is difficult to distinguish these attacks from mesial frontal tonic seizures, but most likely they represent a form of paroxysmal dystonia rather than an epileptic event. Symptomatic paroxysmal movement disorders that manifest with choreoathetosis or dystonia may be seen in addition to the genetically determined varieties.[22] A long-standing, usually congenital fixed neurologic deficit generally is present.

Lateralized painful tonic attacks without impairment of awareness are characteristic of multiple sclerosis.[25] They occur many times a day and, like the other paroxysmal manifestations of multiple sclerosis, appear to be self-limited. They respond well to phenytoin, although they are not likely to be epileptic in nature.

Lugaresi et al.[26] have drawn attention to paroxysmal nocturnal dystonia. The attacks are frequent, stereotyped, unassociated with impairment of awareness, and usually awaken the patient. Some of these patients may occasionally have more obvious seizures; paroxysmal nocturnal dystonia is therefore now considered to be a manifestation of mesial frontal epilepsy and not a sui generis movement disorder.

Myoclonus

Benign essential myoclonus is inherited as an autosomal dominant condition, but its mechanism is poorly understood.[27] The myoclonic jerks may be sporadic or repetitive, and patients speak of being able to relieve them by lying on a flat, hard surface. Occasionally, generalized seizures may be found in association, which raises the question of a relationship to the progressive myoclonus-epilepsies. In some of these disorders, notably Unverricht-Lundborg disease or the renal failure myoclonus syndrome, generalized seizures may occur infrequently and are easily controlled.[28]

Spinal myoclonus usually is associated with a demonstrable and obvious spinal lesion. One boy sustained a mild back injury and later developed violent jerking of the trunk activated by movement. The condition was eventually shown to be a psychogenic movement disorder.

Myorhythmia resembles and is analogous with palatal myoclonus.[29] It is characterized by a high frequency of widespread muscular twitches, more than 100 per minute, in the same range as palatal myoclonus. These are most likely a release phenomenon related to involvement of cerebelloolivary and central tegmental systems.

Startle disease (hyperexplexia) is a dominantly inherited disorder in which, in addition to excessive startle, there are episodes of spontaneous clonus mainly involving the legs, usually occurring at night and lasting up to many minutes.[30-32] The patients also are stiff and may fall without losing consciousness and without being able to protect themselves. This stiffness is most evident in infancy, leading to the erroneous diagnosis of spastic quadriplegia. The stiff baby syndrome may be life-threatening when it occurs in the neonatal period, presumably because of the anoxia that occurs during the attacks. Family members may be affected by a minor form of the disorder characterized by excessive startle; this occurs only during illness or when they are under stress. Sporadic cases also are found. The falling attacks and the episodic clonus often are diagnosed as epileptic.[33]

Hyperexplexia should not be confused with jumping as described by Beard.[34,35] In this disorder, inherited as an autosomal dominant with variable penetrance, excessive startle, echolalia, echopraxia, and forced obedience are the characteristic features. It is analogous to *miryachit* occurring in Siberia,[36] *latah* in Malaysia,[37] "goosey" in the United States,[38] and similar disorders described in different parts of the world. Sometimes a striking cultural overlay exists, which has led to the erroneous conclusion that it represents a learned or acquired behavior.[39] Jumping and its equivalents described in other populations probably represent a genetically specific tic disorder. Excessive startle, echolalia, and echopraxia are known to occur frequently in patients with multiple tics.

When unusual tics resembling myoclonus occur, an epileptic cause may be suspected. An accurate diagnosis can be established from the history and observation of the movements.

Sleep Disorders

The spectrum of non-epileptic sleep disorders is discussed more fully in Chapter 5. Here, a few sleep disorders are highlighted.

Excessive hypnagogic myoclonic jerks sometimes occur,[40] and this increase in physiologic myoclonus may perhaps be related to depression. Nocturnal myoclonus may be associated with restless legs. A family history suggesting dominant inheritance often exists. Not infrequently, children with sleep disorders such as night terrors (*pavor nocturnus*) are referred for consideration of the possibility of epilepsy. In most instances, the diagnosis can be clarified by history. Some relation apparently exists between night terrors and migraine or a family history of migraine, but this association remains to be clarified.

Some patients have nocturnal seizures exclusively, and the differential diagnosis between epilepsy and sleep disorder is difficult. Video monitoring may lead to clarification of the diagnosis.

Sleep drunkenness or rapid eye movement behavior disorder with directed and at times aggressive behavior evokes the possibility of an epileptic mechanism.[41] Here again the diagnosis may be made by history.

Aggressive behavior may occur during postictal confusion and exceptionally during seizures. In that situation, however, the background history of epilepsy is clear.

Frequently, the significance of enuresis is questioned. In the absence of an obvious epileptic disorder in which nocturnal seizures are known to occur and which may lead to urinary incontinence, enuresis should be considered to be non-epileptic.[42]

Diencephalic Syndromes

The diencephalic seizures described by Penfield[43] must be extraordinarily rare. Some attacks that originate in the temporal lobes may have impressive autonomic components, such as piloerection, that may be ipsilateral, contralateral, or bilateral. Other sympathetic manifestations such as a change in color or pupillary dilatation may be seen but have less clear localizing value.

Peduncular hallucinosis, the *syndrome de la calotte pedonculaire de l'Hermitte*, consists of seeing small colored animals or small people, but other content may be present.[44] These episodes are initially almost universally diagnosed as epileptic in nature when they occur in isolation and out of the context of an obvious diencephalic disorder. For instance, a woman with a loculated lateral ventricle and hemiparesis had prolonged attacks in which she saw herself accompanied by two tall thin men with cadaveric hands, dressed in dark suits, one on each side, who attempted to push her into a pit full of shiny, brightly colored, writhing snakes. In another patient who had a suprasellar meningioma removed, hallucinations developed in which she saw herself sitting on the back steps of a typical Montreal house; next to her was a flowerpot full of pink baby mice. This entity of peduncular hallucinosis was largely ignored by English-speaking neurologists until it was clarified by Caplan.[45]

The hallucinations seen in the Kleine-Levin syndrome, petit mal status, and Korsakoff's syndrome are probably also of diencephalic origin. The Kleine-Levin syndrome of hypersomnia, megaphagia, hypersexuality, hallucinations, behavioral disorder, headache, and amnesia has at times been misdiagnosed as petit mal status. It occurs both in adolescent boys and girls. Occasional single attacks occurring in adult men may be related to an encephalitic process.

Fugue States

In absence status, mental impairment varies from the just barely perceptible to stupor.[46] It may develop in patients with active primary generalized epilepsy or, after many years of remission, lead to recurrence of epilepsy in the older age group. It may also arise de novo, particularly in older people. A triggering cerebral disturbance, such as may be caused by maturity-onset diabetes or by benzodiazepine withdrawal, may be responsible for this activation. It may also be triggered by tricyclic antidepressants, metabolic disorders such as hypercalcemia, or severe and less specific diffuse systemic disease.

The EEG in absence status may show some focal changes, and such patients are more difficult to control. There is usually no difficulty in distinguishing this type of absence status from partial complex status. Generalized epileptic discharges associated with a frontal lesion may also produce a picture that is clinically indistinguishable from absence status.[47]

Although amnesia for attacks of absence status often follows, the clinical history, the context in which these episodes occur, and the generalized seizures that often conclude such attacks allow distinction from fugues.

Most fugue states are psychogenic. The longer and more complex the behavior, the more likely this is to be the case.[48]

Amnesia after temporal lobe seizures is most prominent in patients with bitemporal foci, even when the duration is relatively brief. Patients may not get off the bus at the correct stop or walk or ride a bicycle further than originally intended; however, they rarely, if ever, initiate travel or display complex behavior.

Transient global amnesia usually is considered to be related to vascular dysfunction.[49-51] Migraine occasionally produces such attacks, and the confusional migraine of young people produces an indistinguishable clinical picture. The puzzled, baffled behavior with repetitive and stereotyped questioning is characteristic. Much has been written about a possible epileptic cause for transient global amnesia, but this argument was never convincing.

Special Childhood Disorders

Infants or small children occasionally have shuddering attacks in which they may cross the legs as if wanting to void.[52] Generally, these attacks are first considered to be epileptic in nature. They have been shown to be related to essential or familial tremor and to represent an infantile form of this benign disorder.

Alternating hemiplegia of infancy is a condition that begins in the first year of life.[53] The children become miserable, cry, and are upset. This is followed by lateralized hemiparesis or hemiplegia that may last for minutes or hours and fully resolves after sleep. Episodes usually involve both sides alternately, and bilateral episodes may have been originally considered to represent inhibitory epilepsy until their specific nature was recognized. The cause is unknown. Invariably, a history of migraine in the parents, usually the mother, is found. As the children get older, migrainous symptoms are more apparent, but the relationship to migraine is still not entirely clear. Because the disorder is usually first considered to be epileptic, anticonvulsant medication is commonly prescribed. For reasons that are still unclear, it is difficult to wean these children from phenytoin because their attacks become more frequent and severe. Conversely, this drug does not reduce the frequency and severity of attacks when it is first administered. The episodes respond partially to calcium channel blockers such as flunarizine. Many of the children are initially normal, but mental retardation and choreoathetotic or dystonic movement disorder subsequently develop.

Breath-holding spells or vasovagal attacks can lead to anoxic convulsions and thus present a problem in differential diagnosis.[54,55] It is unusual for seizures to be triggered by the stimuli that usually induce vasovagal attacks, and the distinction from epilepsy can be made by obtaining a detailed history of each event. Even if not every episode has been witnessed, sufficient evidence for a syncopal cause often is available. From a physiologic point of view, the final common path, whether it be an epileptic convulsion or an anoxic one, is the same, but the prognosis and treatment differ.

Various Other Disorders

Decerebrate attacks, or cerebellar fits as they used to be called, usually cause no problem in diagnosis because of the context in which they appear.[56] Inexperienced nursing staff occasionally misinterrupt the events as seizures.

Hypoglycemia often is postulated as a cause of seizures by non-neurologic physicians. However, it rarely proves to be the cause of epileptic attacks.

Cataplexy may be misdiagnosed as epileptic drop attacks,[57] which was the case in the wife of a physician whose narcoleptic hypersomnia was interpreted for years as being psychogenic. Her falling attacks initially were diagnosed as being epileptic.

The drop attacks of older people are most likely syncopal, and usually no evidence supports an epileptic cause.

In tertiary syphilis, sometimes without any other symptoms, attacks of abnormal sensation and movement may occur and have an unusual distribution. They have been referred to as *congestive* or *apoplectic attacks* and may have a vascular cause. For instance, attacks may start in one arm, involve that side of the body, and eventually spread to the contralateral side. These attacks, although uncommon, should be considered when the pattern is unusual and does not correspond to somatotopic cortical spread.

Alcoholic blackouts may occur during acute intoxication and usually are not accompanied by withdrawal seizures.[58] Visual hallucinations of the blind (the Charles Bonnet syndrome) and auditory hallucinations of the deaf may also be suspected of having an epileptic cause.[59]

Inhibitory seizures characterized by unilateral nonconvulsive paralysis do occur, although they are rare. This entity has recently been redefined by Fisher.[60]

Unusual Non-Epileptic Psychogenic Attacks

Every generation of neurologists is fascinated by non-epileptic seizures, and every technological advance developed has been applied to the study of these attacks. Their recognition continues to present problems, and they probably constitute the most common paroxysmal event misdiagnosed as epilepsy. We mention only some exceptional forms here, because the differential diagnosis is discussed in Chapters 1–3, 5, and 6.

Patients with non-epileptic seizures are now more sophisticated and better informed, and they have often seen a number of neurologists and psychiatrists. Their seizure patterns are becoming much more sophisticated as well. For instance, a pattern of complex partial seizures, strongly reminiscent of temporal lobe attacks, may be found.[61] Such "pseudotemporal lobe epilepsy" may be more common in patients such as health professionals.

In addition to conversion reactions and malingering, psychogenic attacks may be factitious. Munchausen syndrome may be purely epileptic in its manifestations. The prognosis is far worse than that of non-epileptic seizures related to conversion.[62] Such patients may also present with pseudo–status epilepticus, leading to the use of a great deal of parenteral medication and at times repeated and prolonged anesthesia.

References

1. Gowers WR. Epilepsy and Other Chronic Convulsive Diseases: Their Causes, Symptoms, and Treatment (2nd ed). London: J & A Churchill, 1901.
2. Zivin L, Ajmone-Marsan C. Incidence and prognostic significance of "epileptiform" activity in the EEG of non-epileptic subjects. Brain 1968;91:751.
3. Engel J Jr. Seizures and Epilepsy. Philadelphia: Davis, 1989.
4. Gastaut H, Fischer-Williams M. Electro-encephalographic study of syncope; its differentiation from epilepsy. Lancet 1957;23:1018.
5. Aminoff MJ, Scheiriman MM, Griffin JC, Herre JM. Electrocerebral accompaniments of syncope associated with malignant ventricular arrhythmias. Ann Intern Med 1988;108:791.
6. Lai CW, Ziegler DK. Repeated self induced syncope and subsequent seizure. Arch Neurol 1983;40:820.
7. Von Bernuth G, Bernsau V, Gutheil H, et al. Tachyarrhythmic syncopes in children with structurally normal hearts with and without QY prolongation in the electrocardiogram. Eur J Pediatr 1982;138:206.
8. Driver MV, Selby PJ. Apparent epilepsy due to intermittent ventricular tachyarrhythmia (Romano-Ward syndrome). Electroenceph Clin Neurophysiol 1977;43:289.
9. Fowler HL. Stokes Adams attacks masquerading as epilepsy, case reports. Milit Med 1984;149:680.
10. Keene KL, Melmed CA, Andermann F, Baxter DW. Anoxic seizures due to asthma: a serious complication in adults. Can J Neurol Sci 1981;8:177.
11. Andermann F. Clinical Features of Migraine-Epilepsy Syndromes. In F Andermann, E Lugaresi (eds), Migraine and Epilepsy. Boston: Butterworth, 1987;3–30.
12. Andermann E, Andermann F. Migraine-Epilepsy Relationships: Epidemiological and Genetic Aspects. In F Andermann, E Lugaresi (eds), Migraine and Epilepsy. Boston: Butterworth, 1987;281–291.
13. Gastaut H, Zifkin B. Benign Epilepsy of Childhood with Occipital Spike and Wave Complexes. In F Andermann, E Lugaresi (eds), Migraine and Epilepsy. Boston: Butterworth, 1987;47–81.

14. Bladin PF. The Association of Benign Rolandic Epilepsy with Migraine. In F Andermann, E Lugaresi (eds), Migraine and Epilepsy. Boston: Butterworth, 1987;145–152.
15. Hockaday JM, Whitty CWM. Factors determining the electroencephalogram in migraine: a study of 560 patients according to the clinical type of migraine. Brain 1969;92:769.
16. Panayiotopoulos CP. Difficulties in Differentiating Migraine and Epilepsy Based on Clinical and EEG Findings. In F Andermann, E Lugaresi (eds), Migraine and Epilepsy. Boston: Butterworth, 1987;31–46.
17. Bickerstaff ER. Basilar artery migraine. Lancet 1961;1:15.
18. Golden GS, French JH. Basilar artery migraine in young children. Pediatrics 1975;56:722.
19. Camfield PR, Metrakos K, Andermann F. Basilar migraine, seizures and severe epileptiform EEG abnormalities. Neurology 1978:28:584.
20. D'Alessandro R, Sacquenga T, Pazzaglia P, Lugaresi E. Headache after Partial Complex Seizures. In F Andermann, E Lugaresi (eds), Migraine and Epilepsy. Boston: Butterworth, 1987;237–278.
21. Kertesz A. Paroxysmal kinesigenic choreoathetosis: an entity within the paroxysmal choreoathetosis syndrome. Description of 10 cases, including 1 autopsied. Neurology 1977;2:285.
22. Lance JW. Familial paroxysmal dystonic choreoathetosis and its differentiation from related syndromes. Ann Neurol 1977;2:285.
23. Vaamonde J, Muruzabal J, Artieda J, Obeso JA. Semiological peculiarities of familial paroxystic ataxia (FPA). Mov Dis 1990;5:8.
24. Zasorin NL, Baloh RW, Myers LB. Acetazolamide-responsive episodic ataxia syndrome. Neurology 1983;33:1212.
25. Matthews WB. Tonic seizures in disseminated sclerosis. Brain 1958;81:193.
26. Lugaresi E, Cirignotta F, Montagna P. Nocturnal paroxysmal dystonia. J Neurol Neurosurg Psychiatry 1986;49:375.
27. Prżuntek H, Murh H. Essential familial myoclonus. J Neurol 1983;230:152.
28. Classification of the progressive myoclonus epilepsies and related disorders. Marseilles Consensus Statement. Ann Neurol 1990;28:113.
29. Masucci EF, Kurtzke JF, Saini N. Myorhythmia: a widespread movement disorder. Clinicopathological correlations. Brain 1984;107:52.
30. Andermann F, Keene KL, Andermann E, Quesney LF. Startle disease or hyperexplexia: further delineation of the syndrome. Brain 1980;103:985–997.
31. Andermann F, Andermann E. Startle disease or hyperexplexia [Letter]. Ann Neurol 1984;15:367.
32. Kurczynski TW. Hyperexplexia. Arch Neurol 1983;40:246.
33. Andermann F, Andermann E. Excessive Startle Syndromes: Startle Disease, Jumping and Startle Epilepsy. In S Fahn, CD Marsden, MH Van Woert (eds), Myoclonus. New York: Raven, 1986;321–338.
34. Beard GM. Remarks on jumpers or jumping Frenchmen. J Nerv Ment Dis 1878;5:526.
35. Beard BM. Experiments with jumpers of Maine. Pop Sci Month 1880;18:170.

36. Hammond W. Miryachit: a newly described disease of the nervous system and its analogues. N Y Med J 1884;39:191.
37. Simons RC. Resolution of the latah paradox. J Nerv Ment Dis 1980;168:195.
38. Hardison J. Are the jumping Frenchmen of Maine goosey? JAMA 1980;244:70.
39. Saint-Hilaire MH, Saint-Hilaire JM, Granger L. Jumping Frenchmen of Maine. Neurology 1986;36:1269.
40. Broughton R. Sleep disorders: disorders of arousal. Science 1968;159:1070.
41. Parkes JD. The parasomnias. Lancet 1986;11:1021.
42. Pedley TA. Differential diagnosis of episodic symptoms. Epilepsia 1983;24 [Suppl 1]:S31.
43. Penfield W. Diencephalic autonomic epilepsy. Arch Neurol Psychiatry 1929;22:358.
44. Van Bogaert L. L'hallucinose pédonculaire. Rev Neurol 1927;43:608.
45. Caplan LR. "Top of the basilar" syndrome. Neurology 1980;30:72.
46. Andermann F, Robb P. Absence status: a reappraisal following review of thirty-eight patients. Epilepsia 1972;13:177.
47. Berkovic SF, Andermann F, Aube M, et al. Nonconvulsive confusional frontal status. Epilepsia 1985;26:529.
48. Mesulam MM. Dissociative states with abnormal temporal lobe EEG, multiple personality and the illusion of possession. Arch Neurol 1981;38:176.
49. Fisher CM, Adams RD. Transient global amnesias. Acta Neurol Scand 1964;40:1.
50. Kushner MF, Hauser WA. Transient global amnesia: a case control study. Ann Neurol 1985;18:684.
51. Miller JWS, Yanagihara T, Petersen RC, Klass DW. Transient global amnesia and epilepsy: electroencephalographic distinction. Arch Neurol 1987;44:629.
52. Vanasse M, Bedard P, Andermann F. Shuddering attacks in children: an early clinical manifestation of essential tremor. Neurology 1976;26:1027.
53. Krageloh I, Aicardi J. Alternating hemiplegia in infants: report of five cases. Dev Med Child Neurol 1980;22:784.
54. Lombroso CT, Lerman P. Breath-holding spells (cyanotic and pallid infantile syncope). Pediatrics 1967;39:563.
55. Stephenson JBP. Reflex anoxic seizures (white breath-holding): nonepileptic vagal attacks. Arch Dis Child 1978;53:193.
56. Celesia GG, Andermann F. Some observations on the electrographic correlates of the decerebrate attack. Electroenceph Clin Neurophysiol 1964;16:295.
57. Parkes JD. Narcolepsy. In TL Riley, A Roy A (eds), Pseudoseizures. Baltimore: Williams & Wilkins, 1982;62–82.
58. Goodwin DW, Crane JB, Guze SB. Alcoholic "blackouts": a review and clinical study of 100 alcoholics. Am J Psychiatry 1969;126:191.
59. Asaad G, Shapiro B. Hallucinations: theoretical and clinical overview. Am J Psychiatry 1986;143:1088.
60. Fisher CM. Transient paralytic attacks of obscure nature: the question of nonconvulsive seizure paralysis. Can J Neurol Sci 1978;5:267.

61. Lesser RP. Psychogenic Seizures. In TA Pedly, BS Meldrum (eds), Recent Advances in Epilepsy. New York: Churchill Livingstone, 1985;273–296.
62. Savard G, Andermann F, Teitelbaum J, Lehmann H. Epileptic Munchausen's syndrome: a form of pseudo-seizures distinct from hysteria and malingering. Neurology 1988;38:1628.

CHAPTER 5

Parasomnia Purgatory: Epileptic/Non-Epileptic Parasomnia Interface

Mark W. Mahowald and Carlos H. Schenck

> We dance round in a ring and suppose,
> but the secret sits in the middle and knows.
>
> Robert Frost

Parasomnias are defined as undesirable behavioral, experiential, or autonomic phenomena that occur either exclusively or predominantly during the sleeping state. Advances in the field of sleep disorder medicine in general, and polysomnographic (PSG) monitoring techniques in particular, have allowed the identification and classification of many of the parasomnias. Despite these major advances, a wide variety of clinically impressive and bothersome, but poorly understood, sleep-related behaviors remain in "parasomnia purgatory," awaiting delineation, classification assignment, and treatment. This review addresses the fascinating interface among the nocturnal seizure/disorder of arousal/psychogenic spell borderland and discusses some of these "lost souls."

The former, and simpler, concept that describes most complex motor activities or unusual experiential phenomena arising from sleep as somehow a manifestation of dreaming has been debunked. The discovery of rapid eye movement (REM) sleep, coupled with the ability to perform complex, prolonged physiologic monitoring of patients who have parasomnias, has permitted the identification and classification of many of these sleep disorders.[1] These phenomena, which usually take a behavioral, experiential, or autonomic form, emerging only, or preferentially, during the sleep-

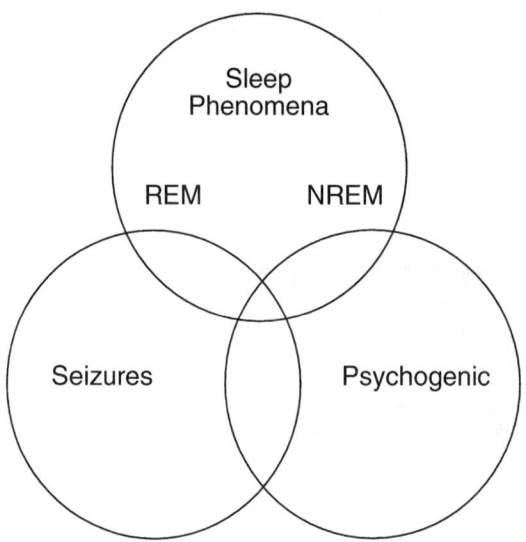

FIGURE 5.1. Overlapping nature of the various parasomnias. (REM = rapid eye movement; NREM = nonrapid eye movement.)

ing state, are commonly encountered in clinical practice and are too often dismissed as "bumps in the night" or as manifestations of underlying psychiatric disorders. The correct diagnosis of most parasomnias leads to effective treatment. However, the diagnosis may be difficult, because many of these disorders masquerade as one another. In some cases, the symptoms appear to represent an already identified parasomnia, when in fact they are due to a currently unidentified condition. In others, a cryptic parasomnia may actually be the trigger for the manifest parasomnia. Unfortunately, a pervasive tendency exists in clinical medicine to make a "definitive" diagnosis, which may result in a frank misdiagnosis, often of a psychiatric disorder (for lack of a better category), when the proper diagnosis would be "unknown etiology."

Four identified parasomnia arenas pose the most difficult diagnostic challenge: (1) disorders of arousal (sleep terrors [ST]/sleepwalking [SW]/sleep drunkenness [SD]/confusional arousals), (2) REM sleep behavior disorder (RBD), (3) atypical nocturnal seizures, and (4) psychogenic phenomena. The disorders of arousal and the RBD are both primary sleep disorders. Although most currently unclassifiable parasomnias fall into one of these groups, it must be kept in mind that other, as-yet unidentified categories await discovery. The overlapping nature of the parasomnias is depicted schematically in Figure 5.1.

For practical, clinical purposes, there are two main categories of parasomnias: (1) primary, which represent phenomena of sleep itself; and (2) secondary, which are physiologic phenomena of other organ systems that occur exclusively or predominantly during the sleeping state. Integral to the understanding of the primary sleep parasomnias is the concept of state dissociation. It is now recognized that we spend our lives in three completely different states of being: wakefulness (W), nonrapid eye movement (NREM) sleep, and REM sleep. Each state is an active, rather than quiescent, process. Although the transition from one state to another usually progresses in an orderly fashion, it is clear that these states may either appear in incomplete forms, with components of one intruding into another, or oscillate rapidly. These mixed, or incompletely declared, states result in bizarre and fascinating clinical behaviors and have served to explain enigmatic conditions that were previously attributed to psychiatric disorders or supernatural phenomena.[2]

Primary Sleep Parasomnias

Disorders of Arousal

The disorders of arousal represent the incomplete intrusion of W into (usually deep) NREM sleep, resulting in the clinical picture of SW or ST (also termed *pavor nocturnus*). SD and confusional arousals are a variation on this theme.[3]

ST/SW are impressive sleep phenomena that tend to arise from stages 3 and 4 slow-wave sleep, therefore tending to occur during the first third of the sleep cycle and rarely during naps. SW is prevalent in childhood (up to 17%), with a peak incidence at 11–12 years of age, and is more common in adults (approximately 3–4% in one study) than has been generally acknowledged.[4–6] The behaviors observed during SW, such as leaving the house, loading shotguns, or driving automobiles, may be extremely complex.[7] One interesting subtype of SW is that of nocturnal bulimia.[8–10] The less common ST is undoubtedly an extreme form of SW. It is frequently initiated by a loud scream associated with symptoms of panic and may be followed by impressive motor activity, such as hitting the wall or running around or out of the bedroom, resulting in bodily injury or property damage. Although affected individuals appear to be awake, they are unable to properly perceive the environment or to exercise proper judgment. Attempts at consolation are often fruitless and may only prolong the confusional state. A common feature of ST/SW is inconsolability during the activity, with amnesia for the event.[11,12] Our own experience runs counter to the dictum that imagery is never remembered.[13] Furthermore, the widely held belief that somnambulism and sleep terrors are benign and do not result in injury is clearly erroneous. The accompanying behaviors may be violent, resulting in considerable injury to the individual or others or damage to the environment.[14]

Another example of NREM/W dissociation is SD, a disturbance of cognition and attention that occurs in the transition between sleep and wakefulness, resulting in the appearance of delirious, complex motor behavior without conscious awareness.[15,16] As with ST/SW, SD is potentiated by prior sleep deprivation or the ingestion of alcohol or sedative/hypnotics before sleep onset.[16] It could be expected to occur more frequently in the setting of chronic sleep fragmentation, as seen in obstructive sleep apnea or in conditions of impaired wake-sleep "boundary control" such as narcolepsy. The pathophysiology of these disorders is not clearly understood, but both genetic and environmental factors are operant. A physiologic process is suggested by (1) the atypical arousal/electroencephalographic (EEG) pattern, suggesting a mixed W/NREM state during the episode; (2) the difference of visual evoked potentials during arousal from slow-wave sleep as compared to those arousals from REM sleep or during wakefulness;[17] and (3) the unusually intense and persistent orienting response to auditory stimuli in ST subjects, indicating a heightened intrinsic excitability of the nervous system.[18]

A conceptual model of disorders of arousal has been proposed based on tonic sleep factors (genetic, developmental, and psychological) and phasic sleep factors (fever, drugs, or arousals due to endogenous or exogenous stimuli such as apnea or seizures).[19] That somnambulism can be induced in normal children by standing them up during slow-wave sleep[20] and that sleep terrors can be precipitously triggered in susceptible individuals by sounding a buzzer during slow-wave sleep[11,21] speaks against these behaviors being the culmination of complex, ongoing sleep mentation. Although it has been said that persistence of these behaviors beyond childhood or their development in adulthood is an indication of significant psychopathology,[22,23] more recent studies indicate that they frequently begin in adulthood and are not usually associated with ongoing or remote psychiatric disorders.[13,24] SW/ST/SD all support the concept of the prolonged simultaneous occurrence or rapid oscillation of sleep (probably NREM) and W.

Treatment of uncomplicated ST/SW is often not necessary. Provision of reassurance and the understanding that the symptoms may diminish with time are often sufficient. The tricyclic antidepressants and benzodiazepines may be effective and should be administered if the behaviors are dangerous to persons or property or are extremely disruptive to family members. Nonpharmacologic treatments, such as hypnosis, progressive relaxation, autogenic training, anticipatory awakening, and psychotherapy, are recommended for long-term management. The avoidance of exogenous triggers, such as drugs, alcohol, and sleep deprivation, is also important.[19,25-27]

As mentioned previously, ST/SW can be triggered by a variety of endogenous or exogenous arousing stimuli. Therefore, some secondary sleep parasomnias, such as obstructive sleep apnea, periodic movements of sleep, gastroesophageal reflux, or nocturnal seizures resulting in arousal, may trigger a clinical event that is, in fact, an ST/SW/SD episode, but the true underlying etiology is yet a different parasomnia (a sleep disorder within a sleep disorder).

Rapid Eye Movement Behavior Disorder

Normally, REM sleep is associated with generalized somatic muscle paralysis (atonia), sparing the diaphragm and extraocular muscles, which may act as a protective measure by preventing the physical enactment of dreams. The chronic RBD disorder in humans (predicted in 1965 by animal experiments[28]) has now been identified. In RBD, the REM-related atonia is absent, incomplete, or interrupted, resulting in dramatic and frequently injurious behavior during dreams. The extensive oneiric (dream) behaviors displayed by these patients are frequently misdiagnosed as manifestations of a seizure or psychiatric disorder. Although usually idiopathic and tending to affect older men, RBD has been associated with a variety of primary neurologic diseases in approximately one-third to one-half of cases. The vast majority of our RBD patients presented to us with the chief complaint of sleep injury (fractures, lacerations, repeated ecchymoses). The patients' attempts to prevent injury—Posey jacket; rope around the waist, tethered to the bed; covering windows with plastic; forming pillow barricades; using sleeping bags (two were destroyed); padded waterbeds; mattress on the floor; sleeping in an empty room—indicate the severity of the motor behavior associated with this condition. Several wives have nearly been strangled by their husbands, who grabbed their necks very tightly during attempted dream enactment. Others sustained blows to the head. Treatment with low-dose bedtime clonazepam is very effective. A similar, but transient, form is seen in toxic-metabolic conditions, induced by medications, or associated with alcohol withdrawal.[29,30]

Common to RBD and ST/SW/SD is the appearance of motor activity occurring independently from waking consciousness. In RBD, the motor behavior correlates with dream imagery, and in ST/SW/SD it often occurs in the absence of (remembered) mentation. It is well known that decorticate experimental and decapitated barnyard animals are capable of performing very complex, integrated motor acts. This ability is explained by the presence of locomotor centers (LMCs), extending from the mesencephalon to the medulla, which are capable of generating complex behaviors without cortical input.[31-35] These areas project to the central pattern generator of the spinal cord, which itself is able to produce complex stepping movements in the absence of supraspinal influence.[36] Such dissociation of the LMCs from the parent state of REM or NREM sleep could explain the presence of complex motor behavior seen in RBD and ST/SW/SD. Dissociation between LMCs and waking consciousness or memory may explain the complex motor activity associated with amnesia that is characteristic of alcohol-induced "blackouts"[37] and with "unconscious" behavior that occurs during complex partial seizures.[38] The dissociation between behavior and consciousness may be related to sleep-related inactivation of attentional or memory systems.[39]

Secondary Sleep Parasomnias

Nocturnal Seizures

Conventional seizures frequently occur during sleep and usually present little diagnostic difficulty. Approximately 10% of patients who experience seizures have them exclusively or predominantly during sleep.[40] However, even the diagnosis of conventional nocturnal seizures may be difficult if the patient has no history of diurnal spells. Both waking and sleep-deprived EEGs may not reveal the diagnosis,[41,42] necessitating all-night PSG study using a full seizure montage, appropriate paper speed, and continuous video recording. Extensive studies have been performed attempting to correlate seizure type with sleep stages, with inconclusive or mixed results. Assertions that generalized seizures tend to occur during the transition between wakefulness and sleep and that focal spikes or seizures prefer REM sleep have been made, but exceptions are numerous.[43–46] It is clear that NREM sleep promotes seizures and that REM sleep can be thought of as an "antiepileptic" state.[47,48] Certain predisposing factors in NREM sleep appear to facilitate epileptic discharges. A relationship may exist between sleep spindles and spike and wave bursts in human epilepsy.[49] There may also be a relationship between the cyclic alternating pattern of "fluctuating cortical excitability" with both epilepsy and sleep disorders.[50–53] One thought-provoking comparison was made between REM sleep and epilepsy.[54]

Atypical nocturnal spells of difficult classification may present with bizarre symptoms that masquerade as either parasomnias or psychiatric conditions. Although not all of these "spells" may represent seizures, their clinical appearance; the fact that they are recurrent, stereotypic, and inappropriate; and the frequent response to anticonvulsant medication warrant tentative inclusion in this category.

Seizures as Recurrent Dreams, Nightmares, or Sleep Tremors/Sleepwalking

Seizures as recurrent dreams, nightmares, or ST/SW have been well described in both adults and children. The diagnosis may be overlooked, because the symptom is simply interpreted as a primary sleep phenomenon.[55–59]

Episodic Nocturnal Wanderings

Episodic nocturnal wanderings indistinguishable by history from ST/SW but responding to anticonvulsants have been described. The patients ambulated, vocalized, and displayed violent behavior during sleep. Not all exhibited waking EEG abnormalities. These may be examples of frontal lobe seizures (see below). The response to anticonvulsant medication and the report of the disappearance of ST after temporal lobectomy for conventional seizure control support an epileptiform etiology.[60-65] Confused, aimless wandering may also be the manifestation of poriomania, a postictal automatism.[66]

Hypnogenic Paroxysmal Dystonia

Hypnogenic paroxysmal dystonia (HPD) is a syndrome characterized by predominantly or exclusively nocturnal episodes of coarse, occasionally violent, movements of the limbs associated with tonic spasms, often occurring multiple times a night. Vocalization or laughter may occur. The scalp EEG between events is normal and during the spells displays only movement artifact, without clear evidence of electrical seizure activity.[67-71] Carbamazepine is often very effective in eliminating these spells.[72] Vigilance level–dependent tonic seizures[73] and familial paroxysmal hypnogenic dystonia[74] may represent variants of HPD. An association with reflex paroxysmal dystonia is reported.[75] Although controversial, more recent investigation has firmly supported an epileptic (possibly frontal lobe in origin) etiology for HPD.[76-82] It may be unilateral[67,71,83-86] and familial.[74] Nocturnal and diurnal paroxysmal dystonia can exist in the same patient, as can reflex and hypnogenic paroxysmal dystonia.

Pure Tonic Seizures with Arousal

Pure tonic seizures with arousal (or paroxysmal polyspike activity with arousal) refer to seizures that present as pure, otherwise unexplained, paroxysmal arousals. Affected individuals generally do not have diurnal seizures and present with complaints of insomnia or excessive daytime sleepiness, or both, resulting from the seizure-induced sleep fragmentation. These arousals may represent the sole manifestation of seizures arising from deep-sited foci.[87] Treatment includes anticonvulsants or sedative/hypnotics (which possibly increase the arousal threshold).[88-92]

Autonomic/Subcortical/Diencephalic Seizures

Autonomic/subcortical/diencephalic seizures may present considerable clinical confusion. The very existence of subcortical seizures has been questioned, but overwhelming experimental and clinical data support this phenomenon. The presence of seizures in anencephaly documents the fact that seizures can arise exclusively from subcortical structures.[93-95] The role of subcortical structures in seizures was the subject of an extensive review.[96] The cerebellum also has been implicated in the genesis of seizures.[97] The autonomic symptoms of seizures may reflect either primary[98-111] or secondary[112,113] involvement of subcortical structures. Isolated autonomic symptoms are a well-documented manifestation of seizures[114–116] and are probably much more common than has generally been suspected. Such seizures could present from sleep with such manifestations as pain,[117] apnea,[118–120] stridor,[121] coughing,[122] choking,[123] emesis,[124–126] laryngospasm,[127,128] chest pain and arrhythmias,[129–132] piloerection,[133] paroxysmal flushing, and localized hyperhidrosis.[134,135] Effective treatment with anticonvulsants, clonidine, bromocriptine/morphine, and beta-adrenergic blocking agents has been reported.[134,136] Failure to consider seizures as the cause of paroxysmal autonomic symptoms has contributed to the underestimation of their prevalence and may prevent diagnosis and appropriate treatment.

The motor manifestations of subcortical seizures may take the form of tonic expression.[137–140] Such activity is reminiscent of HPD and pure tonic seizures with arousal.

Seizures That Present as Isolated, Recurrent Arousals or Awakenings

Seizures that present as isolated, recurrent arousals or awakenings may present as sleep maintenance insomnia with or without resulting excessive daytime sleepiness.[88–92] Some patients with occasional paroxysmal periodic motor attacks during sleep have very frequent (every 20–60 seconds) subclinical arousals, resulting in severe sleep fragmentation.[141] These paroxysmal arousals may be due to deep epileptic foci.[87] The arousal preceding nocturnal seizures may be the initial manifestation of the seizure.[142] Animal studies support the concept of frequent arousals as the manifestation of a seizure.[143] This finding may explain the fact that many patients with epilepsy report frequent, otherwise unexplained, occasionally precipitous nocturnal awakenings.[87,144]

Diagnosis of Nocturnal Seizures

Although exclusively nocturnal seizures may be uncommon, they are routinely misdiagnosed and should never be overlooked as possibly etiologic in *any* sleep-related behavior that is recurrent, stereotyped, or inappropriate, regardless of the specific nature of that behavior. Nocturnal seizures are undoubtedly more common than has generally been realized; however, they are underdiagnosed for two reasons.

The primary reason for underdiagnosis is the all too common misconception that the absence of scalp EEG abnormalities either precludes or speaks against the diagnosis of seizures. It has been repeatedly documented that true electrical seizure activity may have *no* scalp EEG representation. The disturbing concept of scalp EEG/seizure dissociation can be explained by a number of mechanisms:

1. Obliteration of the scalp EEG seizure activity by movement/muscle artifact.[145] Seizures may be accompanied only by diffuse muscle arti-

fact.[146,147] Complex partial seizures whose initial clinical manifestation is dystonia that precedes the surface EEG activity by 5–15 seconds have been reported.[76] The scalp EEG abnormality may be obscured by the attendant motor activity. This is a particular problem if no postictal EEG changes are seen (see No. 4).
2. Simple absence of concomitant scalp EEG manifestations of seizures originating in deeper structures. This phenomenon has been extensively substantiated. Numerous well-documented cases of scalp video-EEG depth electrode seizure disparity have been described.[148–151] The incidence of absent scalp EEG changes *during* clinical complex partial seizures may be as high as 18%.[152] One report describes both clinical auras and subclinical seizures associated with electrical seizure activity detected by depth electrodes but absent even from simultaneously recording subdural electrodes.[153]
3. Generalized amplitude suppression, low-voltage fast activity, or alpha-frequency activity as the scalp EEG manifestation of the seizure. Such EEG activity, if interrupting sleep EEG patterns, may appear to represent medication effect, artifact, or a simple arousal or state change.[138,154–156]
4. The absence of postictal EEG changes.[138] To further complicate matters, clinically apparent postictal behavior may be absent.[157]
5. Sampling error. The difficulty in capturing a clinical or subclinical event may necessitate prolonged monitoring. The fact that in a given subject there may be EEG correlates with some, but not all, clinical seizures underscores the advantage of recording multiple spells.

Another reason for misdiagnosis is the bizarre nature of the clinical manifestations of the seizure, leading to the suspicion of psychiatric disorders or isolated autonomic phenomena (discussed above), which are misattributed to disorders of other organ systems. Possibly the most curious and peculiar behavioral manifestations of seizures are those associated with epileptogenic foci located in the orbital or mesial regions of the frontal lobe. These may be associated with extremely complex motor behavior, including kicking, running, and impressive vocalization (screaming, swearing) with sexual automatisms. The tendency of the spells to cluster spontaneously (with seizure-free intervals that last months) and to be predominately or exclusively nocturnal may erroneously suggest ST/SW or pseudoseizures.[146,156,158–165]

The preservation of consciousness during seizures can occur[151,166] and should not necessarily be taken as evidence for pseudoseizures. Bizarre experiential phenomena may also be the manifestation of seizures: orgasms,[167] hallucinations (autoscopia, which could be confused with hypnagogic hallucinations),[168] obsessions,[169] feelings of ecstasy[170] or embarrassment,[171] crying,[172] laughing,[173] headaches,[174] spitting,[175] vomiting,[176] or cursing.[61] The fact that environmental clues may play a role in the context of psychomotor seizures further enhances the chance of erroneous psychogenic labeling.[177]

It must be remembered that other apparently primary parasomnias may actually be the manifestation of a seizure disorder. These include the rhythmic movement disorder (RMD) and periodic limb movement disorder (PLMD; nocturnal myoclonus). *RMD* refers to a group of behaviors characterized by stereotyped movements (nocturnal rhythmic oscillation of the head or limbs, nocturnal head banging [jactatio capitis nocturna], or body rocking), seen most frequently in childhood and rarely in adults.[178] RMD may be the sole manifestation of a seizure.[179]

PLMD is a common disorder that may be associated with the complaint of either insomnia or excessive daytime sleepiness or that may be identified as an asymptomatic finding on PSG. It is different from conventional myoclonus, which tends to be more rapid and random and to diminish during sleep.[180] It should not be confused with the motor sleep start, a physiologic jerk of all or part of the body that occurs at sleep onset.[181] PLMD is characterized by the periodic (every 20–40 seconds), sustained (0.5–4.0 seconds in duration) contracture of one or both anterior tibialis muscles variably associated with unperceived arousals. Some cases of PLMD are most dramatic, involving all four extremities and the trunk, raising the possibility that, in some instances, these nocturnal movements may in fact represent repetitive myoclonic seizures.

Just as these (and likely other) parasomnias may actually represent seizures, the converse is also true: Nocturnal seizures may be epiphenomena of secondary parasomnias, with the prototypic example being obstructive sleep apnea, which may masquerade as a "nocturnal seizure disorder."[182,183] Diffuse esophageal spasms in infants may also be confused with seizures.[184]

These difficulties in evaluating nocturnal seizures emphasize the necessity of extensive, in-person laboratory monitoring.[185,186] "Ambulatory" EEG monitoring has led to the misdiagnosis of functional psychiatric disease in a number of our patients who were subsequently demonstrated to have bona fide nocturnal seizures. Extensive PSG monitoring using a full scalp EEG montage with a paper speed of at least 15 mm per second is mandatory. Multiple studies may be necessary to capture an event. Continuous audiovisual monitoring and recording with detailed technician observation are imperative. Such studies are best performed in experienced facilities with interpretation by an experienced clinical polysomnographer or electroencephalographer. The treatment of nocturnal seizures is similar to that of diurnal seizures.

Psychiatric Conditions

Formal PSG monitoring has permitted the reassignment of many of the previously mentioned parasomnias from the psychiatric domain. It also has facilitated the objective documentation and verification of psychogenic conditions that arise from the sleeping state.

Dissociative Disorders

Dissociative disorders (DDs) are rare, accounting for only eight (5%) of our series of 150 consecutive adults presenting to a sleep disorders center during a 7.5-year period for evaluation of sleep-related injury/violence. The mean age at referral was 30 years, and 88% of the patients were female. Two individuals fulfilled *DSM-III-R* (*Diagnostic and Statistical Manual of Mental Disorders*, Revised Third Edition) criteria for multiple personality disorder, and the remaining six were diagnosed as DD not otherwise specified but were strongly suspected of having multiple personality disorder. Three of the eight had post-traumatic stress disorder (PTSD) resulting from early life psychic trauma. PSG studies were diagnostic for DD in one-half and supportive of the diagnosis in the rest. A history of sexual abuse in childhood should be aggressively pursued in cases of DD.[187] DD (often with a history of childhood sexual abuse) should always be considered in the differential diagnosis of pseudoseizures.[188] Confirmatory PSG findings include capturing a spell that arises from a period of well-established, fully developed wakefulness without EEG seizure activity. Supportive PSG data are the absence of PSG evidence of seizures, RBD, or ST/SW.[189]

Post-Traumatic Stress Disorder

PTSD as defined in the *DSM-III-R* is associated with prominent sleep disturbances and "nightmares." It may follow any "psychological distressing event that is beyond the range of usual human experience" and is certainly not confined to combat situations. PTSD may be experienced by both adults and children as a sequel to other major psychic trauma, such as natural disasters, catastrophic accidents, or assaults.[190] The associated sleep abnormalities described include poor sleep continuity and light sleep, with "nightmares" occurring during either REM or NREM sleep[191] and repetitive body movements resembling those seen in non-PTSD patients (ST/SW, body rocking, head banging).[192,193] The "dreams" studied in affected combat veterans may arise from all stages of sleep and may demonstrate features of RBD, indicating that they represent neither conventional REM anxiety attacks nor ST.[194] Differentiating between seizures and PTSD may be difficult.[195] An intriguing suggestion has been made that the cardinal waking symptoms of PTSD (heightened startle reflex and flashbacks) may represent dysregulated REM phenomena occurring during W,[193] supporting the concept of state dissociation. No thorough, systematic PSG and psychiatric study describing the sleep physiology in this fascinating group of patients is currently available. Treatment is difficult and includes counseling. Imipramine or alprazolam may be effective.[19] PTSD appears to be a factor in some cases of DD.[189]

Panic Disorder

Although isolated references have been made to the association of panic attacks and sleep, the confusion of terminology (dream anxiety attack, ST, nighttime panic attack) and the striking similarity of symptoms among these disorders urge caution in interpretation.[196–199] A number of patients with diurnal panic disorder (PD) report panic symptoms arising from sleep. It is conceivable that, just as with nocturnal seizures, some individuals may have panic attacks exclusively during the sleeping state or diurnal symptoms may "spill over" into the sleeping state, or vice versa.[200,201] The salient features of nocturnal panic attacks are (1) precipitous arousal from sleep; (2) impressive autonomic symptoms (tachycardia, tachypnea, diaphoresis, mydriasis, tremulousness); and (3) experiential feelings of fear, apprehension, dread, or impending doom. Just as with PTSD, PD occurs in children.[202] The symptoms may be identical to those caused by a number of other conditions (ST/SW, gastroesophageal reflux, obstructive sleep apnea, nocturnal asthma/angina, and seizures with fear/autonomic symptoms), making nocturnal PD one of the most important "lost souls." One report of a patient with precipitous arousals from sleep with features of both PD and seizures, requiring medications for both conditions to control the symptoms, underscores the overlapping nature of many nocturnal events.[203]

Organic neural substrates have been proposed for both PTSD[204] and PD,[205–207] and each has been reported to be the manifestation of seizures.[208,209] DD may also have a psychobiological basis.[210] The fact that environmental events can affect the structure and function of the central nervous system and that the central nervous system displays learning of new neural behaviors[211–217] has important implications for DD, PTSD, and PD. Ever-growing evidence suggests that PTSD is far more common than was previously believed. The history supportive of PTSD may be very difficult to obtain, particularly in children, raising the possibility that PTSD may lurk in the background and play a role in the development of ST/SW, PD, and DD. The finding of organized behavior occurring during EEG-defined NREM sleep—without evidence of arousal—has been reported in young adults by means of operant conditioning and other techniques.[218,219] This finding, coupled with the concept of neural plasticity, raises fascinating questions as to the nature of psychic influences in the genesis of complex sleep behaviors.

Conclusion

A myriad of bizarre parasomnias continue to stalk the borderlands between ST, SW, psychogenic spells, and atypical seizures. It is imperative to maintain an open and inquiring mind as to etiology, rather than feel compelled to assign a specific (and possibly erroneous) diagnosis. Such spells offer a rich source for clinical investigation. As newer techniques of monitoring are developed, and as more experience is gained, our knowledge of sleep will be enriched, and fewer sleep-related events will remain in "parasomnia purgatory."

The impressive overlap of symptoms among these parasomnias mandates the use of exacting diagnostic criteria in published case reporting. The forensic science implications of these occasionally violent or injurious events has been extensively reviewed elsewhere.[14,24,220–223]

Acknowledgments

We acknowledge the ongoing clinical collaboration of Drs. Gerald M. Rosen and Scott R. Bundlie; Jan Schluter, R.N.; and Constance Ullevig, R.N.; the technical assistance of Andrea Patterson, R.EEG.T., R.PSG.T.; and the secretarial assistance of Ms. Traci Oletzke.

This work was supported, in part, by a grant from Hennepin Faculty Associates.

References

1. Mahowald MW, Ettinger MG. Things that go bump in the night—the parasomnias revisited. J Clin Neurophysiol 1990;7:119.
2. Mahowald MW, Schenck CH. Status dissociatus—a perspective on states of being. Sleep 1991;14:69.
3. Nino-Murcia G, Dement WC. Psychophysiological and Pharmacological Aspects of Somnambulism and Night Terrors in Children. In HY Meltzer (ed), Psychopharmacology: The Third Generation of Progress. New York: Raven, 1987;873–879.
4. Klackenberg G. Somnambulism in childhood—prevalence, course and behavior correlates. A prospective longitudinal study (6–16 years). Acta Paediatr Scand 1982;71:495.
5. Bixler EO, Kales A, Soldatos CR, Healey S. Prevalence of sleep disorders in the Los Angeles metropolitan area. Am J Psychiatry 1979;136:1257.
6. Hublin C, Kaprio J, Partinen M, et al. Prevalence and genetics of sleepwalking: a population-based twin study. Neurology 1997;48:177.
7. Mahowald MW, Bundlie SR, Hurwitz TD, Schenck CH. Sleep violence–forensic science implications: polygraphic and video documentation. J Forensic Sci 1990;35:413.
8. Schenck CH, Hurwitz TD, Bundlie SR, Mahowald MW. Sleep-related eating disorders: polysomnographic correlates of a heterogeneous syndrome distinct from daytime eating disorders. Sleep 1991;14:419.
9. Schenck CH, Hurwitz TD, O'Connor KA, Mahowald MW. Additional categories of sleep-related eating disorders and the current status of treatment. Sleep 1993;16:457.

10. Schenck CH, Mahowald MW. Review of nocturnal sleep-related eating disorders. Int J Eating Disorders 1994;15:343.
11. Fisher C, Kahn E, Edwards A, Davis DM. A psychophysiological study of nightmares and night terrors. I. Physiological aspects of the stage 4 night terror. J Nerv Ment Dis 1973;157:75.
12. Fisher C, Kahn E, Edwards A, et al. A psychophysiological study of nightmares and night terrors. III. Mental content and recall of stage 4 night terrors. J Nerv Ment Dis 1974;158:174.
13. Schenck CH, Hurwitz TD, Bundlie SR, Mahowald MW. Sleep-related injury in 100 adult patients: a polysomnographic and clinical report. Am J Psychiatry 1989;146:1166.
14. Mahowald MW, Schenck CH. Complex motor behavior arising during the sleep period: forensic science implications. Sleep 1995;18:724.
15. Guilleminault C, Phillips R, Dement WC. A syndrome of hypersomnia with automatic behavior. Electroencephalogr Clin Neurophysiol 1975;38:403.
16. Roth B, Nevsimalova S, Rechtschaffen A. Hypersomnia with "sleep drunkenness." Arch Gen Psychiatry 1972;26:456.
17. Broughton RJ. Sleep disorders: disorders of arousal? Science 1968;159:1070.
18. Rogozea R, Florea-Ciocoiu V. Orienting reaction in patients with night terrors. Biol Psychiatry 1985;20:894.
19. Mahowald MW, Rosen GM. Parasomnias in children. Pediatrician 1990;17:21.
20. Kales A, Jacobson A, Paulson MJ, et al. Somnambulism: psychophysiological correlates. I. All-night EEG studies. Arch Gen Psychiatry 1966;14:586.
21. Fisher C, Byrne J, Edwards A, Kahn E. A psychophysiological study of nightmares. Monogr J Am Psychoanal Assoc 1970;18:747.
22. Kales JD, Kales A, Soldatos CR. Night terrors. Clinical characteristics and personality factors. Arch Gen Psychiatry 1980;47:1413.
23. Soldatos CR, Kales A. Sleep disorders: research in psychopathology and its practical implications. Acta Psychiatr Scand 1982;65:381.
24. Moldofsky H, Gilbert R, Lue FA, MacLean AW. Sleep-related violence. Sleep 1995;18:731.
25. Hurwitz TD, Mahowald MW, Schenck CH, et al. A retrospective outcome study and review of hypnosis as treatment of adults with sleepwalking and sleep terror. J Nerv Ment Dis 1991;179:228.
26. Sadigh MR, Mierzwa JA. The treatment of persistent night terrors with autogenic training: a case study. Biofeedback Self Regul 1995;20:205.
27. Tobin JDJ. Treatment of somnambulism with anticipatory awakening. J Pediatr 1993;122:426.
28. Jouvet M, Delorme F. Locus coeruleus et sommeil paradoxal. CR Soc Biol 1965;159;895.
29. Mahowald MW, Schenck CH. REM Sleep Behavior Disorder. In MH Kryger, W Dement, T Roth (eds), Principles and Practice of Sleep Medicine (2nd ed). Philadelphia: Saunders, 1994;574–588.

30. Schenck CH, Hurwitz TD, Mahowald MW. REM sleep behavior disorder: a report on a series of 96 consecutive cases and a review of the literature. J Sleep Res 1993;2:224.
31. Mori SH. Integration of posture and locomotion in acute decerebrate cats and in awake, freely moving cats. Progr Neurobiol 1987;28:161.
32. Shik ML, Orlovsky GN. Neurophysiology of locomotor automatism. Physiol Rev 1976;56:465.
33. Grillner S, Dubic R. Control of locomotion in vertebrates: spinal and supraspinal mechanisms. Adv Neurol 1988;47:425.
34. Berntson GG, Micco DJ. Organization of brainstem behavioral systems. Brain Res Bull 1976;1:471.
35. Mogenson GJ. Limbic-motor integration. Progr Psychobiol Physiological Psychology 1986;12:117.
36. Mori S, Nishimura H, Aoki M. Brain Stem Activation of the Spinal Stepping Generator. In JA Hobson, MAB Brazier (eds), The Reticular Formation Revisited. New York: Raven, 1980;241–259.
37. Zucker DK, Austin FM, Branchey L. Variables associated with alcoholic blackouts in men. Am J Drug Alcohol Abuse 1985;11:295.
38. Penfield W, Jasper H. Epilepsy and the Functional Anatomy of the Human Brain. Boston: Little, Brown, 1954.
39. Hobson JA, Schmajuk NA. Brain state and plasticity: an integration of the reciprocal interaction model of sleep cycle oscillation with attentional models of hippocampal function. Arch Ital Biol 1988;126:209.
40. Young GB, Blume WT, Wells GA, et al. Differential aspects of sleep epilepsy. Can J Neurol Sci 1985;12:317.
41. Passouant P. Historical Views on Sleep and Epilepsy. In MB Sterman, MN Shouse, P Passouant (eds), Sleep and Epilepsy. New York: Academic, 1982;1–6.
42. Billiard M, Echenne B, Besset A, et al. All-night polygraphic recordings in the child with suspected epileptic seizures, in spite of normal routine and post-sleep deprivation EEGs. Electroencephalogr Clin Neurophysiol 1981;11:450.
43. Stevens JR, Kodama H, Lonsbury B, Mills L. Ultradian characteristics of spontaneous seizure discharges recorded by radio telemetry in man. Electroencephalogr Clin Neurophysiol 1971;31:313.
44. Martins da Silva A, Aarts JHP, Binnie CD, et al. The circadian distribution of interictal epileptiform EEG activity. Electroencephalogr Clin Neurophysiol 1984;58:1.
45. Sterman MB, Shouse MN, Passouant P. Sleep and Epilepsy. New York: Academic, 1982.
46. Sammaritano M, Gigli GL, Gotman J. Interictal spiking during wakefulness and sleep and the localization of foci in temporal lobe epilepsy. Neurology 1991;41:290.
47. Shouse MN, Siegel JM, Wu FM, et al. Mechanisms of seizure suppression during rapid-eye-movement (REM) sleep in cats. Brain Res 1989;505:271.

48. Shouse MN, da Silva AM, Sammaritano M. Circadian rhythm, sleep, and epilepsy. J Clin Neurophysiol 1996;13:32.
49. Kellaway P, Frost JD Jr, Crawley JW. The Relationship between Sleep Spindles and Spike-and-Wave Bursts in Human Epilepsy. In M Avoli, P Gloor, G Kostopoulos, et al. (eds), Generalized Epilepsy. Neurobiological Approaches. Boston: Birkhauser, 1990;36–48.
50. Terzano MG, Parrino L, Spaggiari MC. The cyclic alternating pattern sequences in the dynamic organization of sleep. EEG Clin Neurophysiol 1988;69:437.
51. Terzano MG, Parrino L, Anelli S, Halasz P. Modulation of generalized spike-and-wave discharges during sleep by cyclic alternating pattern. Epilepsia 1989;30:772.
52. Terzano MG, Parrino L, Garofalo PG, et al. Activation of partial seizures with motor signs during cyclic alternating pattern in human sleep. Epilepsy Res 1991;10:166.
53. Terzano MG, Parrino L, Anelli S, et al. Effects of generalized interictal EEG discharges on sleep stability: assessment by means of cyclic alternating pattern. Epilepsia 1992;33:317.
54. Elazar Z. Normal and abnormal motor functions of reticular formation. Isr J Med Sci 1987;23:84.
55. Epstein AW, Hill W. Ictal phenomena during REM sleep of a temporal lobe epileptic. Arch Neurol 1966;15:367.
56. Boller F, Wright DG, Cavalieri R, Mitsumoto H. Paroxysmal "nightmares." Neurology 1975;25:1026.
57. Snyder CH. Epileptic equivalents in children. Pediatrics 1958;21:308.
58. Epstein AW. Recurrent dreams. Their relationship to temporal lobe seizures. Arch Gen Psychiatry 1964;10:49.
59. Fuster B, Castells C, Etcheverry M. Epileptic sleep terrors. Neurology 1954;4:531.
60. Montplaisir J, Laveriere M, Saint-Hilaire JM, et al. Sleep and temporal lobe epilepsy: a case study with depth electrodes. Neurology 1981;31:1352.
61. Drake MEJ. Cursive and cursing epilepsy. Neurology 1984;34:267.
62. Halbreich U, Assael M. Electroencephalogram with sphenoidal needles in sleepwalkers. Psychiatr Clin 1979;11:213.
63. Spire JP, Maselli R. Episodic nocturnal wandering: further evidence of an epileptic disorder. Neurology 1983;33[Suppl 2]:215.
64. Popoviciu L. Frontier States between Sleep Incidents and Nocturnal Epileptic Attacks. In WP Koella, P Levin, (eds), Sleep 1976. Third European Congress of Sleep Research (Montpellier). Basel, Switzerland: Karger, 1977;65–74.
65. Plazzi G, Tinuper P, Montagna P, et al. Epileptic nocturnal wanderings. Neurology 1995;45[Suppl 4]:A332.
66. Mayeux R, Alexander MP, Benson DF, et al. Poriomania. Neurology 1979;29:1616.
67. Lugaresi E, Cirignotta F. Hypnogenic paroxysmal dystonia: epileptic seizure or a new syndrome? Sleep 1981;4:129.

68. Lugaresi E, Cirignotta F. Nocturnal Paroxysmal Dystonia. In MB Sterman, MN Shouse, P Passouant (eds), Sleep and Epilepsy. New York: Academic, 1982;507–511.
69. Montplaisir J, Godbout R, Rouleau I. Hypnogenic paroxysmal dystonia: nocturnal epilepsy or sleep disorder? Sleep Res 1985;14:193.
70. Silvestri R, De Domenico P, Raffaele M, et al. Hypnogenic paroxysmal dystonia: a new type of parasomnia? Funct Neurol 1988;3:95.
71. Lugaresi E, Cirignotta F, Montagna P. Nocturnal paroxysmal dystonia. J Neurol Neurosurg Psychiatry 1986;49:375.
72. Tatara A, Manni R, Piccolo G. A long-lasting CBZ controlled case of hypnogenic paroxysmal dystonia. Ital J Neurol Sci 1988;9:73.
73. Rajna P, Kundra O, Halasz P. Vigilance level–dependent tonic seizures— epilepsy or sleep disorder? A case report. Epilepsia 1983;24:725.
74. Lee BI, Lesser RP, Pippenger CE, et al. Familial paroxysmal hypnogenic dystonia. Neurology 1985;35:1357.
75. Lehkuniec E, Micheli F, De-Abelaiz R, et al. Concurrent hypnogenic and reflex paroxysmal dystonia. Movement Disord 1988;3:290.
76. Kotagal P, Luders H, Morris HH, et al. Dystonic posturing in complex partial seizures of temporal lobe onset: a new lateralizing sign. Neurology 1989; 39:196.
77. Meierkord H. Epilepsy and sleep. Curr Opin Neurol 1994;7:107.
78. Hirsch E, Sellal F, Maton B, et al. Nocturnal paroxysmal dystonia: a clinical form of focal epilepsy. Neurophysiol Clin 1994;24:207.
79. Sallal F, Hirsch E. Nocturnal paroxysmal dystonia [Letter]. Movement Dis 1993;2:252.
80. Tinuper P, Cerullo A, Cirignotta F, et al. Nocturnal paroxysmal dystonia with short-lasting attacks: three cases with evidence for an epileptic frontal lobe origin of seizures. Epilepsia 1990;31:549.
81. Hirsch E. Abnormal Paroxysmal Postures and Movements during Sleep: Partial Epilepsy or Paroxysmal Hypnogenic Dystonia. In J Horne (ed), Sleep '90. Bochum, Germany: Pontenagle, 1990;471–473.
82. Meierkord H, Fish DR, Smith SJM, et al. Is nocturnal paroxysmal dystonia a form of frontal lobe epilepsy? Movement Disord 1992;1:38.
83. Oguni M, Oguni H, Kozasa M, Fukuyama Y. A case with nocturnal paroxysmal unilateral dystonia and interictal right frontal epileptic EEG focus: a lateralized variant of nocturnal paroxysmal dystonia? Brain Dev 1992; 14:412.
84. Rosenberg RS, Pasternak JF. Nocturnal paroxysmal dystonia resembling tonic-clonic seizures. Sleep Res 1990;19:274.
85. Lapierre O, Montplaisir J, Remillard G. Therapeutic effect of clobazam in nocturnal paroxysmal dystonia: further support for an epileptic etiology. Sleep Res 1991;20A:339.
86. Godbout R, Montplaisir J, Rouleau I. Hypnogenic paroxysmal dystonia: epilepsy or a sleep disorder. A case report. Clin Electroencephalogr 1985; 16:136.

87. Montagna P, Sforza E, Tinuper F, et al. Paroxysmal arousals during sleep. Neurology 1990;40:1063.
88. Niedermeyer E, Walker AE. Mesio-frontal epilepsy. Electroencephalogr Clin Neurophysiol 1971;31:104.
89. Erba G, Cavazzuti V. Pure tonic seizures with arousal. Sleep Res 1981;10:164.
90. Benner RP, Atkinson R. Generalized paroxysmal fast activity: electroencephalographic and clinical features. Ann Neurol 1982;11:386.
91. Peled R, Lavie P. Paroxysmal awakenings from sleep associated with excessive daytime somnolence: a form of nocturnal epilepsy. Neurology 1986; 36:95.
92. Erba G, Ferber R. Sleep disruption by subclinical seizure activity as a cause of increased waking seizures and decreased daytime function. Sleep Res 1983; 12:307.
93. DeMyer W, White PT. EEG in holoprosencephaly (arhinencephaly). Arch Neurol 1964;11:57.
94. Ferguson JH, Levinsohn MW, Derakshan I. Brainstem seizures in hydranencephaly. Neurology 1974;24:1152.
95. Danner R, Shewmon A, Sherman MP. Seizures in an atelencephalic infant. Is the cortex essential for neonatal seizures? Arch Neurol 1985;42:1014.
96. Fromm GH, Faingold CL, Browning RA, Burnham WME. Epilepsy and the reticular formation. The role of the reticular core in convulsive seizures. Neurol Neurobiol 1987;27:1.
97. Harvey AS, Jayakar P, Duchowny M, et al. Hemifacial seizures and cerebellar ganglioglioma: an epilepsy syndrome of infancy with seizures of cerebellar origin. Ann Neurol 1996;40:91.
98. Iacono RP, Hashold BSJ. Mental and behavioral effects of brain stem and hypothalamic stimulation in man. Hum Neurobiol 1982;1:273.
99. Wilson WP, Nashold DS. Epileptic discharges occurring in the mesencephalon and thalamus. Epilepsia 1968;9:265.
100. Andy OJ. Focal thalamic discharges. Neurophysiology 1987;4:254.
101. Grazia Cesa-Bianchi M, Mancia M, Mutani R. Experimental epilepsy induced by cobalt powder in lower brain-stem and thalamic structures. EEG Clin Neurophysiol 1967;22:525.
102. Mayer DJ, Liebeskind JC. Pain reduction by focal electrical stimulation of the brain: an anatomical and behavioral analysis. Brain Res 1974;68:73.
103. Nashold BS, Wislon WP, Slaughter G. The midbrain and pain. Adv Neurol 1974;4:191.
104. Nashold BSJ, Wilson WP. Central pain. Observations in man with chronic implanted electrodes in the midbrain tegmentum. Confin Neurol 1966; 27:30.
105. Kreindler A, Zuckermann E, Steriade M, Chimion C. Electroclinical features of convulsions induced by stimulation of the brainstem. J Neurophysiol 1958;21:430.
106. Weir B. Spikes-wave from stimulation of reticular core. Arch Neurol 1964;11:209.

107. Elazar Z, Feldman Z. Brainstem seizures produced by microinjections of carbachol. Epilepsia 1987;28:463.
108. Penfield W. Diencephalic autonomic epilepsy. Arch Neurol Psychiatry 1929;22:358.
109. Carr-Locke D, Millac P. Diencephalic epilepsy in a patient with agenesis of the corpus callosum confirmed by computerised axial tomography. J Neurol Neurosurg Psychiatry 1977;40:808.
110. Solomon GE. Diencephalic autonomic epilepsy caused by a neoplasm. J Pediatr 1973;83:277.
111. McLean AJ. Autonomic epilepsy. Report of a case with observations at necropsy. Arch Neurol Psychiatry 1934;32:189.
112. Van Buren JM, Ajmone-Marson C. A correlation of autonomic and EEG components in temporal lobe epilepsy. Arch Neurol 1960;3:683.
113. Wannamaker BB. Autonomic nervous system and epilepsy. Epilepsia 1985;26 (Suppl 1):S31.
114. Mulder DW, Daly D, Bailey AA. Visceral epilepsy. Arch Intern Med 1954;93:481.
115. Brown RW, McLeod WR. Sympathetic stimulation with temporal lobe epilepsy. Med J Aust 1973;2:274.
116. Van Buren JM. Some autonomic concomitants of ictal automatism. A study of temporal lobe attacks. Brain 1958;81:505.
117. Trevathan E, Cascino GD. Partial epilepsy presenting as focal paroxysmal pain. Neurology 1988;38:329.
118. Sanmarti FX, Estivial E, Campistol J, et al. Apneic episodes in an infant: exceptional epileptic seizures. Electroencephalogr Clin Neurophysiol 1985;60:16p.
119. Walls TJ, Newman PK, Cumming WJK. Recurrent apnoeic attacks as a manifestation of epilepsy. Postgrad Med J 1981;57:575.
120. Monod N, Peirano P, Plouin P, et al. Seizure-induced apnea. Ann N Y Acad Sci 1988;533:411.
121. Maytal J, Resnick TH. Stridor presenting as the sole manifestation of seizures. Ann Neurol 1985;18:414.
122. Winans HM. Epileptic equivalents, a cause for somatic symptoms. Am J Med 1949;7:150.
123. Brown LW, Fry JM. Paroxysmal nocturnal choking: a newly described manifestation of sleep-related epilepsy. Sleep Res 1988;17:153.
124. Kramer RE, Lüders H, Goldstick LP, et al. Ictus emeticus and electroclinical analysis. Neurology 1988;38:1048.
125. Panayiotopoulos CP. Benign nocturnal childhood occipital epilepsy: a new syndrome with nocturnal seizures, tonic deviation of the eyes, and vomiting. J Child Neurol 1989;4:43.
126. Panayiotopoulos CP. Benign childhood epilepsy with occipital paroxysms: a 15-year prospective study. Ann Neurol 1989;26:51.
127. Ravindran M. Temporal lobe seizure presenting as "laryngospasm." Clin Electroencephalogr 1981;12:139.

128. Amir J, Ashkenazi S, Schonfeld T, et al. Laryngospasm as a single manifestation of epilepsy. Arch Dis Child 1983;58:151.
129. Devinsky O, Price BH, Cohen SI. Cardiac manifestations of complex partial seizures. Am J Med 1986;80:195.
130. Kiok MC, Terrence CF, Fromm GH, Lavine S. Sinus arrest in epilepsy. Neurology 1986;36:115.
131. Gilchrist JM. Arrhythmogenic seizures: diagnosis by simultaneous EEG/ECG recording. Neurology 1985;35:1503.
132. Hockman CH, Mauch HP, Hoff EC. ECG changes resulting from cerebral stimulation. II. A spectrum of ventricular arrhythmias of sympathetic origin. Am Heart J 1966;71:695.
133. Brogna CG, Lee SI, Dreifuss FE. Pilomotor seizures. Magnetic resonance imaging and electroencephalographic localization of originating focus. Arch Neurol 1986;43:1085.
134. Metz SA, Halter JB, Porte DJ, Robertson RP. Autonomic epilepsy: clonidine blockade of paroxysmal catecholamine release and flushing. Ann Intern Med 1978;88:189.
135. Kuritzky A, Hering R, Goldhammer G, Bechar M. Clonidine treatment in paroxysmal localized hyperhidrosis. Arch Neurol 1984;41:1210.
136. Bullard DE. Diencephalic seizures: responsiveness to bromocriptine and morphine. Ann Neurol 1987;21:609.
137. Mutani R, Bergamini L, Fariello R. A case of status epilepticus with tonic expression (so-called "reticular epilepsy"). Epilepsia 1970;11:321.
138. Gastaut H, Roger J, Ouahchi S, et al. An electro-clinical study of generalized epileptic seizures of tonic expression. Epilepsia 1963;4:15.
139. Nathanson M, Krumholz A, Biddle D. Seizures of axial structures. Presumptive evidence for brain stem origin. Arch Neurol 1978;35:448.
140. Egli M, Mothersill I, O'Kane M, O'Kane F. The axial spasm—the predominant type of drop seizure in patients with secondary generalized epilepsy. Epilepsia 1985;26:401.
141. Sforza E, Montagna P, Rinaldi R, et al. Paroxysmal periodic motor attacks during sleep: clinical and polygraphic features. EEG Clin Neurophysiol 1993;86:161.
142. Malow BA, Varma NK. Seizures and arousals from sleep—which comes first? Sleep 1995;18:783.
143. Shouse MN, Langer J, King A, et al. Paroxysmal microarousals in amygdala-kindled kittens: could they be subclinical seizures? Epilepsia 1995;36:290.
144. Hoeppner JB, Garron DC, Cartwright RD. Self-reported sleep disorder symptoms in epilepsy. Epilepsia 1984;25:434.
145. Ralston BL, Papatheodorou CA. The mechanism of transition of interictal spiking foci into ictal seizure discharges. Part II: Observations in man. EEG Clin Neurophysiol 1960;12:297.
146. Ludwig B, Ajmone-Marsan C, Van Buren J. Cerebral seizures of probable orbitofrontal origin. Epilepsia 1975;16:141.

147. Ludwig B, Ajmone-Marsan B, Strauss E, Wada JA. Cerebral seizures of probable orbitofrontal origin. Epilepsia 1987;16:141.
148. Devinsky O, Kelley K, Porter RJ, Theodore WH. Clinical and electroencephalographic features of simple partial seizures. Neurology 1988;38:1347.
149. Mizrahi E. Clinical and neurophysiologic correlates of neonatal seizures. Cleve Clin J Med 1988;56(Suppl 1):S100.
150. Ajmone-Marsan C, Abraham K. Considerations on the use of chronically implanted electrodes in seizure disorders. Confin Neurol 1966;27:95.
151. Morris HHI, Dinner DS, Lüders H, et al. Supplementary motor seizures: clinical and electroencephalographic findings. Neurology 1988;38:1075.
152. Klass DW. Electroencephalographic manifestations of complex partial seizures. Adv Neurol 1975;11:113.
153. Sperling MR, O'Connor MJ. Comparison of depth and subdural electrodes in recording temporal lobe seizures. Neurology 1989;39:1497.
154. Fariello RG, Doro JM, Forster FM. Generalized cortical electrodecremental event. Clinical and neurophysiological observations in patients with dystonic seizures. Arch Neurol 1979;36:285.
155. Delgado Escueta AV, Enrile Bacsal F, Treiman DM. Complex partial seizures on closed-circuit television and EEG: a study of 691 attacks in 79 patients. Ann Neurol 1982;11:292.
156. Brenner RP, Atkinson R. Generalized paroxysmal fast activity: electroencephalographic and clinical features. Ann Neurol 1982;11:368.
157. Williamson PD, Spencer SS. Clinical and EEG features of complex partial seizures of extratemporal origin. Epilepsia 1986;27(Suppl 2):S46.
158. Tharp B. Orbital frontal seizures. An unique electroencephalographic and clinical syndrome. Epilepsia 1972;13:627.
159. Williamson PD, Spencer DD, Spencer SS, et al. Complex partial seizures of frontal lobe origin. Ann Neurol 1985;18:497.
160. Waterman K, Purves SJ, Strauss E, Wada JA. An epileptic syndrome caused by mesial frontal lobe seizure foci. Neurology 1987;37:577.
161. Quesney LF, Krieger C, Leitner C, et al. Frontal Lobe Epilepsy: Clinical and Electrographic Presentation. In RJ Porter, RH Mattson, AA Ward Jr, M Dam (eds), Advances in Epileptology: XVth Epilepsy International Symposium. New York: Raven, 1984;503–508.
162. Geier S, Bancaud J, Talairach J, et al. The seizures of frontal lobe epilepsy. A study of clinical manifestations. Neurology 1977;27:951.
163. King DW, Smith JR. Supplementary sensorimotor area epilepsy in adults. Adv Neurol 1996;70:285.
164. Chauvel P, Kleimann F, Vignal JP, et al. The Clinical Signs and Symptoms of Frontal Lobe Seizures. In HH Jasper, S Riggio, PS Goldman-Rakic (eds), Epilepsy and the Functional Anatomy of the Frontal Lobe. New York: Raven, 1995;115–126.
165. Williamson PD. Frontal Lobe Epilepsy. Some Clinical Characteristics. In HH Jasper, S Riggio, PS Goldman-Rakic (eds), Epilepsy and the Functional Anatomy of the Frontal Lobe. New York: Raven, 1995;127–152.

166. Matsuo F. Partial epileptic seizures beginning in the truncal muscles. Acta Neurol Scand 1984;69:264.
167. Calleja J, Carpizo R, Berciano J. Orgasmic epilepsy. Epilepsia 1988;29:635.
168. Devinsky O, Feldmann E, Burrowes K, Bromfield E. Autoscopic phenomena with seizures. Arch Neurol 1989;46:1080.
169. Andy OJ. Seizures and obsessions. J Clin Neurophysiol 1987;4:257.
170. Cirignotta F, Todesco CV, Lugaresi E. Temporal lobe epilepsy with ecstatic seizures (so-called Dostoevsky epilepsy). Epilepsia 1980;21:705.
171. Devinsky O, Hafler DA, Victor J. Embarrassment as the aura of a complex partial seizure. Neurology 1982;32:1284.
172. Luciano D, Devinsky O, Perrine K. Crying seizures. Neurology 1993;43:2113.
173. Armstrong SC, Watters MR, Pearce JW. A case of nocturnal gelastic epilepsy. Neuropsychiatry Neuropsychol Behav Neurol 1990;3:213.
174. Laplante P, Saint-Hilaire JM, Bouvier G. Headache as an epileptic manifestation. Neurology 1983;33:1493.
175. Hecker A, Andermann F, Rodin EA. Spitting automatism in temporal lobe seizures. Epilepsia 1972;13:767.
176. Panayiotopoulos CP. Benign Childhood Epilepsy with Occipital Paroxysms. In F Andermann, A Beaumanoir, L Mira, et al. (eds), Occipital Seizures and Epilepsy in Children. London: John Libbey, 1993;151–164.
177. Forster FM, Liske E. Role of environmental clues in temporal lobe epilepsy. Neurology 1963;13:301.
178. Thorpy MJ, Glovinsky PB. Parasomnias. Psychiatr Clin North Am 1987; 10:623.
179. Guilleminault C, Silvestri R. Disorders of Arousal and Epilepsy during Sleep. In MB Sterman, MN Shouse, PP Passouant (eds), Sleep and Epilepsy. New York: Academic, 1982;513–531.
180. Mano T, Shiozawa Z, Sobue I. Extrapyramidal Involuntary Movements during Sleep. In R Broughton (ed), Henri Gastaut and the Marseilles School's Contribution to the Neurosciences, vol EEG, Suppl No. 35. Amsterdam: Elsevier, 1982;431–442.
181. Parkes JD. The parasomnias. Lancet 1986;2:1021.
182. Cirignotta F, Zucconi M, Mondini S, et al. Cerebral anoxic attacks in sleep apnea syndrome. Sleep 1989;12:400.
183. Wyler AR, Weymuller EAJ. Epilepsy complicated by sleep apnea. Ann Neurol 1981;9:403.
184. Wyllie E, Wyllie R, Rothner AD, Morris HHI. Another paroxysmal disorder in the differential diagnosis of seizures in infants: diffuse esophageal spasms. Ann Neurol 1988;24:328.
185. Aldrich MS, Jahnke B. Diagnostic value of video-EEG polysomnography. Neurology 1991;41:1060.
186. Mahowald MW. Diagnostic testing: sleep disorders. Neurol Clin 1996;14:183.
187. Chu JA, Dill DL. Dissociative symptoms in relation to childhood physical and sexual abuse. Am J Psychiatry 1990;147:887.

188. Shen W, Bowman ES, Markand ON. Presenting the diagnosis of pseudoseizure. Neurology 1990;40:756.
189. Schenck CH, Milner D, Hurwitz TD, et al. Dissociative disorders presenting as somnambulism: polysomnographic, video and clinical documentation (8 cases). Dissociation 1989;2:194.
190. American Psychiatric Association. Diagnostic and Statistical Manual of Mental Disorders (3rd ed). Washington, DC: American Psychiatric Association, 1987.
191. Friedman M. Toward a rational pharmacotherapy for posttraumatic stress disorder: an interim report. Am J Psychiatry 1988;145:281.
192. Lavie P, Hertz G. Increased sleep motility and respiration rates in combat neurotic patients. Biol Psychiatry 1979;14:983.
193. Ross RJ, Ball WA, Sullivan KA, Caroff SN. Sleep disturbance as the hallmark of posttraumatic stress disorder. Am J Psychiatry 1989;146:697.
194. Hefez A, Metz L, Lavie P. Long-term effects of extreme situational stress on sleep and dreaming. Am J Psychiatry 1987;144:344.
195. Stewart JT, Bartucci RJ. Posttraumatic stress disorder and partial complex seizures. Am J Psychiatry 1986;143:113.
196. Lesser IM, Poland RE, Holcomb C, Rose DE. Electroencephalographic study of nighttime panic attacks. J Nerv Ment Dis 1985;173:744.
197. Grunhaus L, Birmaher B. The clinical spectrum of panic attacks. J Clin Psychopharmacol 1985;5:93.
198. Hauri P, Friedman M, Ravaris CL. Sleep in patients with spontaneous panic attacks. Sleep 1989;12:323.
199. Mellman TA, Uhde TW. Electroencephalographic sleep in panic disorder. Arch Gen Psychiatry 1989;46:178.
200. Mellman TA, Uhde TW. Sleep panic attacks: new clinical findings and theoretical implications. Am J Psychiatry 1989;146:1204.
201. Craske MG, Barlow DH. Nocturnal panic. J Nerv Ment Dis 1989;177:160.
202. Herskowitz J. Neurologic presentations of panic disorder in childhood and adolescence. Dev Med Child Neurol 1986;28:617.
203. Dantendorfer K, Frey R, Maierhofer D, Saletu B. Sudden arousals from slow wave sleep and panic disorder: successful treatment with anticonvulsants—a case report. Sleep 1996;19:744.
204. Kolb LC. A neurophysiological hypothesis explaining posttraumatic stress disorders. Am J Psychiatry 1987;144:989.
205. Reiman EM. The quest to establish the neural substrates of anxiety. Psychiatr Clin North Am 1988;11:295.
206. Gorman JM, Liebowitz MR, Fyer AJ, Stein J. A neuroanatomical hypothesis for panic disorder. Am J Psychiatry 1989;146:148.
207. Reiman EM, Raichle ME, Mintun MA, et al. Neuroanatomical correlates of a lactate-induced anxiety attack. Arch Gen Psychiatry 1989;46:493.
208. Wall M, Tuchman M, Mielke D. Panic attacks and temporal lobe seizures associated with a right temporal lobe arteriovenous malformation: case report. J Clin Psychiatry 1985;46:143.

209. Ghadirian AM, Gauthier S, Bertrand S. Anxiety attacks in a patient with a right temporal lobe meningioma. J Clin Psychiatry 1986;47:270.
210. Putnam FW. Diagnosis and Treatment of Multiple Personality Disorder. New York: Gilford, 1989.
211. Edelman GM. Neural Darwinism. New York: Basic Books, 1987.
212. Reiser MF. Mind, Brain, Body—Toward a Convergence of Psychoanalysis and Neurobiology. New York: Basic Books, 1984.
213. Kandel ER. Environmental Determinants of Brain Architecture and of Behavior: Early Experience and Learning. In ER Kandel, JH Schwartz JH (eds), Principles of Neural Science. New York: Elsevier/North Holland, 1981;620–632.
214. Iriki A, Pavlides C, Keller A, Asanuma H. Long-term potentiation in the motor cortex. Science 1989;245:1385.
215. Aoki C, Siekevitz P. Plasticity in brain development. Sci Am 1988;259:56.
216. Lipton SA. Growth factors for neuronal survival and process regeneration. Implications in the mammalian central nervous system. Arch Neurol 1989; 46:1241.
217. Snider WD, Johnson EMJ. Neurotropic molecules. Ann Neurol 1989;26:489.
218. Granda AM, Hammack JT. Operant behavior during sleep. Science 1961; 333:1485.
219. Ogilvie RD, Wilkinson RT, Allison S. The detection of sleep onset: behavioral, physiological, and subjective convergence. Sleep 1989;12:458.
220. Guilleminault C, Kushida C, Leger D. Forensic sleep medicine and nocturnal wanderings. Sleep 1995;18:721.
221. Guilleminault C, Moscovitch A, Leger D. Forensic sleep medicine: nocturnal wandering and violence. Sleep 1995;18:740.
222. Broughton RJ, Shimizu T. Sleep-related violence: a medical and forensic challenge. Sleep 1995;18:727.
223. Mahowald MW, Schenck CH. Medical-legal aspects of sleep medicine. Neurol Clin 1999;17:215.

CHAPTER 6

Non-Epileptic Seizures in Children

Frank J. Ritter and Prakash Kotagal

Non-epileptic seizures (NES) have been the focus of many reviews.[1-10] It is not known how often non-epileptic paroxysmal events occur in children. During the first 2 years of life, prospective epidemiologic studies suggest that approximately one in four (26.6%) infants have at least one paroxysmal event that could be mistaken for a seizure.[11] With increasing use of simultaneous video-electroencephalography (EEG), the magnitude of the problem of NES in childhood is becoming clearer. NES occur in 10–20% of children referred to epilepsy centers for the evaluation of uncontrolled epilepsy.[12-15] In children who are neurologically or mentally abnormal, some reports claim that as many as 30–60% of paroxysmal non-epileptic events are misdiagnosed and treated as epilepsy.[16-21] Some of these children have both non-epileptic and epileptic seizures. In this group, staring episodes, head drops, brief jerks, and repetitive self-stimulatory or stereotypic behaviors are the most frequent types of events misdiagnosed as seizure. An abnormal EEG is not diagnostic of epilepsy and may be misleading, resulting in unnecessary treatment or medication toxicity. Epileptiform discharges (spikes, spike wave) occur in 3.5–5.0% of routine EEGs in healthy children who do not have epilepsy.[12,22-26] Common problems that lead to the misinterpretation of the EEG may contribute to the misdiagnosis of epilepsy.[27,28]

NES should be considered in all children with epilepsy that is refractory to treatment. This is especially true if the seizures are frequent or show no response to the manipulation of anti-epileptic medications, or both. In some cases, increasing doses of anti-epileptic medications may actually increase the frequency of occurrence of NES.[29]

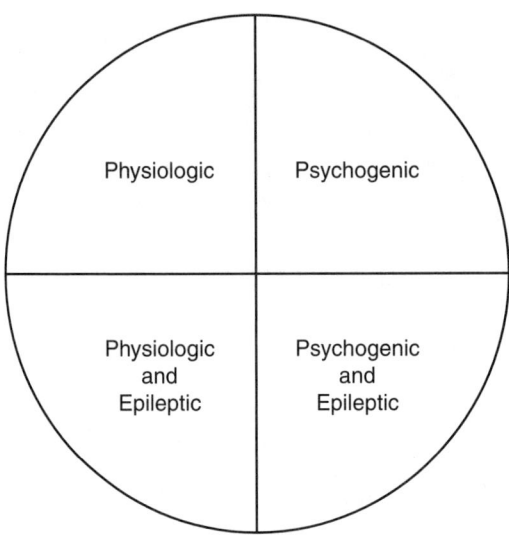

FIGURE 6.1. Non-epileptic seizures in children.

NES in children can be divided into four categories: (1) physiologic NES (e.g., breath-holding spells), (2) mixed epileptic seizures and physiologic NES, (3) psychogenic NES (e.g., conversion reactions), and (4) mixed epileptic seizures and psychogenic NES (Figure 6.1). Some of the paroxysmal events in childhood that may be confused with epilepsy are reviewed here.

Physiologic Events

Benign Myoclonus

Benign myoclonus of early infancy usually has its onset between 3 and 9 months of age.[30–32] These infants appear to have tonic-myoclonic seizures of the axial muscles with or without involvement of the limbs. Mostly head, neck, and upper extremities are involved in episodes that occur while the infants are awake. The episodes occur in flurries and may cluster around sleep times, especially when awakening from sleep. Some infants have been described as having as many as 30–40 clusters of myoclonus per day. The infants are otherwise normal. The EEG is normal, even while the events are being recorded. These episodes usually resolve by the time the patient is 2 years of age. This type of benign myoclonus can also occur in sleep. These episodes have been reported as occurring in infants who also had infantile spasms.[16] These types of mixed physiologic NES and epileptic seizures can only be differentiated by careful evaluation of video-EEG.

Other important types of infantile myoclonus include (1) opsoclonus-myclonus associated with encephalopathy and occult neuroblastoma[33,34] and (2) metabolic disorders such as hypoglycemia and biotinidase deficiency.[35,36]

Alternating Hemiplegia of Childhood

Alternating hemiplegia of childhood has an age of onset between 10 days and 1 year. The majority of infants have the first episode before age 6 months.[37] The initial episodes are brief (30 seconds to 3 minutes) unilateral tonic posturing, often associated with nystagmus toward the tonic side and autonomic changes. The first few episodes are usually not associated with hemiplegia. Parents frequently describe the infant as appearing to be in pain. Within 2–6 months, the episodes are followed by a brief hemiparesis, which is often mistaken for a postictal Todd's paralysis.

The hemiparesis alternates sides; occasionally, both sides are affected within the same episode. These episodes increase in frequency, severity, and duration over the next few years, plateau, and then decrease, but they never totally resolve. When the episodes of paresis are prolonged, they are associated with swallowing difficulties, drooling, choking, and slurred speech. The children recover completely after sleep, but the hemiparesis may return within 20 minutes of awakening. Fatigue, extreme emotion, or excitement often triggers the episodes. The children are usually hypotonic, and their development is delayed. Choreoathetotic movements and ataxia are uniformly seen as the episodes progress. Approximately one-fourth of the children also have epileptic seizures, which are not associated with the hemiplegic episodes. The hemiplegic episodes may occur as often as every 48 hours but are usually less frequent, occurring one or two times a week and rarely less frequently than once a month. The EEG is normal between attacks. During an episode of hemiplegia, the EEG is slow over the contralateral hemisphere. Other laboratory studies are unrevealing. The prognosis is poor.

Spasmus Nutans

Spasmus nutans usually has its onset between 4 and 12 months. Typically it begins with episodes of head nodding, with nystagmus and "head tilt" or torticollis occurring later in the course. Infants are awake and alert during the episode. This disorder usually resolves in 1 to 2 years but has been reported to persist up to 8 years of age. Development is normal, and the EEG does not show epileptiform discharges. Mass lesions of the optic chiasm or third ventricle can cause similar symptoms, and neuroimaging is therefore recommended.[38–41]

Gastroesophageal Reflux (Sandifer's Syndrome)

Gastroesophageal reflux (Sandifer's syndrome) can have its onset at any time in childhood, but most of the symptoms mistaken for seizure occur in infancy. The infant or child suddenly stiffens, usually with the head deviated to one side. Although awake, infants generally do not respond or have a marked decrease in responsiveness. These episodes can result in significant apnea in some infants. The episodes mimic tonic adversative seizures. They frequently are associated with eating and occasionally occur without any apparent precipitating factor. Most of these infants have a history of spitting up frequently. The EEG is normal. The episodes may resolve spontaneously but, depending on associated symptoms, medical or surgical treatment may be necessary.[42-44]

Neonatal Hyperexplexia

Neonatal hyperexplexia is extremely rare but important because, if unrecognized and untreated, it can be fatal. Neonates or infants have repeated myoclonic jerks and intermittently have sustained tonic spasms. The latter may be life-threatening, with apnea due to contraction of the respiratory muscles. These episodes may be startle (touch or acoustic) precipitated or spontaneous. Longer life-threatening episodes can be stopped by forcible flexion of the head and legs toward the trunk. Symptoms usually spontaneously improve over months to years. Clonazepam is of benefit, but it does not always stop the prolonged spasms. Forced flexion has been the most effective treatment. Development is eventually normal.[45]

Infantile Masturbation

Infantile masturbation events are commonly brought to the attention of the pediatrician but occasionally present to the neurologist as epilepsy. Episodes may begin as early as 2 to 3 months of age. The episodes do not involve obvious rubbing of the genitalia or copulatory movements. They are frequently described as sudden onset of stiffening, most frequently rigid lower extremities or stereotypic rhythmic activity, often accompanied by irregular breathing, facial flushing, and diaphoresis. The episodes usually last less than a minute but occasionally are more prolonged.[46,47]

Shuddering Attacks

Shuddering attack episodes may have their onset in infancy, from 8 months through childhood (10–12 years). These are sudden episodes of relatively high-frequency tremor (8–12 Hz), with the head and trunk postured and the elbows and knees abducted. The episodes are brief, only a few seconds, but happen many times a day (up to hundreds). The episodes look like someone has poured cold water down the back. Development and the EEG are normal. These episodes usually spontaneously resolve in late childhood. They have been associated with essential tremor in adults.[48,49]

Benign Paroxysmal Vertigo

The onset of benign paroxysmal vertigo is usually between 1 and 3 years of age. Children may appear frightened and may cry out for help. They are unsteady, may cling to their parents, or may lie very still on the floor. The vast majority of children have episodes that last less than 5 minutes, and they occasionally last only a few seconds. Pallor, sweating, or vomiting may occur but is not common. Frequency of the episodes is usually between one and four per month. Occasionally, episodes may cluster. Consciousness is preserved. Caloric testing of vestibular function is reported to be abnormal in most of these children. The episodes tend to spontaneously resolve in most patients by the time they are 4 or 5 years of age. Antihistamines may be helpful for some of these children but, in general, no treatment is necessary.[50,51]

Breath-Holding Spells

The incidence of breath-holding spells with loss of consciousness is 4.6%. The highest incidence occurs between 7 and 12 months of age. These spells usually spontaneously resolve by 4 years of age, although rarely they are observed after the age of 6 years. A familial incidence of 25% has been reported. Two types of breath-holding spells are described: cyanotic and pallid.

The cyanotic type of breath-holding spell comprises the vast majority of these episodes. They are always provoked. Frustration, anger, pain, sudden fright, or minor injuries are the most common precipitating events. Such spells begin with a long period of crying (16–60 seconds), then the infant becomes cyanotic, holds the breath in expiration and, after a period of 25–30 seconds, becomes rigid and opisthotonic. If the apneic phase lasts longer, twitching or frankly clonic movements of the extremities occur. The apnea ends by gasping, proceeding toward normal respiration; the infant then resumes normal activity. Rarely, the infant is drowsy for a few hours.

The pallid type of breath-holding spells also has been called *vagotonia, type II hypoxic crisis,* and *reflex anoxic cerebral crisis with syncope and vagal hypersensitivity.* These episodes are always provoked. Sudden frights and minor injuries, especially blows about the head, are the most common precipitating factors. Crying is usually brief, if at all, and breath holding is not commonly observed. A few seconds after provocation, the infant's eyes roll back and the infant stiffens, perhaps jerks once or twice, wakes briefly, and then falls asleep. An after-pallor is frequently seen. The female to male ratio of this type of episode is 2:1. These episodes result from excessive vagal tone causing asystole. After 15 seconds of asystole, depending on the patient's age, an anoxic seizure often occurs. These spells may reoccur in adolescents as syncope proceeded by an aura. Anemia and iron deficiency have been reported as abnormal laboratory findings in infants with breath-holding spells. Other investigators did not confirm this report, however, and no controlled studies of iron therapy exist. The ocular compression test, a special procedure in the EEG laboratory, is positive in 60–75% of infants with pallid breath-holding spells, 25% of those with the cyanotic type, and 7% of normal infants.

The best therapy is reassurance that the infant is not able to control these spells, that they are not harmful, and that they eventually will be outgrown. When they occur, the parent should leave the infant alone, that is, not pick up the child. Fussing over the infant is reported to increase the frequency of events.

Finally, the treatment of the pallid type with atropine, 0.01 mg/kg not to exceed 0.4 mg per day, is not benign. Parents must be cautioned against hypothermia, central nervous system toxicity, dry mouth, and possible gastrointestinal irritation.[52–55]

Night Terrors

Night terrors are reported to occur in 3% of all prepubertal children. The usual onset is between 2 and 4 years of age, and they tend to resolve at approximately 12 years of age. The episodes start suddenly, with the child typically sitting upright and screaming. Wide-open eyes with pupils dilated, tachycardia, increased muscle tone, and diaphoresis are typical. There may be unintelligible vocalization. The child is unresponsive to consolation; continued effort may worsen autonomic and motor activity. If the child can be awakened, he or she is usually confused and has no recall or only limited, fragmented recall of events. The episodes tend to occur in the first third of sleep. They need to be distinguished from complex partial seizures of frontal origin.[56–58]

Cardiac Arrhythmias

Cardiac arrhythmias can lead to syncope. Loss of consciousness may appear to be precipitous. Failure to recognize the long-QT syndrome may be fatal. The long-QT syndrome frequently has its onset of symptoms in early to mid-childhood. The mean age of onset of symptoms is 10.7 ± 7.6 years, with a range of 1.5–39.0 years of age. The Ramono-Ward autosomal dominant type is the most common and is linked to chromosome 11. Sudden death occurs in 0.5% of individuals with long-QT syndrome per year who are not treated. Approximately 5% have episodes of aborted sudden death. The mean age of death is 16.5 years of age for females and approximately 8 years of age for males. The arrhythmia should be considered in all children who have episodes of loss of consciousness associated with exercise or emotional stress.[59–62]

Other Types of Physiologic Non-Epileptic Seizures

Other types of physiologic NES include movement disorders—for example, paroxysmal choreoathetosis and dyskinesias, tics, catalepsy, and arid paroxysmal dystonia.[63] These disorders are more completely discussed in Chapter 4.

Munchausen Syndrome by Proxy

Munchausen syndrome by proxy is a form of child abuse. The child's parent (98% of the time it is the biological mother) reports a seizure. The seizures are recurrent and, if treated, are refractory. Frequently, the child is taken from physician to physician looking for "someone who can help." Usually no one other than the parent can confirm the seizures, although many people may see the child immediately after the episodes. The child may be postictal or drowsy due to the mechanism the parent has used to precipitate the appearance of illness (e.g., suffocation, poison, or insulin). The frequent seizures do not occur in the parents' absence. Frequently, the physical findings do not correlate well with the historical information and the case is puzzling. A family history of unexplained deaths of children or unexplained brain damage may exist. The parent is usually extremely attentive, likes to become familiar with the hospital personnel, and often works to be involved as part of the "treatment team."[64] This disorder is more completely discussed in Chapter 18.

Conversion Reaction

The conversion reaction is the most common type of psychogenic NES in childhood. Psychogenic NES of this type usually begins in mid-childhood, with an average onset at approximately 12 years of age.[12,14,15,65] Conversion reactions account for approximately 2% of pediatric neurology inpatients.[63,66,67] With the exceptions of headache and pain, NES are the most common neurologic conversion symptom.[68-70] Before the age of 10 years, male and female headache symptoms are equally frequent but, after the age of 12 years, a female predominance emerges. Family dysfunction, family communication difficulties, and stress are almost uniformly present, although a history of these problems is denied in 88% of the cases. Although common in adults, *la belle indifférence* is infrequent in childhood. Sexual abuse, incest, learning disabilities, and poor peer relationships are commonly considered as precipitants of the reaction. Most of the children have psychogenic NES that mimic either complex partial or convulsive seizures. Children with psychogenic NES also have epileptic seizures. When children have both epileptic seizures and NES, the NES almost always resemble the epileptic seizures. Once the diagnosis of psychogenic NES is made and appropriate intervention undertaken, the episodes tend to resolve. Outcomes in children appear to be more favorable than in adults.[5,71-75]

Psychogenic Non-Epileptic Etiologies

There is no doubt that adolescents in particular can exhibit the full spectrum of psychogenic non-epileptic etiologies discussed in Chapter 1. One disorder of particular interest is the reinforced behavior pattern seen in the cognitively impaired, often multiply handicapped child. These children have unconsciously learned to produce seizure-like episodes that result in secondary gain from the environment. As such, these events do not represent an underlying psychological conflict but rather a learned behavior disorder. The patient recognizes the NES as a powerful way to control the environment, and the patient is paradoxically reinforced for this behavior by the caregiver or others. A simple, direct behavioral modification program is the most reasonable way to approach this disorder.

Nonetheless, undifferentiated somatoform disorder and somatization disorder, malingering, panic disorder, hypochondriasis, depersonalization, psychotic disorder, associated disorder not otherwise specified, and post-traumatic stress disorder can all be seen, especially in the adolescent patient (as is discussed more thoroughly in Chapter 1). As was previously emphasized, before age 12, these psychogenic etiologies, with the exception of reinforced behavior pattern and Munchausen by proxy, are rare. The physiologic non-epileptic etiologies predominate (Figure 6.2).

Prevalence of Pediatric Non-Epileptic Seizures

NES are commonly encountered in pediatric neurology practices. Up to 25% of children referred to the pediatric neurologist have NES. Of 842 children evaluated in the pediatric epilepsy monitoring unit at Cleveland Clinic from 1989 to 1995, 199 (23.6%) were diagnosed to have non-epileptic events; these were recorded in 168 (20%) patients. Of these 168 patients, 35 (20.8%) had epilepsy in addition to their non-epileptic events. It is important that these events be diagnosed correctly so that the children are not placed on anti-epileptic medications needlessly while other etiologies go untreated. A well-taken history often leads to the correct diagnosis. Some parents bring videotapes of these events to the clinician that may be quite helpful. In other cases, documentation of these episodes with prolonged video-EEG monitoring is required. We now discuss the actual clinical presentations and evaluation of the more common NES seen in the pediatric epilepsy monitoring unit.

Case Studies of Differential Diagnosis and Evaluation of Non-Epileptic Seizures in Children

Case 1

Presentation

This 11-year-old boy presented with a 1-year history of events consisting of staring and unresponsiveness of 3- to 5-minute duration. During some of

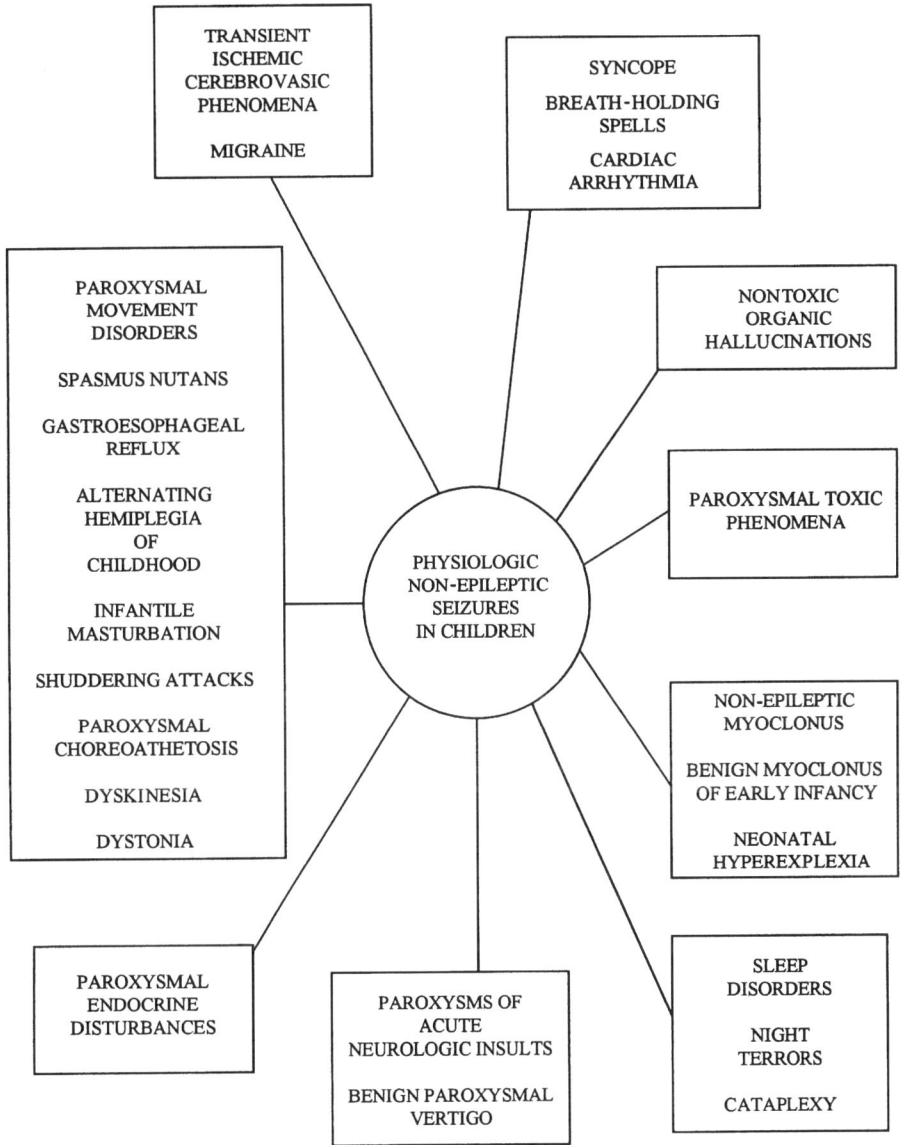

FIGURE 6.2. Spectrum of physiologic non-epileptic seizures in children.

these events, he would close or roll his eyes, nod his head, become limp, fall down, and have jerking movements of the limbs. These were longer events, lasting up to 10 minutes. He had no history of tongue biting or incontinence. Neurologic examination was normal. Routine EEG and magnetic resonance imaging (MRI) of the brain were normal.

Evaluation

The patient underwent 5 days of video-EEG monitoring. No interictal epileptiform abnormalities were noted. One episode of staring with unresponsiveness and six episodes with eye rolling and thrashing about were recorded. Ictal EEG was normal in all the episodes. Psychosocial history revealed no history of physical or emotional trauma. The child had witnessed a classmate have a grand mal seizure, subsequently receiving a lot of attention. The patient also received extra attention from family members after he began having the spells.[76,77]

Case 2

Presentation

A 7-month-old male infant had a 10-day history of "spells," which consisted of brief jerking of the extremities, without eye and/or head movement or loss of consciousness, occurring two to three times a day. Routine EEG and computed tomographic scan of the brain were normal.

Evaluation

Video-EEG monitoring for 2 days was performed. No interictal epileptiform abnormalities were seen. Four clusters of these spells consisting of a quick jerk of the upper extremities and trunk were recorded, during which no EEG change was evident. The child was discharged on no anti-epileptic medication. Events gradually diminished after the age of 18 months and ceased after 21 months.[30]

Case 3

Presentation

This 21-month-old boy presented with a history of seizures from the age of 6 months, during which he would hold his breath, lose consciousness, and then arch his back. This spell was followed by generalized convulsive movements that lasted 1–2 minutes and as long as 12 minutes. His appearance was pale at onset, becoming cyanotic later in the episode. Anger, frustration, or minor trauma usually brought these seizures on, especially when he was tired. Such episodes occurred approximately once a month at first. At the time he was evaluated, the episodes were occurring one to two times a day. The convulsive movements did not respond to a trial of carbamazepine (Tegretol).

Evaluation

On atropine elixir, the episodes were somewhat less frequent and were not followed by convulsive activity, but this treatment had to be discontinued due to side effects. Prolonged video-EEG monitoring showed no interictal epileptiform discharges. Five typical episodes were recorded, during which EEG became markedly suppressed followed by diffuse slowing. No cardiac asystole was seen during these events. Over time, the episodes gradually diminished in frequency and severity and have not been noted since age 6 years.[51,78]

Case 4

Presentation

A 16-month-old female infant presented with episodes that occurred from 7 months of age. She would tense up and have a fine tremor of the whole body accompanied by a change in facial expression that lasted approximately 5–15 seconds. Developmental milestones were normal, as were physical and neurologic examination. Routine EEG and MRI scan of the brain were also normal. The patient had been placed on valproic acid without benefit.

Evaluation

Video-EEG monitoring showed normal interictal EEG without any epileptiform discharges. Three typical episodes were recorded. No ictal pattern was noted on EEG. She was taken off valproic acid and did quite well. Episodes have gradually diminished in frequency. She is now 4 years old and has episodes once in 2–3 weeks. Development remains normal.[48,49,79]

Case 5

Presentation

A 2.5-year-old boy was brought in by his parents for evaluation of "spells" noted from the age of 8 months. During these spells, he was noted to have arrest of activity, staring, and repetitive blinking and was apparently unresponsive for 30–60 seconds. He also had episodes in which he would suddenly fall down limply for no apparent reason. He would cry and then get up quickly. Each of these seizures occurred two to three times a week. His development was proceeding normally, and examination showed no abnormalities. Routine EEG and MRI scan of the brain were normal.

Evaluation

During video-EEG monitoring, no definite interictal epileptiform discharges were seen. Several episodes of repetitive eye blinking were recorded, with no corresponding ictal pattern on EEG. During these episodes, the patient appeared to be normally responsive. Follow-up 6 months later indicated no more episodes of body jerks or falling noted since discharge.[73,75]

Case 6

Presentation

A 6-year-old boy had nighttime episodes in which he woke up crying and screaming, often 75–120 minutes after he went to sleep. He had up to three episodes in a night, 30 minutes to 2 hours apart. His parents would find him sitting up in bed, usually with his eyes open, but not aware of their presence. He might have a scared expression and rock his body back and forth. He has become more violent and aggressive (nondirected). He has also run downstairs and attempted to leave the house. He has no precipitating factors and no medical problems. There was no antecedent physical or emotional trauma; the boy was hospitalized twice in 3 months before the onset of these events. Family history was negative, and physical and neurologic examinations were unremarkable.

Evaluation

A polysomnogram combined with video-EEG monitoring was performed, and no episodes were recorded. Subsequently, the parents were able to capture a typical event on home video. The boy is now 7 years old. Episodes are much milder; he may cry out or sit up in bed, or both, once in 2–3 months.[80–82]

Case 7

Presentation

A 5-year-old boy had a history of holding his breath and making thrashing movements since he was 18 months of age. From 8 months of age, his parents noted that he would rock his body while falling asleep. He also has had episodes during which he appeared to hold his breath for 30–60 seconds, followed by a loud exhale. He then rocked his body or banged his head on the pillow for 1–5 minutes before falling asleep. These episodes occurred one to 15 times a night.

Evaluation

Routine EEG and overnight video-EEG monitoring showed no abnormalities or recorded events. Prolonged video-EEG monitoring was performed for 3 days, and several episodes were recorded. No change was noted in the EEG during these episodes. Polysomnography revealed a moderate degree of obstructive sleep apnea with an apnea plus hypopnea index of 20. After adenotonsillectomy, the apneas have disappeared; however, the head-banging/body-rocking episodes, although less prominent, continued until the last follow-up at age 7.5 years.[57]

References

1. Devinsky O, Thacker K. Nonepileptic seizures. Neurol Clin 1995;13:299.

2. Alper K. Nonepileptic seizures. Neurol Clin 1994;12:153.
3. Fisher RS. Imitators of Epilepsy. New York: Demos, 1994.
4. Sakamoto A, Holthausen H, Noacthar S. Diagnosis of Pseudoepileptic Seizures. In P Wolf (ed), Epileptic Seizures and Syndromes. London: John Libbey, 1994.
5. Rowan AJ, Gates JR. Non-Epileptic Seizures. Boston: Butterworth–Heinemann, 1993.
6. Morrell MJ. Differential diagnosis of seizures. Neurol Clin 1993;11:737.
7. Gram L, Johannessen SE, Osterman M, Sillanpää M. Pseudoepileptic Seizures. Bristol, PA: Wrightson Biomedical, 1993.
8. Sassower K, Duchowny M. Psychogenic Seizures and Non-Epileptic Phenomena in Childhood. In O Devinsky, WH Theodore (eds), Epilepsy and Behavior. New York: Wiley-Liss, 1991;223–235.
9. Paranzatelli MR, Pedley TR. Differential Diagnosis in Children. In M Dam, L Gram (eds), Comprehensive Epileptology. New York: Raven, 1990;423–447.
10. Stephenson JBP. Fits and faints. Clin Dev Med 1990;109:1.
11. Reerink JD, Peters ACB, Verloove-Vanhorick SP, et al. Paroxysmal phenomena in the first two years of life. Dev Med Child Neurol 1994;37:1099.
12. Metrick ME, Ritter FJ, Gates JR, et al. Nonepileptic events in childhood. Epilepsia 1991;32:322.
13. Duchowny M, Resnick JJ, Deray MJ, Alvarez LA. Video EEG diagnosis of repetitive behavior in early childhood and its relationship to seizures. Pediatr Neurol 1998;4:162.
14. Dreifuss FE, Holmes GL, Sackellares JC. Epilepsy and Pseudoseizures in Childhood. Advances in Epileptology XII. New York: Raven Press, 1981; 323–327.
15. Holmes G, Sackellares JC, McKiernan J, et al. Evaluation of childhood pseudoseizures using EEG telemetry and video tape monitoring. J Pediatr 1980; 97:554.
16. Donat JF, Wright FS. Clinical imitators of infantile spasms. J Child Neurol 1992;7:395.
17. Donat JF, Wright FS. Episodic symptoms mistaken for seizures in the neurologically impaired child. Neurology 1990;40:156.
18. Brunquell S, Fahn S, Eisenberg M, et al. Differentiation of epileptic from nonepileptic head drops in children. Epilepsia 1990;31:401.
19. Neill JC, Alvarez N. Differential diagnosis of epileptic versus pseudoseizures in disabled persons. Appl Res Ment Retard 1986;7:285.
20. Holmes GL, McKeever M, Russman BS. Abnormal behavior or epilepsy? Use of long-term EEG and video monitoring with severely to profoundly mentally retarded patients with seizures. Am J Ment Defic 1983;87:456.
21. Najarajan L, Bye AM. Staring episodes in children analyzed by telemetry. J Child Neurol 1992;7:35.
22. Autret A, Lucas B, Degiovanni E, et al. A note on the occurrence of unusual electroencephalographic sleep patterns in selected normal children. J Child Neurol 1992;7:422.
23. Cavazutti GB, Capella L, Nalin A. Longitudinal study of epileptiform EEG patterns in normal children. Epilepsia 1980;21:43.

24. Mattson R. Electroencephalographic (Polygraphic) Studies in the Diagnosis of Non-Epileptic Seizures. In JR Gates, AJ Rowan (eds), Non-Epileptic Seizures. Boston: Butterworth–Heinemann, 1993;85–92.
25. Ramsay RE, Cohen A, Brown MC. Co-existing Epilepsy and Non-Epileptic Seizures. In JR Gates, AJ Rowan (eds), Non-Epileptic Seizures. Boston: Butterworth–Heinemann, 1993;47–54.
26. Okubo Y, Matsura M, Asai T, et al. Epileptiform EEG discharges in healthy children: prevalence, emotional and behavioral correlates and genetic influences. Epilepsia 1994;35: 832.
27. Drury I, Beydoun A. Pitfalls of EEG interpretation in epilepsy. Neurol Clin 1993;11:857.
28. Mizrahi EM. Avoiding the pitfalls of EEG interpretation in childhood epilepsy. Epilepsia 1991;32:322.
29. Trimble MR. Pseudoproblems, pseudoseizures. Br J Hosp Med 1983;29:326.
30. Lombroso CT, Fejerman N. Benign myoclonus of early infancy. Ann Neurol 1987;1:138.
31. Dravert C, Giraud N, Bureau M, Roger J. Benign myoclonus of early infancy or benign non-epileptic infantile spasms. Neuropediatrics 1986;17:33.
32. Resnick TJ, Moseh SL, Perotta L, Chambes HJ. Benign neonatal sleep myoclonus. Arch Neurol 1986;43:255.
33. Kinsbourne M. Myoclonic encephalopathy of infants. J Neurol Neurosurg Psychiatry 1962;25:271.
34. Solomon GE, Chutorian AM. Opsoclonus and occult neuroblastoma. N Engl J Med 1968;279:475.
35. Aicardi J. Myclonic epilepsies of infancy and childhood. Adv Neurol 1986; 43:11.
36. Bressman S, Fahn S, Eisenberg M, et al. Biotin-responsive encephalopathy with myoclonus, ataxia and seizures. Adv Neurol 1986;43:119.
37. Andermann F, Aicardi J, Vigevamo F. Alternation Hemiplegia of Childhood. New York: Raven, 1995.
38. Norton E, Cogan, D. Spasmus nutans: a clinical study of 20 cases followed two years or more since onset. Arch Ophthalmol 1954;52:442.
39. Hoefnagal D, Biery B. Spasmus nutans. Rev Med Child Neurol 1968;10:32.
40. Jayalaksmi P, McNair STF, Tucher SH, Schaffer DG. Infantile nystagmus: a prospective study of spasmus nutans, congenital nystagmus and unclassified nystagmus of infancy. J Pediatr 1970;77:177.
41. King RA, Nelson LB, Wagner RS. Spasmus nutans. Arch Ophthalmol 1986;104:1501.
42. Herbst JJ, Minton SD, Book LS. Gastroesophageal reflux causing respirator distress and apnea in newborn infants. J Pediatr 1979;95:763.
43. Herbst JJ. Gastroesophageal reflux. J Pediatr 1981;98:859.
44. Bray PF, Herbst JJ, Johnson DD, et al. Childhood gastroesophageal reflux: neurologic and psychiatric syndromes mimicked. JAMA 1977;237:1342.
45. Pascotto A, Coppola G. Neonatal hyperexplexia: a case report. Epilepsia 1992;33:817.

46. Fleisher DR, Morrison A. Masturbation mimicking abdominal pain or seizures in young girls. J Pediatr 1990;116:810.
47. Wulff CH, Ostergaard K, Storm K. Epileptic fits or infantile masturbation? Seizures 1992;1:1199.
48. Holmes G, Russman BS. Shuddering attacks. AAJDC 1986;140:72.
49. Vanasse M, Bedard P, Anderson F. Shuddering attacks in children: an early clinical manifestation of essential tremor. Neurology 1976;26:1027.
50. Dunn DW, Snyder CH. Benign paroxysmal vertigo of childhood. Am J Dis Child 1976;130:1099.
51. Basser LS. Benign paroxysmal vertigo of childhood. Brain 1964;87:141.
52. Lombrosso CT, Lerman P. Breath-holding spells (cyanotic and pallid infantile syncope). Pediatrics 1967;39:453.
53. Abe K, Oda N, Amatomi M. Natural history and predictive significance of head banging, head rolling and breath-holding spells. Dev Med Child Neurol 1984;26:644.
54. Holowach J, Thurston DL. Breath-holding spells and anemia. N Engl J Med 1963;268:21.
55. Gauk EW, Kidd L, Prichard JS. Mechanism of seizures associated with breath-holding spells. N Engl J Med 1963;268:1435.
56. Sheldon SH. Parasomnias. In SH Sheldon, AZ Golbin (eds). Pediatric Sleep Medicine. Philadelphia: Saunders, 1992;119–135.
57. Mahowald MW, Schenck CH. Parasomnia Purgatory: The Epileptic/Non-Epileptic Parasomnia Interface. In JR Gates, AJ Rowan (eds), Non-Epileptic Seizures. Boston: Butterworth–Heinemann, 1993;123–139.
58. Williamson PD. Psychogenic Non-Epileptic Seizures and Frontal Seizures: Diagnostic Considerations. In JR Gates, AJ Rowan (eds), Non-Epileptic Seizures. Boston: Butterworth–Heinemann, 1993;55–72.
59. Vincent MD, Timothy KW, Leppert M, Keating M. The spectrum of symptoms and QT intervals in carriers of the gene for the long-QT syndrome. N Engl J Med 1992;327:846.
60. Moss AJ. Molecular genetics and ventricular arrythmias. N Engl J Med 1992;327:885.
61. Rutter N, Southall DP. Cardiac arrhythmias misdiagnosed as epilepsy. Arch Dis Child 1985;60:54.
62. Pignata C, Faring G, Andria G, DelGiudice E. Prolonged Q-T interval syndrome presenting as idiopathic epilepsy. Neuropediatrics 1983;14:2325.
63. Kinast J, Erenbeag G, Rothner D. Paroxysmal choreoiathetosis: report of five cases and review of the literature. Pediatrics 1980;65:74.
64. Driefuss FF. Munchausen Syndrome by Proxy. In JR Gates, AJ Rowan (eds), Non-Epileptic Seizures. Boston: Butterworth–Heinemann, 1993;203–207.
65. Wyllie E, Friedman D, Rothner AD, et al. Psychogenic seizures in children and adolescents: outcome after diagnosis by ictal video and electroencephalographic recording. Pediatrics 1990;85:480.
66. Siegel M, Barthel RP. Conversion disorders on a child psychiatric consultation service. Psychosomatics 1986;27:201.

67. Goodwin J, Simms J, Bergman R. Hysterical seizures: a sequel to incest. Am J Orthopsychiatry 1979;49:698.
68. Schneider S, Rice DR. Neurologic manifestations of childhood hysteria. J Pediatr 1979;94:153.
69. Maloney MJ. Diagnosing hysterical conversion reactions in children. J Pediatr 1980;97:1016.
70. Bangash JH, Worley GM, Kandt R. Hysterical conversion reactions mimicking neurological disease. AJCD 1988;142:1203–1206.
71. Gross M. Incestuous rape: a cause for hysterical seizures in four adolescent girls. Am J Orthopsychiatry 1979;49:704.
72. Silver LB. Conversion disorder and pseudoseizures in adolescence: a stress reaction to unrecognized and untreated learning disabilities. J Am Acad Child Psychiatry 1982;21:508.
73. Wyllie E, Friedman D, Lüders H, et al. Outcome of psychogenic seizures in children and adolescents compared with adults. Neurology 1991;421:742.
74. Finlayson R, Lucas AR. Pseudoepileptic seizures in children and adolescents. Mayo Clin Proc 1979;54:83.
75. Fenton GA, Gibbons VP, Pratt GD, Kotagal S. Characteristics and outcome of psychogenic seizures in children. Ann Neurol 1990;28:470.
76. Bleasel A, Kotagal P. Paroxysmal nonepileptic disorders in children and adolescents. Semin Neurol 1995;15:203.
77. Jeavons P. Non-Epileptic Attacks in Childhood. In C Rose (ed), Research Progress in Epilepsy. London: Pitman, 1983.
78. Emery B. Status epilepticus secondary to breath-holding and pallid syncopal spells. Neurology 1990;40:859.
79. Sallustro F, Atwell C. Body rocking, head banging and head rolling in normal children. Pediatrics 1978;93:704.
80. Keith P. Night terrors: a review of the psychology, neurophysiology and therapy. J Child Psychiatry 1975;3:477.
81. Fisher C, Kahn B, Edwards A, Davis D. A psychophysiological study of nightmares and night terrors. The suppression of stage 4 night terrors with diazepam. Arch Gen Psychiatry 1973;28:252.
82. Dimauro F, Emery B. The natural history of night terrors. Clin Pediatr 1987;26:5505.

CHAPTER 7

Part Summary: Neurologic Aspects of Non-Epileptic Seizures in the Adult and Pediatric Patient

John R. Gates

In this section on the neurologic aspects of non-epileptic seizures, we find that we made significant progress during the 1990s. As discussed in Chapter 1, we now have a better idea of the epidemiology and a classification scheme for this spectrum of disorders. We can now comfortably divide non-epileptic seizures into physiologic and psychogenic seizure types and appropriately retire the pejorative terms *pseudoseizure, hysterical seizure,* and *fit.*

Our epidemiologic data, although limited, suggest an incidence of non-epileptic seizures in at least 5% of the total epilepsy population. The female to male seizure ratio is fairly consistently observed as 4:1 in adults and 2:1 in children. As discussed by all the authors in this section, the spectrum of non-epileptic and physiologic seizures is quite large. As is thoroughly discussed in Chapters 4–6, non-epileptic seizure paroxysmal events can occur in syncope, movement disorders, non-epileptic myoclonus, startle phenomenon, migraine, unique disorders in infants and children, cerebrovascular disease, sleep disorders, toxic-metabolic or infectious states, and diencephalic brain stem disorders and in a spectrum of miscellaneous disorders. Syncope can be especially problematic, because it can cause increased prolactins and is associated with automatisms.

TABLE 7.1
Neurologic Aspects of Non-Epileptic Seizures

Accepted terms for non-epileptic seizure
  Physiologic
  Psychogenic
Retired terms for non-epileptic seizure
  Pseudoseizure
  Hysterical seizure
  Fit

As discussed in Chapters 2–6, recurrent stereotyped and inappropriate events may be a seizure. Electroencephalography with a video record is needed to record multiple typical events to render a definitive diagnosis. An integrated, multidisciplinary approach to diagnosis appears to be preferred. Humility on the part of the epileptologist and clinic neurophysiologist is always prudent. Epilepsy and non-epileptic seizures can coexist, with an observation of approximately 30%. Not all unusual epileptic events are frontal in origin. Temporal seizures can also have unusual manifestations, as can seizures from other cortical sites. Nonetheless, suggestive features exist to differentiate epileptic atypical events from non-epileptic seizures. Atypical predominantly frontal epileptic events are brief, often occurring several times a day with rapid recovery.

As discussed in Chapter 6, children offer unique challenges, especially in their early years. Several unique disorders, such as jitteriness, shuddering, esophageal reflux, breath-holding attacks, or alternating hemiplegia, require specific diagnostic acumen.

In summary, we have learned much since 1990 about the neurologic aspects of non-epileptic seizures; however, we have much more to clarify.

PART II

Psychological and Neuropsychological Evaluation of the Patient with Non-Epileptic Seizures

CHAPTER 8

Use of Neuropsychological Testing to Differentiate Neurologic from Non-Neurologic Disorders

John A. Walker

The general question discussed in this chapter is the following: Can neuropsychological testing differentiate organic from nonorganic conditions, beginning with the assumption that a large number of patients with nonepileptic seizures might be considered not to have an organic disorder, compared to patients with epilepsy who do have an organic disorder? In the clinical setting, a common task for the neuropsychologist is to differentiate neurologic from non-neurologic disorders.[1] Probably one-half of my time is spent doing this in patients who do not have epilepsy, considering, for example, questions of dementia versus depression in elderly patients or in individuals who have acquired immunodeficiency syndrome; questions about an emotional disorder versus a neurologic disorder; or, in patients who have known neurologic disorders, the question of how much of the neurologic disorder accounts for this patient's performance and how other elements of performance might be better accounted for by emotional problems. In California, where one-half of the lawyers in the United States practice, this differentiation of organic from nonorganic conditions can have significant impact in legal cases. It also has an impact in worker's compensation cases, and certainly at the individual patient level, it has an impact on the treatment and the quality of their lives.[2,3] Thus, can we borrow the logic of how neuropsychologists use differential diagnostic situations and apply that to the specific situation of non-epileptic seizures?

Neuropsychological Test Components

The components of neuropsychological testing include an interview, cognitive kinds of neuropsychological tests, and emotional kinds of neuropsychological tests. In making a differential diagnosis in a patient, the interview sometimes can be absolutely critical. It is the best opportunity to find out how patients feel about what is going on and what kinds of problems they have. The physical testing is just a small snapshot of performance. The real question is: How are the patients doing in everyday life? In information gathering, it is ideal to get corroboration from other kinds of sources. Using only neuropsychological testing, for example, without its being put into the context of the patient, is probably akin to reading an electroencephalogram without ever seeing the patient or knowing the clinical history. One would not get very far in making a diagnosis of non-epileptic seizures in taking that approach and or in just using test scores without placing the patient in context.

The other components of neuropsychological testing are cognitive and emotional tests. The focus here is on three very simple tests that have some utility in the differential diagnosis of neurologic versus non-neurologic patients: the Oral Fluency Test, the Rey Auditory Verbal Learning Test, and the finger-tapping speed test. It must be emphasized that a large number of other kinds of cognitive tests could be done, as well as a large amount of emotional testing. The Beck Depression Inventory, a simple 21-item self-completed questionnaire about symptoms of depression, and the Minnesota Multiphasic Personality Inventory (MMPI) are emphasized here.[4]

The Oral Fluency Test is a very simple test that takes 60 seconds per trial. The instructions to the patient are brief: Tell the examiner all the words you can think of for the next 60 seconds that start with a particular letter (proper names and trivial changes are not allowed). Usually, three trials with a variety of different letter triads are used—for example, C, F, and L or F, A, and S. Variations on this theme also are possible—for example, asking the person to generate instances of categories such as animals. Typically, patients can generate considerably more instances of a category than they can with a single initial letter. Simple testing, 3 minutes of performance by the patient, can yield helpful information about how that person is solving a problem under time pressure.

The Rey Auditory Verbal Learning Test is another test that has a long tradition in neuropsychology. Patients are read a 15-item list of common words and are given five trials to see how well they can acquire that list. Next there is a distraction trial with another list of 15 words to give the patients a chance to forget the first list and see how well they can concentrate on the new list; then, as soon as one trial of that distracter list is done, patients are given a recall of the first list to see how well they can maintain that first list and how much confusion they have between the two lists. Finally, in the way that the author uses it, a recognition trial is given immediately in which the person is given 15 words from the first list intermixed with 15 words they have not heard at all; the tester sees how well the person can simply say, "Yes, I heard that word," or "No, I didn't hear that word." The Rey Auditory Verbal Learning Test has been used so widely that probably a thousand different variations exist of how different practitioners use it.

The finger-tapping test is another simple test. The person is asked to tap a little lever with the first finger of each hand. The author usually alternates between the two hands—left, right, left, right, left, right—and generally takes approximately five trials until some stable performance is reached. In this setting, the patient is not given much rest in between so that, without a lot of breaks, most patients fatigue just slightly as they go through repeated trials.

There are some important caveats about neuropsychological testing, not only for differential diagnosis of any kind of patient, but particularly for patients with non-epileptic seizures. These include a reminder that the test only samples behavior and that the short period that the practitioner spends with the patient is just a small slice of their life and may or may not be representative of how that patient performs in everyday life. The behavior measured usually is reactive; that is, the task is presented to the person, who has to respond. Again, this may or may not adequately measure problems in everyday life. The practitioner makes inferences about what that observed behavior means in terms of brain function, status in everyday life, and so forth, but these are just inferences. Two psychologists can certainly disagree about what those particular inferences might be. We assume for differential diagnosis that patients with brain injury perform differently than those without brain injury, and this assumption must be recognized for what it is. Probably more important, tests that are intact may be as telling as tests that are impaired, and it is that pattern of what is impaired and what is intact that often leads to the crucial diagnosis. Summary scores may not be as useful as details of performance, and unanswered questions arise about their reliability and validity for differential diagnosis. That is, unlike the setting of telemetry-based monitoring for non-epileptic seizures versus epileptic seizures, if the practitioner decides that a patient has a conversion disorder, there is no independent way to know if he or she is correct, which can present a real problem.

Case Examples

Case 1

The following are some case examples of how this logic can be applied in differential diagnosis. Patient 1 was a 39-year-old female attorney who had no loss of consciousness when a parking gate garage closed, hitting her on the head. She remembered the event very well. There was a question of hemifacial spasm afterward, but she was able to work her usual job as a high-powered attorney for several weeks after the injury. Slowly, her performance eroded over time to the point that her husband said that a good day for her consisted of getting from her bed to the couch. (Of course, a lawsuit was pending in this case.) This woman was able, nonetheless, to spend more than 5 hours in my office for an interview and testing. A few other things about her background also are relevant. She had been a very aggressive, hard-working person on the partnership track and in the past 2 years had finally conceived and delivered her first child. The child was approximately 6 months old at the time of her mother's injury, and the patient had returned part-time to work. Also around the time of her injury, her husband had quit his job as an insurance executive and was concentrating on the music career that he always wanted. At this time, the patient was collecting approximately $180,000 a year from a disability policy based on her injury.

The following are some of the patient's test scores: On the oral fluency test for the letter "C," she gave 18 words, 17 with "F," and 18 with "L," for a total of 53, better than the 96th percentile (although she was so disabled that she could barely get out of bed every day). Her Rey Auditory Verbal Learning Test trials were six on the first trial, then eight, then 10, then 13, and then 14 of the 15 words on successive trials, which again is a very fine performance, average to above average. With distracter trials she got six, and after that distracter she could still recall 13 of the 15 words on the list; on recognition trials, she correctly classified the words she had heard and the words she had not heard. More interesting, perhaps, in looking at this woman's results, is her performance on the tapping test. She started out with 26, then went up to 38, then down to 23, 29, 26, 28, 27, and so forth. A similar pattern emerged with her nondominant left hand. The question is raised of whether this woman was putting out maximum performance on a test in which she was instructed to tap as fast as possible until she was told that her 10 seconds were up. Her Beck depression score was mildly elevated but, on her MMPI, she had a typical conversion V pattern—that is, the scale 1 hypochondriasis and scale 3 hysteria were elevated, whereas depression was low. Her other scales were below 70. Of note, it took her more than 30 days to return the MMPI in the mail, with a cover letter from her husband stating that this 500-item yes/no questionnaire had been extremely difficult for her to complete and had to be done in tiny blocks because she became fatigued so easily from the stresses of the test.

In this case, the patient's history and what she is able and not able to do in everyday life contrast quite markedly with her performance on some aspects of cognitive testing. The testing shows that she is entirely intact, but some elements of her performance suggest that she is not giving a full effort, for whatever reason. The best diagnosis for her is probably a conversion disorder, although residual questions about frank malingering still exist.

Case 2

Patient 2 was a 47-year-old male folk artist. He lived very marginally in San Francisco and collected scraps of cardboard from the street and painted on those scraps of cardboard. This is described as "folk art" in the art community, done by someone who is untrained yet has fairly decent skills. He was living in a residential hotel in San Francisco when a fire broke out. Although no one else was injured in the fire, he chose to jump from his third-story window rather than wait for the fire department to arrive. He fractured his right leg but did not lose consciousness, although he fell and hit his head. He was given the diagnosis of postconcussive syndrome by neuropsychologists who tested him because of the fact that he had struck his head and had a laceration. When he hit the ground (and broke his leg), he didn't realize it, tried to stand up and run, but then fell down, hitting his head. Thus, he hit his head from a few feet away, not from the three-story fall. His lifetime of artwork, 25 years or so of cardboard painting and more than a thousand paintings, was lost, but not in the fire. The apartment management company apparently lost them or refused to let him have access to them. He had a lawsuit pending for more than $3 million for his lifetime of lost artwork.

In evaluating his performance on the Rey Auditory Verbal Learning Test, the first thing that is obvious is that he started at six and did not get higher than nine by the fifth trial, a very flat curve. He started out more or less at an average level but never improved beyond that. Interestingly, he said 13 of the 15 words at least once in those five trials. After the distraction, he could still only recall seven. He lost some from his maximum of nine, but in the recognition trial, all the words were there with the exception of one. This performance is perfectly average on recognition trials and a very poor performance on learning trials, suggesting a discrepancy between what he could generate back and what he was able to demonstrate had gotten into his head. Like patient 1, on the tapping test he was extremely erratic. When that was called to his attention, some of his fastest scores came toward the end of the trial, even with sustained tapping. His Beck Depression Score was fairly low, although mildly depressed. He certainly had experienced some degree of emotional trauma in the fire; he had recurrent dreams about fires and difficulty in sleeping. A genuine emotional problem appeared to be triggered by the fire, but mainly he was angry at the management company for the loss of his artwork. Furthermore, there appeared to be some elaboration on his test performance.

Case 3

Patient 3 was a 50-year-old female postal carrier. She had a loss of consciousness when, as she was walking down the street, a temporary fence blew over onto her, knocked her to the ground, and gave her some relatively minor orthopedic injuries. Other background information includes the following: She was a single mother of five children who were now teenagers and adults. She had had a variety of low-level jobs until she finally landed a job as a letter carrier for the post office a few years earlier. She had always been a workaholic; she worked 10- to 12-hour days for the post office with lots of overtime pay. She had had a very tough childhood. She felt she really had to be responsible for herself and her family and that she could not depend on anyone else. The injury appeared to disrupt her feelings about herself and her ability to live up to them.

She showed some interesting patterns on the Oral Fluency Test. She did quite poorly even with education correction, receiving a score of 26 that places her in the low-average range (probably a normal score for her). She had dropped out of school in the tenth grade and had always been an indifferent student. Interestingly, however, when given the opportunity to generate instances of animals, she could think of only six, although she came up with more than that on several of the letters. It appears at least that something was going on that was not organic. On the Rey Auditory Verbal Learning Test, she started with only three and had a maximum of four. She said only five of the 15 words at least once, and after distraction she could recall only one word plus an intrusion from the previous list. On the recognition trial she said "yes" to only four of the 15 words that had been read, and correctly rejected 14 of the 15 that had not been read. This performance is, objectively, extremely poor and, in some people's hands, would certainly suggest a severe amnestic kind of disorder. Interestingly, this woman went to work every day for the post office, got back and forth, and managed the details of her life and her household effectively. On the recognition testing, she said yes to only two of the five words that she said at least once and said yes to 2 of the 10 that she herself had never said. This pattern is interesting in that it would be unexpected in most patients with a significant amnestic disorder. On digit span and block span, she was very restricted, being able only to follow a block span of 2. To clarify, a block span consists of repeating some blocks that are laid out on a little board, tapping the blocks from the same sequence as the examiner taps them, or starting backward and retracing the path. Even when the task for digit span was simplified to area codes, or the block span task was simplified to tapping three blocks that happened to be in a line, she was not able to do this forward or backward. This is very suggestive of poor effort. On tapping, testing was stopped after a few trials because it was obvious that the patient was not giving full effort. With her dominant right hand she tapped only seven times and dropped down to five, and with her left hand she tapped six times and dropped down to four. Her Beck depression score was very high; she was given a diagnosis of post-traumatic stress disorder and depression.

Case 4

Patient 4 was a 54-year-old female school bus driver who, while checking under the hood of her school bus, bumped the rod that held the hood. It hit her on the head and shoulder. She had no loss of consciousness, felt a little bit stunned, and continued on her route for several hours. At the time she was seen a few years later, she had severe complaints of decreased cognition, was anxious if left alone, felt that she could not navigate in space very well, and was basically homebound and had a lawsuit pending. Her performance on the Rey Auditory Verbal Learning Test showed that she was very erratic. She started at five, got to nine in the middle, but dropped down to seven, although she said 13 of the 15 words. With recognition testing, her performance was intact, showing that that information had gotten through. On the tapping test, she actually got faster and faster with repeated trials, quite distinctly different than one sees in the typical patient who is giving maximal effort. Her Beck depression score was 17 out of 63. The diagnosis for her was anxiety disorder with some elaboration.

Conclusions

All of these cases illustrate that in a differential diagnosis situation, which has significance in these instances for lawsuits and certainly has relevance to what we are trying to accomplish in patients with non-epileptic seizures. The actual scores from IQ tests and other kinds of tests that these patients were given were probably not as critical as particular details of their performance on some of these simpler tests in which patients do not necessarily know how they are supposed to perform. Cognitive testing can provide a real advantage because practitioners can break through some of the barriers that patients might otherwise have to more obvious emotional testing. Then practitioners are able to see how individuals perform when they are challenged by what is superficially a relatively simple task but is in many respects a very rich method of exploring what the patient's performance really means. From this, at some point one starts to understand what the patient is all about and what might be done to assist him or her.

Neuropsychological test utility for differential diagnosis applies to non-epileptic seizures as well. Some tasks disclose better than others whether a patient has non-epileptic seizures, and tests of general ability, such as IQ tests, may not be nearly as useful as tests of concentration, memory, motor speed, and language. It is critical to keep in mind that patients' test results should be examined *in the context of their life and their interview*. Furthermore, when we strip away all that information, looking just at the raw scores, we are likely to misclassify people because some patients that we see for differential diagnosis are going to test much better than patients with an organic disorder. That has been one of the kinds of logic we used in trying to think about non-epileptic seizures compared to epileptic seizures. However, many patients test worse, or test differently, than if they had an organic pattern. If we collapse these two groups of patients together, we may not see any difference between them and patients with organic disorders.

In conclusion, it seems that the classification scheme of organic versus psychiatric really tests our stereotypes about these two categories, and we must be aware that some patients are certainly not going to be prototypical. The classification is very much confounded when the organic patient has significant emotional overlay, and many patients with epilepsy certainly have that. It is also confounded when the psychiatric patient has some coexisting organic disorder.

The following are the four key issues that neuropsychological testing needs to accomplish if it is going to become useful in distinguishing epileptic seizures from non-epileptic seizures:

1. Do patients with epileptic and non-epileptic seizures differ because of the presence or absence of organic brain injury? There is a subset of patients with brain injury and non-epileptic seizures, but this is not true for the majority of patients with non-epileptic seizures.
2. A more important question is whether neuropsychological testing distinguishes the *populations* of patients with epileptic seizures versus those with non-epileptic seizures or if it can better classify *individuals*. Again, we must begin to recognize that patients with non-epileptic seizures are at least as heterogeneous as those with epileptic seizures. Consequently, the challenge of differentiating populations becomes much greater.
3. If we can recognize that an individualized approach to diagnosis offers some advantages, we may not only be better able to diagnose but also to generate better treatment strategies.
4. The patterns (not the scores) of neuropsychological test performance may help to suggest classification schemes for subgroups of patients with non-epileptic seizures. Do the patterns of neuropsychological test performance also suggest different treatment strategies for those subgroups?

All of these questions are what we need to wrestle with over the next few years.

References

1. Lezak MD. Neuropsychological Assessment (3rd ed). Oxford: Oxford Press, 1995;319.
2. McMahon EA, Satz P. Clinical Neuropsychology: Some Forensic Applications. In SB Filskov, TJ Bell (Eds), Handbook of Clinical Neuropsychology. New York: John Wiley and Sons, 1981;686–701.
3. Taylor RL. Distinguishing Psychological from Organic Disorders. New York: Springer-Verlag, 1990;158–175.
4. Sprem O, Strauss E. A Compendium of Neuropsychological Tests. New York: Oxford University Press, 1998.

CHAPTER 9

Cognitive and Psychological Functioning in Patients with Non-Epileptic Seizures

*Sara J. Swanson, Jane A. Springer,
Selim R. Benbadis, and George L. Morris III*

Non-epileptic seizures (NES) have been attributed to both emotional disorders[1-5] and organic brain dysfunction.[6-8] The most common psychological diagnosis for patients with NES is conversion disorder with seizures or convulsions based on *DSM-IV* (*Diagnostic and Statistical Manual of Mental Disorders*, Fourth Edition) criteria.[9,10] However, given the significant degree of cognitive impairment found in this group, brain impairment also has been considered important in the pathogenesis of NES.[11] In this chapter, the cognitive and psychological correlates of NES are examined.

Literature Review

Personality and cognitive tests have been used in the differential diagnosis of NES patients. Although differences between patients with epileptic seizure (ES) and NES have been fairly consistently observed on the Minnesota Multiphasic Personality Inventory (MMPI),[8,12,13] neuropsychological differences between these two groups have not been consistently reported.[14-17] Both ES and NES groups show a high rate of impairment on neuropsychological batteries. This finding has led to the view that organic brain dysfunction may contribute to the development of NES. An alternate explanation is that the cognitive impairment observed in NES patients is a result of severe psychiatric disturbance. In this chapter, the notion that neuropsychological impairment in NES patients can be accounted for by the greater psychopathology in this population relative to patients with ES is examined by comparing the personality and cognitive profiles of three groups of patients, those diagnosed with (1) ES, (2) NES, and (3) somatoform disorders without seizures.

Psychological Features of Non-Epileptic Seizures

The MMPI[18] is the most commonly used objective personality inventory for evaluating the behavioral or psychological features of NES.[19] Using the MMPI, Wilkus et al.[8] derived a set of configural rules that were found to correctly classify 80–90% of both ES and NES patients. According to these rules, patients are classified as having NES if one of the following is true: (1) Scale 1 (hypochondriasis) or scale 3 (hysteria) is 70 or higher and one of the two highest points, excluding scales 5 (masculinity/femininity) and 0 (social introversion); (2) scale 1 or scale 3 is 80 or higher, even though not among the highest points; and (3) scale 1 and scale 3 are both higher than 59 and at least 10 points higher than scale 2 (depression). The third rule describes a "conversion V" profile. These authors noted that the mean configuration of the clinical scales for the NES group was a conversion V and that the mean ES group profile showed an elevation on scale 2 (depression) relative to scales 1 and 3. Across studies, significant mean scale elevation differences between ES and NES groups are typically reported for scales 1, 2, 3, 4 (psychopathic deviate), and 8 (schizophrenia), with the NES group scoring higher or in a more pathologic direction.[8,17,20,21]

No differences between MMPI profiles were found in one study, which compared NES and generalized seizure patients,[7] and only 37% of the NES patients were correctly classified using the MMPI configural rules. However, these authors excluded all NES patients without bilateral motor involvement. To examine this contradictory finding further, Wilkus and Dodrill[17] subgrouped patients according to their seizure semiology. They found that NES patients with prominent affective and limited motor expression during seizures could be differentiated from ES patients on the MMPI, but NES patients with limited affective and primarily motor expression could not be differentiated from ES on the MMPI. Given the poor classification rate for this latter group, these authors suggested using prolactin levels to distinguish genuine generalized tonic-clonic seizures from NES with significant motor manifestations. In general, when results of patient classification were examined across studies,[22] it was concluded that two of three NES and three of four

ES patients are correctly classified using the MMPI decision rules. However, Dodrill et al.[22] note that the error rate is such that the MMPI should not be considered diagnostic of NES. Although no single profile is produced by NES patients, the typical profile suggests excessive somatic concern, conversion of psychological distress into physical symptoms, and use of repression or denial as a coping mechanism (consistent with elevations on scales 1 and 3). The utility of the MMPI or MMPI-2 in the psychological evaluation and differential diagnosis of NES patients is generally accepted.

Cognitive Dysfunction in Non-Epileptic Seizures

Application of comprehensive neuropsychological batteries have not differentiated NES from ES when patient groups are matched for level of education, age, and gender.[8] NES patients show high rates of cognitive impairment with impairment indices that are comparable to those of patients with documented ES. For example, 46% of the neuropsychological test scores for an NES group were outside of the normal range, compared to 51% for a matched ES group.[8] Consistent with these results, in a separate study, an impaired Halstead-Reitan Impairment Index was found in 42% of NES patients.[7] Furthermore, no differences were noted between NES and ES groups on measures of intelligence, presence of lateralized brain dysfunction, presence of an abnormal neuropsychological evaluation, or pattern of neuropsychological impairment.[14,23] In a study in which an NES group outperformed an ES group on neuropsychological measures, the groups differed significantly in their years of education (the NES group had 2 more years of education than the ES group). Although the group differences were likely due to the lack of demographic matching, it is noteworthy that the NES group performance was still considered borderline impaired, with 45% of the test scores outside the normal range. Consequently, it has been postulated that organic brain disease may contribute to the occurrence of NES. However, psychiatric illness and emotional disturbance are associated with cognitive impairment, and this alone may account for the cognitive problems reported in NES patients.

Neuropsychological Impairment Associated with Psychiatric Disorders

Some psychiatric disorders, particularly those of a chronic nature, may be as likely to disrupt neuropsychological functions as are some organic conditions.[24,25] A variety of cognitive abilities, primarily involving attention, memory, executive functions, motor abilities, and mental tracking, appear to be reduced in psychiatric patients.[26] Specific performance patterns have been associated with different psychiatric patient groups. For example, patients with mood disorders commonly demonstrate impaired attention and concentration, efficiency of mental processing, and retrieval abilities.[27] Among patients with schizophrenia, there is a prevalence of executive deficits[28] as well as attentional and psychomotor dysfunction.[29] In general, attention and concentration deficits are common among most types of psychiatric patients.

The term *aprosexia* has been used to refer to the nonspecific neurobehavioral disorder that is associated with mild impairment of new learning and other cognitive tasks demanding attention.[30] It is thought to be secondary to psychological disturbance (e.g., depression, apathy, anxiety, withdrawal) but can also be associated with medication or mild metabolic effects. NES patients have significant psychiatric complaints and are commonly diagnosed with other psychiatric disorders in addition to conversion disorder (e.g., mood disorders).[5,31] Thus, cognitive dysfunction among NES patients may well be related to their significant psychiatric symptoms and associated nonspecific attentional difficulties.

Qualitative evidence that the neuropsychological impairment in NES patients may be secondary to attentional disturbance has been reported by Brown et al.[16] They found the NES patients to have unusual performance patterns, such as recalling more information after a delay than immediately, showing significant intratest and intertest scatter, and demonstrating more impairment on testing than would be anticipated given the patient's level of daily functioning. These authors concluded that the lack of group differences between ES and NES patients on neuropsychological measures was due to the effects of psychiatric disturbance of the NES group rather than organic factors. In a separate study, greater conversion V elevations on the MMPI were associated with more impairment on the Halstead-Reitan Impairment Index in NES patients.[7] This result can be interpreted as evidence that the etiology of NES is multifactorial, or it can be viewed as evidence that the cognitive dysfunction observed in NES patients is related to the increased psychopathology found in these individuals.

Original Investigation

The objective of the present investigation was to determine why no neuropsychological differences are found between the profiles of matched NES and ES patient groups. Four hypotheses were tested. One possible explanation for the lack of cognitive differences between NES and ES groups is that the ES group is comprised of patients with both left and right seizure foci. Neuropsychological profiles of these two seizure groups may, in effect, negate each other because one tends to show more verbal and the other more visual spatial deficits.[32–36]

Hypothesis 1: No cognitive differences are found between matched groups of ES and NES patients because the ES group includes patients with both left and right seizure foci. If the ES group is separated by hemisphere of seizure onset, then the NES group will perform better than the right ES group on visual spatial measures and better than the left ES group on verbal tests.

Hypothesis 2: If no between-group differences are found between the NES group and the right or left ES patients, then the lack of cognitive differences between the groups can be accounted for by the more severe psychopathology in NES patients, which may be sufficient to disrupt performances on cognitive tasks. It is predicted that the NES group will score significantly higher (in a more pathologic direction) on the MMPI than the ES group and show more evidence of psychiatric problems based on history of psychiatric hospitalization and use of psychotropic medication.

Hypothesis 3: If increased psychiatric disturbance in NES patients accounts for the lack of difference between NES and ES groups on neuropsychological testing, then there should also be no difference between a control group of non-epileptic patients with somatoform disorders and patients with ES or NES on cognitive testing.

Hypothesis 4: If psychiatric disturbance contributes to cognitive dysfunction, then the number of elevated scales on the MMPI should correlate positively with the number of impaired cognitive tests. Furthermore, there should be greater evidence of attentional disturbance on cognitive testing in the NES group relative to the ES group.

The subjects for this study were (1) 15 patients with a right temporal seizure focus, (2) 15 patients with a left temporal seizure focus, (3) 15 NES patients, and (4) 11 patients with somatoform disorder without seizures or convulsions. All ES patients had medically intractable partial epilepsy and were left-hemisphere dominant for language based on the intracarotid sodium amobarbital (Amytal) test.[37–39] Seizures were documented by long-term video-electroencephalographic (EEG) monitoring, and all ES patients subsequently underwent either left or right temporal lobectomy, with good postoperative seizure control. NES and psychiatric patients had no history of significant neurologic event or disease. Those with histories of mild head injuries without loss of consciousness or post-traumatic amnesia were not excluded. Diagnosis of NES required demonstration of discrete ictal events unassociated with EEG changes based on inpatient long-term video-EEG monitoring. Events could consist of either motor phenomena (focal or generalized), unresponsiveness, or both. No patient with subjective phenomena only (possible auras) was diagnosed as having NES. Patients with both NES and ES were excluded. The somatoform disorder group consisted of six patients with undifferentiated somatoform disorder, two with somatization disorder, two with conversion disorder (without seizures), and one with pain disorder with psychological factors based on

TABLE 9.1
Demographic Data for Patients with Seizures

Group	Right ES	Left ES	NES	Somatoform
N	15	15	15	11
Gender (male/female)	4/11	4/11	4/11	2/9
Age	34.1	38.2	34.6	37.2
Education	13.1	13.7	12.0	13.0

ES = epileptic seizure; NES = non-epileptic seizure.

DSM-IV. All subjects had an IQ of 70 or higher on the Wechsler Adult Intelligence Scale-Revised. The four groups did not differ significantly on demographic variables, including age, education, and gender (Table 9.1).

The independent variable was grouped (right ES, left ES, NES, or somatoform). Dependent neuropsychological variables (Table 9.2) included measures of intelligence, memory, attention, and verbal, visual spatial, executive, and motor and sensory functions. In addition, an aggre-

TABLE 9.2
Cognitive Domains and Neuropsychological Tests

Cognitive Domain	Neuropsychological Test
Intellectual abilities	Wechsler Adult Intelligence Scale-Revised[41]
Verbal memory	Logical Memory I and II Subtests of the Wechsler Memory Scale-Revised[42]
	Selective Reminding Test[43]
Nonverbal memory	Visual Reproduction Subtests of the Wechsler Memory Scale-Revised[42]
	7/24 Spatial Recall Test[44]
Language	Boston Naming Test[45]
	Sentence Repetition[46]
	Tokens Test[46]
Visual/spatial	Judgment of Line Orientation[47]
	Facial Recognition Test[47]
Attention/concentration	Symbol Digit Modalities Test[48]
Executive functions	Wisconsin Card Sorting Test[49,50]
	Controlled Oral Word Association Test[46]
	Trail-Making Tests A and B[51]
Motor	Grooved Pegboard Test[52]
	Finger-Tapping Test[53]
	Grip Strength Test[53]
Sensory	Sensory-Perceptual Examination[54]
Personality	Minnesota Multiphasic Personality Inventory[18]

gate measure based on the proportion of impaired scores was calculated. Impaired tests were defined as scores that were 1.5 standard deviations below measured full-scale IQ. Dependent psychological measures included the MMPI clinical scales, ego strength, hysteria subscales, total number of significantly elevated scales on the MMPI, and the MMPI configural rules. The MMPI hysteria subscales include Hy1 (denial of social anxiety), Hy2 (need for affection), Hy3 (lassitude-malaise), Hy4 (somatic complaints), and Hy5 (inhibition of aggression). It was thought that ES and NES groups would differ on Hy4 because this subscale measures the tendency toward conversion of symptoms. Further description of the Hy subscales can be found in Green.[40]

History of psychiatric hospitalization and present use of psychotropic medication were examined using the chi-square test. In addition, history of physical and sexual abuse and number of perpetrators of abuse were assessed in the NES group. This information was not reliably obtained during the interviews with the ES groups and, therefore, no between-group comparisons could be made. Analysis of variance by group was conducted on the seizure, MMPI, and neuropsychological variables. A .01 significance level was adopted given the large number of dependent variables. Within the NES group, correlation coefficients were calculated between seizure and psychiatric variables and between number of elevated scales on the MMPI and the proportion of impaired neuropsychological tests.

When the ES and NES groups were compared, no differences were seen in seizure frequency, proportion of each group using antiepileptic medication (79% of the NES patients were using antiseizure medication), and average number of anti-epileptic medications prescribed. Significant differences were found in age at onset of recurrent seizures and duration of the seizure disorder ($p = .003$ for both). Consistent with previous reports,[11,55] average age of seizure onset for the NES group was significantly later (27.9 years) than for either the left ES (17.1 years) or the right ES group (13.0 years).

On testing of hypotheses 1 and 3, no group differences were found between the left ES and NES groups on verbal tests or between right ES and NES groups on visual spatial tests. All other neuropsychological variables (including the proportion of impaired neuropsychological tests and the presence of lateralized deficits) did not differ significantly between these three groups. Likewise, no significant differences were found between the psychiatric control group or NES and ES groups on any of the neuropsychological variables. Intellectual quotients and proportion of impaired tests for each group are shown in Table 9.3. The only exception was that the somatoform group was significantly less likely to show lateralized deficits than were the right and left seizure groups.

On testing of hypothesis 2, NES and somatoform patients were found to have more severe psychopathology and emotional disturbance relative

TABLE 9.3
Mean (and Standard Deviations) for Selected Neuropsychological Data for Patients with Seizures

Group	Right ES	Left ES	NES	Somatoform
WAIS-R				
Verbal comprehension DQ	93 (11.6)	92 (7.7)	90 (13.4)	97 (13.5)
Perceptual organization DQ	96 (12.6)	99 (8.6)	92 (10.3)	100 (8.3)
Full-scale IQ	91 (10.0)	94 (10.0)	89 (9.6)	96 (8.0)
Percent of impaired tests	8.5 (8.0)	9.3 (6.7)	8.2 (5.1)	4.3 (5.7)

DQ = developmental quotient; ES = epileptic seizure; NES = non-epileptic seizure; WAIS-R = Wechsler Adult Intelligence Scale-Revised.

to the epilepsy groups. The NES and somatoform patients scored significantly higher (in a more pathologic direction) on scale 1 (hypochondriasis) ($p = .0003$) and scale 3 (hysteria) ($p = .0005$) than both seizure groups (Figure 9.1). The NES group scored lower (in a more pathologic direction) on ego strength ($p = .03$) than the seizure groups. On the hysteria subscales, the NES and somatoform groups scored higher on subscales Hy3 and Hy4, which are associated with lassitude-malaise and somatic complaints with conversion of affect, respectively, but did not score significantly higher on Hy1, Hy2, and Hy5 (Table 9.4). The NES and somatoform groups had significantly greater numbers of clinically elevated scales on the MMPI than did the left ES group.

Given the absence of cognitive and psychological differences between the two seizure groups, patients with left and right seizure foci were combined into a single ES group. Using the MMPI configural rules, 80% of the patients with ES and 61% of the NES patients were correctly classified. In this sample, rule 2 (hypochondriasis or hysteria is 80 or higher) was the most specific for NES because none of the ES patients was misclassified using this rule (Figure 9.2).

The average number of psychiatric hospitalizations was greatest for the NES group relative to the two seizure groups and the somatoform group. Also, a significantly greater percentage of the NES group (46%) had been hospitalized for psychiatric reasons compared to the left ES group (0%). No between-group differences were found for the left seizure focus (0%), right seizure focus (18%), and somatoform disorder group (11%) in

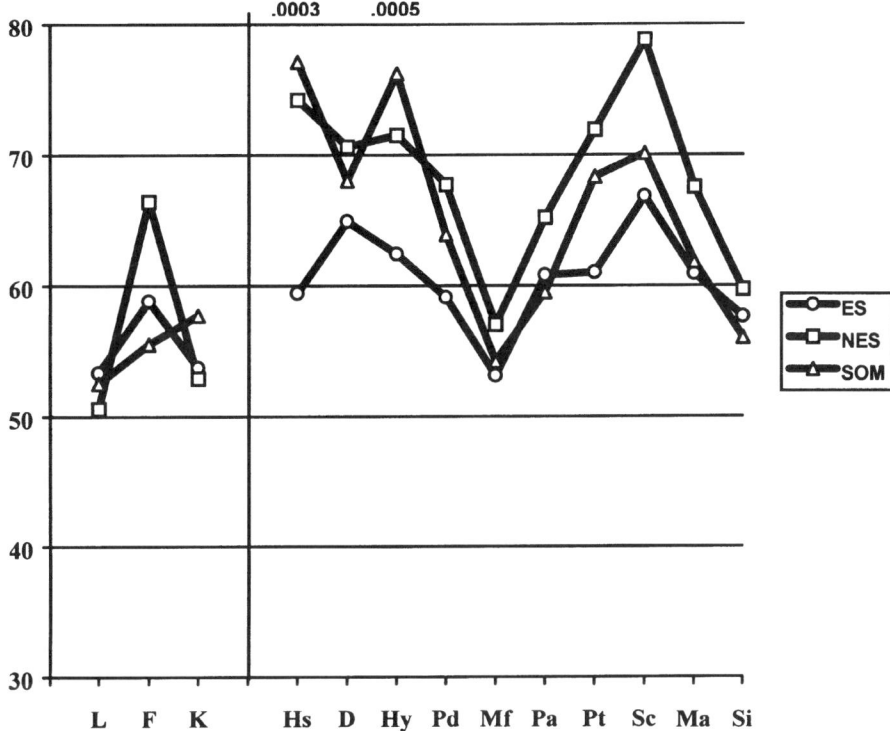

FIGURE 9.1. Average Minnesota Multiphasic Personality Inventory (MMPI) profiles for patients with non-epileptic seizures (NES), epileptic seizures (ES), and somatoform disorders (SOM). The left and right ES are combined because they did not differ on the MMPI. Scales: D = depression; F = infrequency; Hs = hypochondriasis; Hy = hysteria; K = defensiveness; L = lie; Ma = mania; Mf = masculinity/femininity; Pa = paranoia; Pd = psychopathic deviate; Pt = psychasthenia; Sc = schizophrenia; Si = social introversion.

rates of psychiatric hospitalization. The percentage of the NES group using psychotropic medication (62%) was significantly higher than that of both seizure groups (left, 0%; right, 18%) but not significantly different than that of the somatoform group (25%). Large numbers (55%) of NES patients reported histories of physical (45%) or sexual abuse/assault (18%) occurring either in childhood or adulthood.

On testing of hypothesis 4, no significant group differences were found on any of the attentional measures, including the attention/concentration developmental quotient derived from the Wechsler Adult Intelligence Scale (Revised), failures to maintain set on the Wisconsin Card Sorting Test, and the Oral Symbol Digit Modalities Test. Correlational analyses within the NES group revealed no relationship between proportion of impaired tests and number of elevated scales on the MMPI.

TABLE 9.4
Hysteria Subscales

Group	Right ES*	Left ES*	NES*	Somatoform*
Hy1: denial of social anxiety	46.7 (9.8)	51.4 (9.7)	50.6 (12.6)	52.9 (13.5)
Hy2: need for affection	55.5 (9.8)	56.5 (11.1)	54.8 (12.4)	62.0 (11.0)
Hy3: lassitude-malaise	60.7 (12.2)[a,b]	55.9 (7.3)[c,d]	70.5 (15.4)[a,c]	68.2 (13.7)[b,d]
Hy4: somatic complaints	59.6 (12.1)[a,b]	54.2 (11.4)[c,d]	65.5 (11.2)[a,c]	68.5 (12.2)[b,d]
Hy5: inhibition of aggression	50.0 (12.0)	52.5 (8.6)	50.5 (7.9)	47.6 (8.6)

ES = epileptic seizure; NES = non-epileptic seizure.
*Means with the same letters in superscript are significantly different from each other.

In the present study, no differences in the cognitive profiles of matched ES and NES patients were found, even when the patients were divided into groups with either left or right seizure foci. This suggests that the lack of group differences between ES and NES cannot be accounted for by the heterogeneity in the cognitive profiles of the ES group. As predicted,

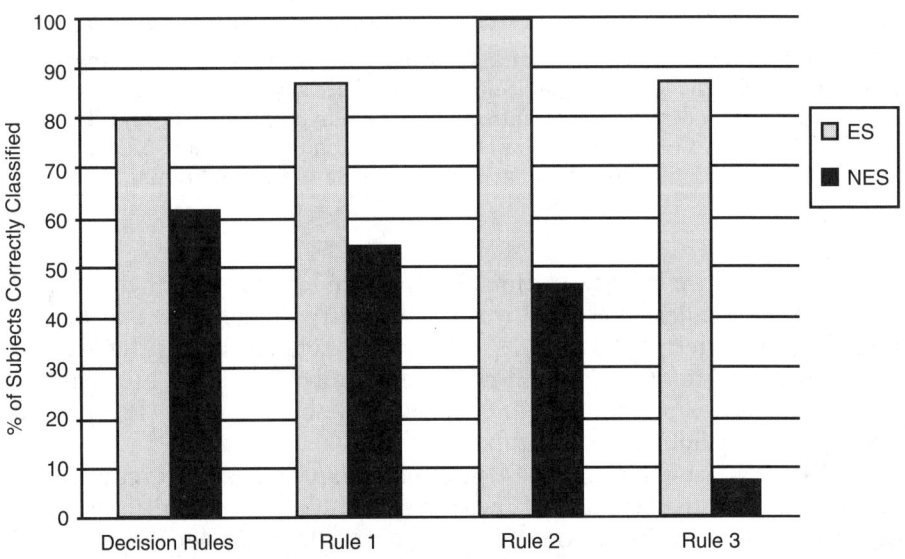

FIGURE 9.2. Minnesota Multiphasic Personality Inventory (MMPI) decision rule. Percent of patients with non-epileptic seizures (NES) and epileptic seizures (ES) correctly classified by MMPI configural rules.

evidence of increased psychiatric symptomatology in the NES group was found, because significantly more (nearly one-half) had been hospitalized for psychiatric reasons and a majority reported histories of physical or sexual abuse. In addition, the NES patient group had significantly higher MMPI scores on scales 1 (hypochondriasis) and 3 (hysteria) and on MMPI hysteria subscales Hy3 (lassitude-malaise) and Hy4 (somatic complaints). This MMPI profile suggests multiple somatic complaints, which may represent conversion of affective distress into physical symptoms. These data suggest that examination of the hysteria subscales may be useful for differential diagnosis of potential NES patients. Thus, the hypothesis that the NES group shows more significant psychiatric disturbance than temporal lobe epilepsy patients was supported. The significantly greater psychopathology in the NES group relative to the ES group is noteworthy because seizure patients in general are known to be at increased risk for psychiatric difficulties.[56]

Based on the present study and past reviews of MMPI studies[19] in NES patients, the MMPI configural rules proposed by Wilkus and coauthors are a useful adjunct to neurologic and psychiatric evaluation in the differential diagnosis of NES, but should not be used as a basis for clinical decision making because using these rules results in a large number of both false-positives and false-negatives. Rule 2 (scale 1 or 3 is 80 or higher, even if not among the highest points) was the most specific to NES in our sample because no ES patients were misclassified using this rule. However, this finding may vary depending on the ES population selected. For example, Hermann[14] found that rules 1 and 2 misclassified 24% and 10%, respectively, of 92 epilepsy surgery candidates, whereas the lowest false-positive rate for ES patients was found using rule 3 (the conversion V).

Neuropsychological discrimination between NES and ES groups was not possible. Furthermore, even when a psychiatric control group of patients with somatoform disorders was included, no cognitive test differentiated the groups. Thus, the psychiatric disturbances in the NES and somatoform groups may be sufficient to impair performance on cognitive testing such that organic brain impairment does not have to be invoked as a pathogenetic mechanism. Although no differences were found among groups on measures of attention in the present study, mild reductions in attentional functioning may occur in individuals within each group for different reasons, such as medication side effects, interictal abnormalities in the ES groups, cognitive effects of seizures, and psychiatric disturbance. The mechanism by which psychiatric dysfunction may contribute to impaired test performances could be variable effort and nonspecific attentional disturbance that interferes with effortful tasks, memory, and mental processing speed. For example, Binder and coauthors[12] reported that measures of exaggeration of cognitive impairment and disability application status were specific to NES patients and suggested suboptimal effort. This was interpreted as evidence of symptom embellishment associated with the histrionic personality style that may be seen in NES patients. Although the present study suggests that there may not be organic brain dysfunction in NES patients despite their poor performance on cognitive tests, it does not exclude the possibility that brain impairment can contribute to the development of NES. For example, Wilkus and colleagues[8] reported high rates of neurologic events in their NES group. Neurologic events that reduce cognitive functioning may contribute to the development of NES by further eroding coping skills and adaptive abilities. Our group differed in that NES patients were selected who were without history of brain injury or neurologic disease. Future research might compare cognitive and psychological profiles of NES with and without histories of neurologic insults.

Finally, differences between the neuropsychological profiles of NES and ES may be observed qualitatively rather than quantitatively. For example, the recognition memory performance of NES patients on the California Verbal Learning Test was notable for a negative response bias compared to a positive response bias in a group of ES patients with a left temporal seizure focus.[15] The negative response bias was interpreted as possibly associated with a tendency toward psychological denial in the NES group. Further research may elucidate the role of neuropsychological assessment in the diagnosis of NES by using cluster analysis to identify the potential spectrum of cognitive profiles that exists in this population.

References

1. Alper K, Devinsky O, Perrine K, et al. Psychiatric classification of nonconversion nonepileptic seizures. Arch Neurol 1995;52:199–201.
2. Bowman ES. Etiology and clinical course of pseudoseizures: relationship to trauma, depression, and dissociation. Psychosomatics 1993;34:333–342.
3. Devinsky O, Thacker K. Nonepileptic seizures. Neurol Clin 1995;13:299–319.
4. Porter RJ. Diagnosis of Psychogenic and Other Nonepileptic Seizures in Adults. In O Devinsky, WH Theodore (eds), Epilepsy and Behavior: Frontiers of Clinical Neuroscience. New York: Wiley-Liss, 1991;237–249.
5. Roy A, Barris M. Psychiatric Concepts in Psychogenic Non-Epileptic Seizures. In AJ Rowan, JR Gates (eds), Non-Epileptic Seizures. Boston: Butterworth–Heinemann, 1993;143–151.
6. Lelliott PT, Fenwick P. Cerebral pathology in pseudoseizures. Acta Neurol Scand 1991;83:129–132.
7. Vanderzant CW, Giordani B, Berent S, et al. Personality of patients with pseudoseizures. Neurology 1986;36,664–668.
8. Wilkus RJ, Dodrill CB, Thompson PM. Intensive EEG monitoring and psychological studies of patients with pseudoepileptic seizures. Epilepsia 1984;25:100–107.
9. Alper K, Devinsky O, Perrine K, et al. Nonepileptic seizures and childhood sexual and physical abuse. Neurology 1993;43:1950–1953.

10. Gates JR, Mercer K. Nonepileptic events. Sem Neurol 1995;15:167–174.
11. Sackellares JC, Giordani B, Berent S, et al. Patients with pseudoseizures: intellectual and cognitive performance. Neurology 1985;35:116–119.
12. Binder LM, Salinsky MC, Smith S. Psychological correlates of psychogenic seizures. J Clin Exp Neuropsychol 1994;16:524–530.
13. Henrichs TF, Tucker DM, Farha J, Novelly RA. MMPI indices in the identification of patients evidencing pseudo seizures. Epilepsia 1988;29:184–187.
14. Hermann BP. Neuropsychological Assessment in the Diagnosis of Non-Epileptic Seizures. In AJ Rowan, JR Gates (eds), Non-Epileptic Seizures. Boston: Butterworth–Heinemann, 1993, 221–232.
15. Bortz JJ, Prigatano GP, Blum D, Fisher RS. Differential response characteristics in nonepileptic and epileptic seizure patients on a test of verbal learning and memory. Neurology 1995;45:2029–2034.
16. Brown MC, Levin BE, Ramsy RE, et al. Characteristics of patients with nonepileptic seizures. J Epilepsy 1991;4:225–229.
17. Wilkus RJ, Dodrill CB. Factors affecting the outcome of MMPI and neuropsychological assessments of psychogenic and epileptic seizure patients. Epilepsia 1989;30:339–347.
18. Hathaway SR, McKinley JC. The Minnesota Multiphasic Personality Inventory Manual (revised). New York: Psychological Corporation, 1951.
19. Hermann BP, Connell BE. Neuropsychological Assessment in the Diagnosis of Nonepileptic Seizures. In TL Bennett (ed), The Neuropsychology of Epilepsy. New York: Plenum, 1992;59–70.
20. Loring DW. Relationship between Quality of Life Variables to Personality Factors in Patients with Epilepsy and NES. Paper presented at Non-Epileptic Seizures: A Consensus Conference on Diagnosis and Treatment, Bethesda, MD, April 1996.
21. Wurzman LP, Matthews CG. The Borderlands of Epilepsy: Explorations with the MMPI. Paper presented at International Neuropsychological Society, Pittsburgh, 1982.
22. Dodrill CB, Wilkus RJ, Batzel LW. The MMPI as a Diagnostic Tool in Non-Epileptic Seizures. In AJ Rowan, JR Gates (eds), Non-Epileptic Seizures. Boston: Butterworth–Heinemann, 1993;211–219.
23. Wyler AR, Hermann BP, Blumer D, Richey ET. Pseudo-Pseudoepileptic Seizures. In AJ Rowan, JR Gates (eds), Non-Epileptic Seizures. Boston: Butterworth–Heinemann, 1993;73–84.
24. Lezak MD. Neuropsychological Assessment (3rd ed). New York: Oxford University, 1995.
25. Yozawitz A. Applied Neuropsychology in a Psychiatric Center. In I Grant, KM Adams KM (eds), Neuropsychological Assessment of Neuropsychiatric Disorders. New York: Oxford University, 1986;121–146.
26. Jaeger J, Berns S, Tigner A, Douglas E. Remediation of neuropsychological deficits in psychiatric populations: rationale and methodological considerations. Psychopharmacol Bull 1992;28:367–390.
27. Cullum CM, Heaton RK, Nemiroff B. Neuropsychology of late-life psychoses. Psychiatr Clin North Am 1988;11:47–59.

28. Jaeger J, Douglas E. Neuropsychiatric rehabilitation for persistent mental illness. Psychiatr Q 1992;63:71–94.
29. Russell JD, Roxanas MG. Psychiatry and the frontal lobes. Aust N Z J Psychiatry 1990;24:113–132.
30. Hamsher KS. Specialized Neuropsychological Assessment Methods. In G Goldstein, M Hersen (eds), Handbook of Psychological Assessment. New York: Pergamon, 1984;235–256.
31. Bowman ES, Markand ON. Psychodynamics and psychiatric diagnoses of pseudoseizure subjects. Am J Psychiatry 1996;153:57–63.
32. Hermann BP, Wyler AR, Richey ET, Rea JM. Memory function and verbal learning ability in patients with complex partial seizures of temporal lobe origin. Epilepsia 1987;28:547–554.
33. Jones-Gotman M, So N, Andermann F, et al. Memory and cognition in bitemporal epileptic patients undergoing depth electrode studies [Abstract]. Epilepsia 1989;30:713.
34. Loring DW, Lee GP, Martin RC, Meador KJ. Material-specific learning in patients with partial complex seizures of temporal lobe origin: convergent validation of memory constructs. J Epilepsy 1988;1:53–59.
35. Moore PM, Baker GA. Validation of the Wechsler memory scale–revised in a sample of people with intractable temporal lobe epilepsy. Epilepsia 1996;37:1215–1220.
36. Saling MM, Berkovic SF, O'Shea MF, et al. Lateralization of verbal memory and unilateral hippocampal sclerosis: evidence of task-specific effects. J Clin Exp Neuropsychol 1993;15:608-618.
37. Binder JR, Swanson SJ, Hammeke TA, et al. Determination of language dominance using functional MRI: a comparison with the Wada test. Neurology 1996;46:978–984.
38. Loring DW, Meador KJ, Lee GP, King DW. Amobarbital Effects and Lateralized Brain Function: The Wada Test. New York: Springer-Verlag, 1992.
39. Wada J, Rasmussen T. Intracarotid injection of sodium Amytal for the lateralization of cerebral speech dominance. J Neurosurg 1960;17:266–282.
40. Green RL. MMPI-2/MMPI. An Interpretive Manual. Boston: Allyn and Bacon, 1991.
41. Wechsler D. Wechsler Adult Intelligence Scale–Revised Manual. New York: Psychological Corporation, 1981.
42. Wechsler D. Wechsler Memory Scale–Revised Manual. San Antonio, TX: Psychological Corporation, 1987.
43. Buschke H. Selective reminding for analysis of memory and learning. J Verbal Learning Verbal Behav 1973;12:543–550.
44. Rao SM, Hammeke TA, McQuillen MP, et al. Memory disturbance in chronic progressive multiple sclerosis. Arch Neurol 1984;41:625–631.
45. Kaplan EF, Goodglass H, Weintraub S. The Boston Naming Test (2nd ed). Philadelphia: Lea & Febiger, 1983.
46. Benton AL, Hamsher KS. Multilingual Aphasia Examination. Iowa City, IA: AJA Associates, 1989.

47. Benton AL, Hamsher KS, Varney NR, Spreen 0. Contributions to Neuropsychological Assessment. New York: Oxford University, 1983.
48. Smith A. Symbol Digit Modalities Test Manual (revised). Los Angeles: Western Psychological Services, 1982.
49. Berg EA. A simple objective treatment for measuring flexibility in thinking. J Gen Psychol 1948;39:15–22.
50. Heaton RK. Wisconsin Card Sorting Test Manual. Odessa, FL: Psychological Assessment Resources, 1981.
51. Army Individual Test Battery. Manual of Directions and Scoring. Washington, DC: War Department Adjutant General's Office, 1944.
52. Klove H. Clinical Neuropsychology. In FM Forster (ed), Medical Clinics of North America. New York: Saunders, 1963.
53. Spreen O, Strauss E. A Compendium of Neuropsychological Tests. New York: Oxford University, 1991.
54. Boll TJ. The Halstead-Reitan Neuropsychological Battery. In SB Filskov, TJ Boll (eds), Handbook of Clinical Neuropsychology. New York: Wiley-Interscience, 1981.
55. Desai BT, Porter RJ, Penry JK. Psychogenic seizures: a study of 42 attacks in six patients, with intensive monitoring. Arch Neurol 1982;39:202–209.
56. Swanson SJ, Rao SM, Grafman J, et al. The relationship between seizure subtype and interictal personality: results from the Vietnam head injury study. Brain 1995;118:91–103.

CHAPTER 10

Neuropsychological Performance and Cognitive Complaints in Epileptic and Non-Epileptic Seizure Patients

Gail L. Risse, Sharon L. Mason, and D. Kent Mercer

The neuropsychological status of patients diagnosed with non-epileptic seizures (NES) has been a controversial topic. Debate has centered on two questions: (1) Can cognitive deficits be identified in the NES population compared to patients with documented seizure disorders?; and (2) What is the etiology of this impairment if it indeed exists? Consideration of etiology has been complicated by the psychiatric symptomatology of these patients as well as by the nature and severity of their non-epileptic seizures. In this chapter, the current status of this debate is reviewed and some new data from the Minnesota Epilepsy Group are presented that examine the cognitive performance and Minnesota Multiphasic Personality Inventory (MMPI) profiles of NES patients in the context of their own cognitive complaints.

In general, it has been difficult to demonstrate significant differences in cognitive performance between groups of patients with NES and those with epileptic seizures (ES). Although some reports have described significantly higher group scores on general intellectual[1] and memory measures[2] for NES cases, these studies have been criticized for failure to match subjects from the two seizure groups on important factors such as age and level of education or failure to include a non-neurologic control group. Furthermore, even when NES patients have outperformed ES patients, their mean scores typically have fallen below the normal range.

A majority of studies have reported no significant differences in the cognitive profiles of patients with non-epileptic versus epileptic diagnoses,[3–8] with both groups demonstrating impairment on at least some measures. Wilkus et al.[3] compared the performance of 25 patients with documented seizures to 25 clearly diagnosed NES patients on the Wechsler Adult Intelligence Scale (WAIS) and the Neuropsychological Battery for Epilepsy. Patients from the two groups were matched for age, gender, and level of education. The two groups did not differ significantly on any measures in the battery; however, a similar proportion of scores from each group (approximately 50%) fell outside of normal limits. The authors concluded that the performance of both groups was suggestive of brain dysfunction. In a follow-up study, Wilkus and Dodrill[4] compared the performance of patients with partial and generalized seizures to that of NES patients and again found no significant differences as long as the groups were matched for age, gender, and education. However, when NES patients and those with generalized seizures were not matched for level of education, ES patients scored significantly lower than patients in the NES group. Similarly, Hermann[7] reported abnormal neuropsychological profiles in 100% of epilepsy patients and 83% of patients with NES in his sample, again suggesting the possibility of underlying brain dysfunction in both the NES and ES groups.

A more recent study by Binder et al.[8] also noted significant neuropsychological impairment in both patients with NES and ES compared to control subjects. However, these authors assert that apparent neuropsychological impairment in the NES group is related to emotional factors based on significantly lower scores on a motivational measure, the Portland Digit Recognition Test, and group differences in MMPI patterns. They suggest that neuropsychological abnormalities are not pathognomonic of brain dysfunction in the NES population. This theory is intuitively appealing given that a primary psychiatric diagnosis is appropriate in a majority of patients with NES. Our clinical experience with this population has repeatedly reinforced the observation that NES patients view themselves as cognitively impaired and that this self-perception is intimately related to their psychiatric status. The data below describe the cognitive complaints, cognitive performance, and MMPI profiles of a group of patients from the Minnesota Epilepsy Group identified with NES.

Methods

Patient Selection

Non-Epileptic Seizure Patients

NES patients who participated in the Minnesota Epilepsy Group study were selected from a population of patients undergoing comprehensive evaluation on the inpatient epilepsy unit. All patients had undergone video-electroencephalographic (EEG) monitoring and seizure-like episodes that failed to show an EEG correlate had been documented in all cases. In addition, all of the patients selected for the NES group met the *DSM-IV* (*Diagnostic and Statistical Manual of Mental Disorders*, Fourth Edition) criteria for conversion disorder. This was not an exclusionary diagnosis; some patients also met criteria for other psychiatric diagnoses, including mood, anxiety, and personality disorders. In addition, all NES subjects had obtained a full-scale intelligence quotient (FSIQ) of greater than 75.

Epilepsy Control Patients

Patients selected for the epilepsy control group also underwent inpatient evaluation on the epilepsy unit. They had a primary diagnosis of epilepsy that had been confirmed by video-EEG monitoring. These patients did not have structural lesions of the brain (excluding mesial temporal sclerosis) and did not have any other diagnosed neurologic disorders. Not all patients had evidence of lateralized seizure onset. They had no history of brain surgery and no history or suspicion of NES. All of the patients in the epilepsy control group also had FSIQs of greater than 75. Patients with psychiatric histories or current psychiatric symptomatology were not excluded from the epilepsy control group except for those with NES. This group of patients represented an almost consecutive series of inpatient admissions to the epilepsy unit excluding NES cases.

Patient Demographics

Patient demographics are presented in Table 10.1. There were 43 patients in the NES group, including 10 men and 33 women. The mean age was 35.1 years, the mean education level was 13.1 years, and the mean FSIQ was 93.4. There were also 43 patients in the epilepsy control group. The mean age of this group was 32.7, with 16 men and 27 women. Mean level of education was 13.3 years, and mean FSIQ was 93.7. Thus, the two groups were well matched. IQ range for both groups was borderline to bright normal.

TABLE 10.1
Demographics of Patients Studied in the Non-Epileptic Seizure and Epilepsy Seizure Groups

Group	Number	Age	Gender	Education	FSIQ
NES	43	35.1	10 M, 33 F	13.1 yrs	93.4
ES	43	32.7	16 M, 27 F	13.3 yrs	93.7

ES = epileptic seizures; FSIQ = full-scale intellience quotient; NES = non-epileptic seizures.

Cognitive Complaints

All patients were routinely asked about their own perceptions of cognitive difficulty during the neuropsychological interview. Questions were open ended and designed to elicit patients' own description of their deficits (i.e., "Have you been having any difficulty with your thinking?"). Positive responses were noted, and the complaints were grouped into four primary areas: memory, attention/concentration, confusion, and language deficits. All other cognitive complaints were classified under miscellaneous. Eighty-four percent of NES patients and 67% of ES patients had complaints in at least one area of function. Difficulty with memory function was the most common complaint for both groups, with 60% of the patients in each group describing some type of memory difficulty (Table 10.2).

In the areas of attention/concentration, confusion, and language deficits, NES patients had more complaints than did patients with epilepsy. A total of 33% of ES patients and 16% of NES patients had no cognitive complaints.

Neuropsychological Test Battery

The neuropsychological test battery was designed to evaluate a broad range of intellectual abilities in patients with epilepsy. A selected sample of data

TABLE 10.2
Percent of Patients from Non-Epileptic Seizure and Epileptic Seizure Groups Reporting Impaired Cognitive Function in Each Area

Group	Memory	Attention/ Concentration	Confusion	Language	Miscellaneous	None
NES	60	23	12	16	9	16
ES	60	9	0	12	9	33

ES = epileptic seizures; NES = non-epileptic seizures.

from this battery is reported in this chapter. Procedures were selected that addressed patients' complaints, as well as problems that NES patients have been reported to experience. The following measures were included:

Intellectual ability
    Wechsler Adult Intelligence Scale-Revised (WAIS-R)
Attention/concentration
    WAIS-R Digit Span
    Serial Digit Learning
Verbal memory
    Wechsler Memory Scale-Revised
        Logical Memory (immediate and delayed)
    Verbal Selective Reminding Test (Buschke)
        Acquisition
        Long-term storage
        Consistent long-term retrieval
        Delayed recall
        Delayed recognition
Nonverbal memory
    Nonverbal Selective Reminding Test
        Long-term storage
        Consistent long-term retrieval
        Delayed recall
Executive functions
    Wisconsin Card Sorting Test
    Associative Fluency
        Controlled Oral Word Association
        Design Fluency
Motor functions
    Grooved Pegboard

Results

Mean performance levels for the NES and ES groups for all neuropsychological measures are presented in Table 10.3. The performance of both groups was compared using standard two-sample t tests and was found to be very similar across measures.

In general, the mean performance of NES patients was slightly higher than that of ES patients across tasks, although most comparisons were not statistically significant. Two measures showed a consistently higher performance by the NES group. These included word fluency, on which the NES mean score was in the high-average range on the Controlled Oral Word Association Test whereas the ES mean score was in the lower-average range, and Design Fluency, on which the NES group performed in the above-average range whereas the ES group was in the average range. On one measure, the

TABLE 10.3
Mean Scores for Non-Epileptic Seizure and Epileptic Seizure Groups on Neuropsychological Measures

Test	NES	ES	Significance
Digit span			
(scaled score)	8.6	10.0	$p < .01$
WMS-R			
Logical memory			
Immediate	11.0	10.5	NS
Delayed	8.8	7.7	NS
Verbal SRT			
LTS (standard score)	88.4	81.6	NS
CLTR (standard score)	82.4	81.6	NS
Delayed recall (%)	71.2	67.7	NS
Nonverbal SRT			
LTS (standard score)	87.8	85.7	NS
CLTR (standard score)	89.6	85.6	NS
Delayed recall (%)	60	61	NS
COWAT (%ile)	59	39	$p < .001$
Design Fluency (raw)	16.4	12.2	$p < .01$
WCST			
Categories	5.0	5.0	NS
% total errors	27.4	27.8	NS
% perservative errors	34	27	NS
Grooved Pegboard			
Right hand (%ile)	37.7	39.5	NS
Left hand (%ile)	40.9	35.4	NS

CLTR = consistent long-term retrieval; COWAT = Controlled Oral Word Association Test; ES = epileptic seizure; LTS = long-term storage; NES = non-epileptic seizure; NS = not significant; SRT = Selective Reminding Test; WCST = Wisconsin Card Sorting Test; WMS-R = Wechsler Memory Scale-Revised.

Digit Span subtest from the WAIS-R, the ES group performed significantly higher than the NES group. For all other measures in the test battery, no significant differences were found in the performance of the two groups. Overall scores ranged from the low-average to the above-average range. There was a tendency for the NES group to perform at a somewhat higher level than the epilepsy patients on measures of verbal learning and retention. This is particularly notable, because a majority of patients in both groups complained of poor memory functioning. Mean performance by the NES patients as a group did not fall below the low-average range in any instance. Thus, there appears to be a striking absence of significant cognitive impairment in this group of NES patients with an average-range IQ. Indeed, our control group of ES patients, who also have mean IQ scores in the low-average range, also fail to demonstrate significant cognitive impairment on a majority of measures.

Personality Assessment with the Minnesota Multiphasic Personality Inventory 2

Use of the MMPI as a potential diagnostic tool in differentiating NES from ES patients has been explored in a number of previous studies.[3,8-16] An extensive review of this literature was presented by Dodrill et al.[17] and focused on the effectiveness of applying specific decision rules to the MMPI profile configuration.[3] According to this method, patients were classified with NES if they met one or more of the following profile criteria: (1) The T score on scale 1 (hypochondriasis) or scale 3 (hysteria) is 70 or higher, and either scale 1 or 3 is one of the two highest clinical scales (disregarding the masculinity/femininity and social introversion scales); (2) scale 1 or 3 is 80 or higher, even though not among the two highest clinical scales; or (3) scales 1 and 3 are both higher than 59, and both are at least 10 points higher than scale 2 (depression). These authors report "hit rates" as high as 80% in identifying NES patients, although the risk of misclassification (particularly if epilepsy patients are classified with NES) is as high as 12-27% in published reports.[17] In any case, these studies underscore the frequency with which physical symptoms are endorsed in this population, raising concerns about the validity of self-reported neuropsychological impairment in NES patients.

We compiled MMPI-2 data on a subset of patients from our NES and ES groups to compare to previous studies that used the MMPI.

Patient Selection

A total of 33 patients from the NES group and 27 patients from the ES group completed the MMPI-2. Cases were excluded if the L or K scales were greater than 70 or the F scale was greater than 100.

Results

Composite profiles for the MMPI-2 clinical scales are presented in Figure 10.1. Scales 1, 2, and 3 (hypochondriasis, depression, and hysteria) are all clinically elevated in the NES group. T score differences between the two groups are statistically significant for hypochondriasis and hysteria ($p < .0001$). No other scales were significantly elevated, and no other differences were seen between the two groups. This profile is similar to that previously described by Dodrill et al.[17] on the MMPI except that they reported a clinical elevation on scale 8 (schizophrenia) for the NES group. Our composite profile is also remarkably similar to that described in another study using the MMPI-2.[8] When the Wilkus et al.[3] decision rules were applied to our data (adjusted for the MMPI-2), MMPI-2 scores successfully classified 58% of NES patients and 70% of epilepsy patients.

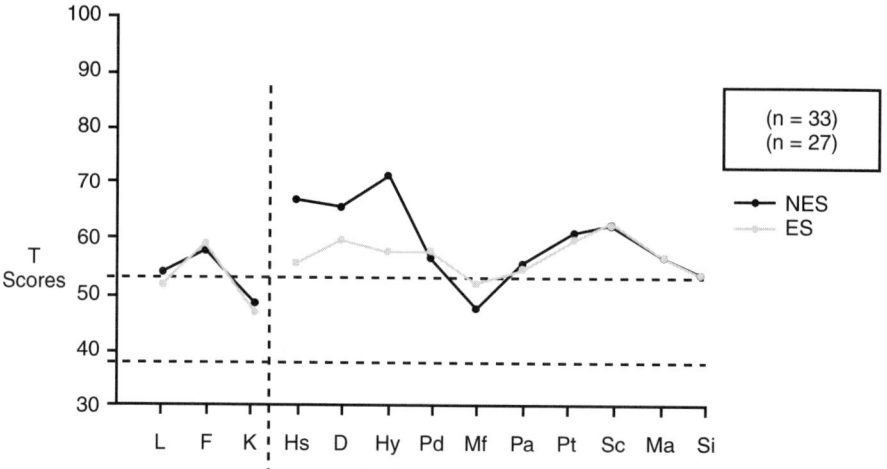

FIGURE 10.1. Minnesota Multiphasic Personality Inventory 2 (MMPI-2) validity and clinical scales. Scales: D = depression; F = infrequency; Hs = hypochondriasis; Hy = hysteria; L = lie; K = defensiveness; Ma = mania; Mf = masculinity/femininity; Pa = paranoia; Pd = psychopathic deviate; Pt = psychasthenia; Sc = schizophrenia; Si = social introversion. (ES = epileptic seizures; NES = non-epileptic seizures.)

The two seizure groups in our sample were further compared on the Harris-Lingoes subscales for depression and hysteria (Figures 10.2 and 10.3). No significant differences were seen between the two groups on any depression subscale, although the NES group showed a slight clinical elevation on D3, which is physical malfunctioning. On the hysteria subscales, the NES group showed clinical elevation on Hy3 (lassitude-malaise) and Hy4 (somatic complaints), endorsing symptoms that deny good health, describe weakness and fatigue, indicate difficulty with concentration, and involve various somatic complaints, including pain, fainting spells, dizziness, nausea, poor vision, and others. Actuarial data[18] on these subscales suggest that individuals with similar profiles are likely to use repression and conversion of affect. The differences between the NES and ES mean scores on these two subscales are statistically significant ($p < .01$). It must be emphasized that these data portray aggregate scores that may obscure more normal profiles in individual cases and more deviant patterns in others, reflecting considerable diversity in this population. Of course, composite profiles cannot form a basis for designing individual treatment plans. Nonetheless, this process helps focus attention on those areas of psychopathology that are, on average, most frequently associated with the diagnosis of NES.

In our population, the NES MMPI-2 data are compatible with the incidence of cognitive complaints in the absence of significant neuropsychological impairment.

Neuropsychological Performance and Cognitive Complaints 147

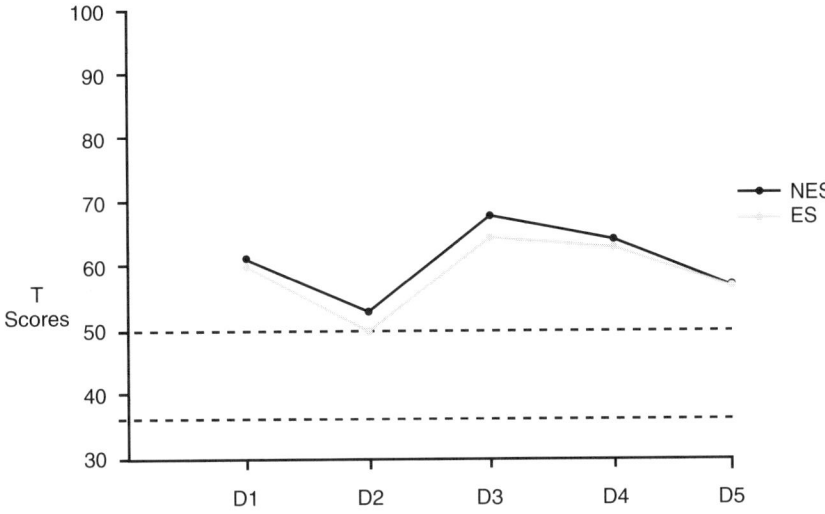

FIGURE 10.2. Minnesota Multiphasic Personality Inventory 2 (MMPI-2) depression subscales. (D1 = subjective depression; D2 = psychomotor retardation; D3 = physical malfunctioning; D4 = mental dullness; D5 = brooding; ES = epileptic seizures; NES = non-epileptic seizures.)

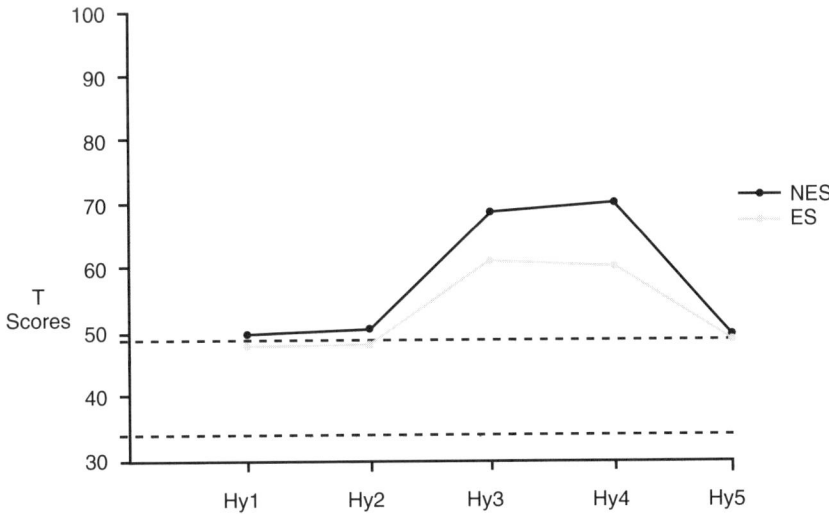

FIGURE 10.3. Minnesota Multiphasic Personality Inventory 2 (MMPI-2) hysteria subscales. (ES = epileptic seizures; Hy1 = denial of social anxiety; Hy2 = need for affection; Hy3 = lassitude-malaise; Hy4 = somatic complaints; Hy5 = inhbition of aggression; NES = non-epileptic seizure.)

Discussion

These data, describing the composite cognitive and personality profiles of patients with NES, argue against significant neurologic dysfunction in this population. All of our NES cases had unambiguous, EEG-confirmed non-epileptic events and met criteria for *DSM-IV* psychiatric diagnoses.

The average neuropsychological performance of these patients was within normal limits and highly discrepant with the patients' description of their own functioning. Failure to identify significant differences between NES and ES group performance might be reasonably attributed to several factors. First, in this and in similar comparison studies, it is highly likely that averaged scores in the ES group underestimate the extent of cognitive impairment because of the heterogeneous nature of this population. Patients with a generic diagnosis of "epilepsy" (even when broken down by seizure type) are not likely to demonstrate a single, consistent pattern of cognitive impairment. Rather, specific cognitive deficits, when present, tend to reflect focal areas of brain dysfunction that correlate with the patients' seizures. Test batteries designed to yield overall indices of "brain damage" are of little value in delineating the specific cognitive effects of a focal seizure disorder. Thus, if patients were grouped by anatomic seizure focus, these individuals might be more likely to demonstrate specific cognitive deficits compared to those with NES, although Swanson et al. (see Chapter 9) did not uncover this difference in their study. Secondly, patients with NES as symptoms of a conversion disorder may be more likely to produce intellectual profiles that underestimate their actual abilities. These patients often appear to be invested in their own dysfunction, both physical and cognitive, and although evidence of overt malingering may be lacking, they could be prone to symptom exaggeration and reduced motivation during test performance, suggesting that more measures of symptom validity would be helpful in identifying the etiology of impaired neuropsychological performance in this population.

As noted earlier, other investigators have attributed neuropsychological impairment in NES patients to emotional rather than neurologic factors based on MMPI/MMPI-2 performance, results on the Portland Digit Recognition Test, and psychiatric history.[8,15] Our data support this conclusion because we also observed a high level of endorsement of physical and cognitive complaints by NES patients in the absence of significant cognitive deficits. It is also possible that yet another variable, such as limited attention/concentration (whether a primary condition or secondary to a psychiatric disturbance, such as depression), may be the basis of self-reported cognitive complaints in some NES patients. This is particularly plausible in view of our data indicating lower mean scores among NES than ES patients on a measure that is sensitive to sustained attention, as well as data presented by Hempel (see Chapter 14) indicating that a significant proportion of pediatric NES patients evidence poor attention.

Although a definitive diagnosis of NES remains contingent on the results of video-EEG monitoring, the neuropsychological assessment and MMPI profiles of these patients may contribute to a broader understanding of this disorder and enable the design of viable treatment options. The continued psychological and neuropsychological investigation of this population for both diagnostic and treatment purposes is well justified.

References

1. Sackellares JD, Giordani B, Berent S, et al. Patients with pseudoseizures: intellectual and cognitive performance. Neurology 1985;35:116–119.
2. Novelly RA. Cerebral Dysfunction and Cognitive Impairment in Non-Epileptic Seizure Disorders. In AJ Rowan, JR Gates (eds), Non-Epileptic Seizures. Boston: Butterworth–Heinemann, 1993;221–232.
3. Wilkus RJ, Dodrill CB, Thompson PM. Intensive EEG monitoring and psychological studies of patients with pseudoepileptic seizures. Epilepsia 1984:25;100–107.
4. Wilkus RJ, Dodrill CB. Factors affecting the outcome of MMPI and neuropsychological assessments of psychogenic and epileptic seizure patients. Epilepsia 1986;27(Suppl 2):S124–S129.
5. Brown MC, Levin BE, Ramsay RE, et al. Characteristics of patients with nonepileptic seizures. J Epilepsy 1991;4:225–229.
6. Hermann BP, Connell BE. Neuropsychological Assessment in the Diagnosis of Nonepileptic Seizures. In TL Bennett (ed), The Neuropsychology of Epilepsy. New York: Plenum, 1992;58–70.
7. Hermann BP. Neuropsychological Assessment in the Diagnosis of Non-Epileptic Seizures. In AJ Rowan, JR Gates (eds), Non-Epileptic Seizures. Boston: Butterworth–Heinemann, 1993;221–232.
8. Binder LM, Kindermann SS, Heaton RK, Salinsky MC. Neuropsychologic impairment in patients with nonepileptic seizures. Arch Clin Neuropsychol 1998;13:513–522.
9. Shaw DJ. Differential MMPI performance in pseudo-seizure epileptic and pseudo-neurologic groups. J Clin Psychol 1966;22:271–275.
10. Finlayson RE, Lucas AL. Pseudoepileptic seizures in children and adolescents. Mayo Clin Proc 1979;54:83–87.
11. Vanderzant CW, Giordani B, Berent S, et al. Personality of patients with pseudoseizures. Neurology 1986;36:664–668.
12. Henrichs TF, Tucker DM, Farha J, et al. MMPI indices in the identification of patients evidencing pseudoseizures. Epilepsia 1988;29:184–187.
13. Barrash J, Gates JR, Heck DG, et al. MMPI subtypes among patients with nonepileptic events. Epilepsia 1989;30:730–731.

14. Drake ME, Pakalnis A, Phillips BB. Neuropsychological and psychiatric correlates of intractable pseudoseizures. Seizure 1992;1:11–13.
15. Binder LM, Salinsky MC, Smith SP. Psychological correlates of nonepileptic seizures. J Clin Exp Neuropsychol 1994;16:524–530.
16. Kalogjera-Sackellares D, Sackellares JC. Analysis of MMPI patterns in patients with psychogenic pseudoseizures. Seizure 1997;6:419–427.
17. Dodrill CB, Wilkus RJ, Batzel LW. The MMPI as a Diagnostic Tool in Non-Epileptic Seizures. In AJ Rowan, JR Gates (eds), Non-Epileptic Seizures. Boston: Butterworth–Heinemann, 1993;211–219.
18. Green RL. MMPI-2/MMPI: An Interpretive Manual. Boston: Allyn and Bacon, 1991.

CHAPTER 11

Depression and Anxiety in Patients with Non-Epileptic versus Epileptic Seizures

Nancy Donofrio, Kenneth Perrine, Kenneth R. Alper, and Orrin Devinsky

Mood disorders are common among patients with both epileptic seizures and non-epileptic seizures (NES), and a number of different instruments exist to measure these mood symptoms. We compared 99 patients with complex partial epilepsy (CPE) (right CPE = 51, left CPE = 48) and patients with non-epileptic seizures (NES = 85) on the Hamilton Anxiety Scale, the Hamilton Depression Scale, the Beck Anxiety Inventory, and the Beck Depression Inventory. On preplanned orthogonal contrasts, NES patients reported significantly more anxiety and depression than the combined (left and right) CPE patients on both the Hamilton scales and the Beck inventories ($F = 5.59$, $p < .02$). However, the disparity between NES patients and CPE patients was significantly greater ($F = 5.59$, $p < .02$) on the clinician-rated Hamilton scales than on the self-report Beck inventories. NES patients may minimize self-reported mood disorders that are more evident when assessed by clinician ratings. Self-report inventories may result in falsely ruling out psychiatric symptomatology in NES patients.

Background

Mood disorders are common among seizure patients. Two-thirds of patients with complex partial seizures report a depressive disorder at or after their original seizure onset.[1] Possible sources of anxiety are the aura, interictal or postictal stages, or reactive mood state to seizures.[2] However, anxiety may occur more frequently with an older age of seizure onset, indicating possible adjustment difficulties.[3] Anxiety may also result directly from a simple partial seizure or panic attack.[2] These affective symptoms may actually be attributable to biological factors, yet are frequently overlooked by the physician.[2]

Mood disorders also occur in patients with NES, who may have significant stress, anxiety, conflict, and depression and score significantly higher than epilepsy patients on measures of affective symptoms.[4,5] The incidence of depression and anxiety in patients with NES may be increased with comorbid psychiatric diagnoses. These may include dependent personality traits, anxiety disorders, mood disorders, and dissociative disorders.[4]

It is necessary to distinguish reactive or psychological symptoms of panic and anxiety from the biological symptoms of epilepsy.[4] Mood disorders may differ between NES and epilepsy patients, and different patterns of mood symptoms may help to differentiate the two groups. The present study compares patients with NES to those with epileptic seizures on self-report and clinician ratings of depression and anxiety to determine if NES patients experience different patterns of these psychiatric symptoms than do epilepsy patients. We hypothesized that patients with NES would show significantly higher levels of disturbed mood than would epilepsy patients.

Method

Subjects were drawn from a review of all patients from 1990 to 1992 who were undergoing video-electroencephalographic (EEG) monitoring at our comprehensive epilepsy center for differential diagnosis, medication adjustment, or surgery evaluation. Patients who had completed all of the psychiatric measures and had a definitive diagnosis of NES or unilateral complex partial seizures were included in the study. There were 99 patients diagnosed with complex partial seizures (CPE right onset = 51, left onset = 48) documented by epileptiform activity on video-EEG at ictal onset of clinical seizures. The CPE group was restricted to those patients with temporal lobe pathology. There were 85 patients with NES, determined by absence of EEG changes at ictal onset of spontaneous events as well as by positive response to saline provocation.[6] The NES patient group consisted of those patients diagnosed with conversion as well as nonconversion NES. Conversion NES was diagnosed in patients who met *DSM-IV (Diagnostic and Statistical Manual of Mental Disorders*, Fourth Edition) criteria for conversion disorder. Nonconversion NES included patients with anxiety disorders, somatization disorder, and psychotic disorders.[7] No significant differences were seen between the three groups in age at evaluation, education, history of inpatient or outpatient psychiatric hospitalizations, history of psychiatric medications, or gender. A significant difference in age of seizure onset did exist, such that patients with NES were significantly older at age of chronic seizure onset (mean [M] = 24.4 years, standard deviation [SD] = 2.9 years) than those with right complex partial seizures (M = 16.8 years, SD = 2.2 years) and left complex partial seizures (M = 14.9 years, SD = 2.1 years).

Procedure

The Hamilton Anxiety Scale, the Hamilton Depression Scale, the Beck Anxiety Inventory, and the Beck Depression Inventory were used to assess affective disturbances. All inventories were administered during inpatient video-EEG monitoring. The Beck scales are self-report inventories completed by the patient. The Hamilton anxiety and depression scales were completed by the same neuropsychiatrist (KA), who was blind to all diagnoses.

The Beck Anxiety Inventory[8] is a 21-item, self-administered scale measuring anxiety that has high reliability and validity.[9] The Beck Depression Inventory is a similar self-administered scale of 21 items assessing depression that has also demonstrated good reliability and validity.[10] Items on both inventories are presented on a four-point scale.

The Hamilton instruments consist of a 14-item anxiety scale and a 27-item depression scale. Good reliability and validity have been demonstrated for both the anxiety scale[11] and the depression scale.[12]

To compare the magnitude of elevations among the four scales, raw scores on the four inventories were transformed to standard scores (SS) on an IQ metric (M = 100, SD = 15) using means and SDs reported in validity and reliability studies[9] according to the formula SS = 100 + 15 × ([raw score − M]/SD).

Analyses

Data were analyzed with a one-way (patient group: right CPE, left CPE, NES) repeated measures (test) analysis of variance (ANOVA). Preplanned orthogonal contrasts tested the right and left CPE group versus the NES group. These analyses were performed on the transformed standard scores to directly compare the mood tests.

Results

Correlations (r) among the tests (Table 11.1) ranged from $r = 0.37$ to $r = 0.77$ ($p < .0001$). The highest correlation was between the two Hamilton scales ($r = 0.77$); the two Beck inventories were significantly correlated, but to a lesser magnitude ($r = 0.47$). Moderate correlations were found between the two depression scales ($r = 0.58$) and between the two anxiety scales ($r = 0.50$).

TABLE 11.1
Correlations among Psychiatric Measures*

	Ham A	Ham D	Beck A	Beck D
Ham A	1.0	0.77	0.50	0.47
Ham D	—	1.0	0.37	0.47
Beck A	—	—	1.0	0.47
Beck D	—	—	—	1.0

Beck A = Beck Anxiety Scale; Beck D = Beck Depression Scale; Ham A = Hamilton Anxiety Scale; Ham D = Hamilton Depression Scale.
*All correlations significant at $p < .0001$.

The ANOVA for the four tests showed a significant effect for patient group (F = 4.73, $p < .01$). NES patients reported more mood disturbance across the four tests than did the CPE patients. The repeated measures term was significant (F = 90.63, $p < .0001$), indicating differences among the tests. The interaction of tests by patient group was not significant. We found no significant differences between the right CPE and left CPE groups across the four tests.

Collapsed across patient groups, the Hamilton scales were significantly different from the Beck inventories (F = 130.57, $p < .0001$). Patients showed more mood disturbance on the clinician-rated Hamilton scales than on the self-report Beck inventories. On the preplanned orthogonal contrasts, NES patients reported significantly more anxiety and depression than the combined (left and right) CPE patients on both the Hamilton scales and the Beck inventories (F = 5.59, $p < .02$). However, the disparity between NES patients and CPE patients was significantly greater (F = 5.59, $p < .02$) on the clinician-rated Hamilton scales than on the self-report Beck inventories (Table 11.2).

TABLE 11.2
Raw Score Test Means for Complex Partial Epilepsy Patients versus Non-Epileptic Seizure Patients

Test	CPE	NES
Hamilton scales		
Anxiety	11.45	14.79
Depression	10.77	13.67
Combined	11.11	14.23
Beck scales		
Anxiety	15.38	17.48
Depression	11.0	11.89
Combined	13.19	14.69

CPE = complex partial epilepsy; NES = non-epileptic seizures.

Discussion

Results confirm previous reports that depression and anxiety are more prevalent in NES patients than in epilepsy patients.[5] The two groups showed significant differences across all four measures of mood disturbance. Additional analyses revealed higher levels of depression and anxiety in all patients as rated by a clinician on the Hamilton scales than on the self-report Beck inventories, especially for NES patients.

Although NES patients appeared significantly more anxious and depressed than epilepsy patients on all measures, the disparity between the groups was much greater on the clinician-rated Hamilton scales than on the self-report Beck inventories. NES patients demonstrate more overt anxiety and depression than epilepsy patients when assessed by a clinician. NES patients may use repression to minimize their conscious experience of mood disturbance,[4] resulting in lower levels of mood disturbance on self-report measures but greater mood disturbance on scales with clinician ratings. These patients may under-report their feelings of depression and anxiety to a greater extent than do epilepsy patients, or clinicians may overestimate mood symptoms in NES patients on rating scales.

In addition to administration differences between the Hamilton scales and the Beck inventories, the Hamilton Depression Scale and the Beck Depression Inventory measure different aspects of depression.[13] The moderate correlation found between the two depression inventories supports this finding. The Hamilton Depression Scale assesses more somatic symptoms, whereas the Beck Depression Inventories assess more cognitive symptoms of depression. For this reason, the Beck Depression Inventory can be considered a more accurate measure of depression in a medical environment, in which somatic manifestations of illness may be elevated and consequently misinterpreted as mood-based depression.[13] On the other hand, scores on the Beck Depression Inventory may be lowered in this setting due to the possibility that the psychological needs of the patient may be satisfied by the secondary gain provided in the inpatient treatment.

The NES patients may report more somatic signs (on the Hamilton) than cognitive signs of depression (on the Beck), suggesting that they acknowledge somatic signs of depression although they lack or repress the cognitive signs. Consequently, these somatic signs of depression or psychiatric illness may be incorrectly attributed to medical causes, possibly leading to diagnostic studies and medical treatment.

Anxiety can be divided into two factors, psychic anxiety and somatic anxiety.[14] The Beck Anxiety Inventory evaluates the subjective, neurophysiologic, autonomic, and panic symptoms of anxiety. The Hamilton anxiety scales take a more global approach, evaluating clinically observable psychic and somatic anxiety.[15] The broad range of assessed anxiety symptoms may result in greater elevations of Hamilton scores as compared to Beck scores.

The mood symptoms experienced by epilepsy patients and NES patients may be attributable to different factors. All patients included in the study were involved in intensive treatment at a tertiary care center for poorly controlled epilepsy. In CPE patients, the epilepsy may cause significant mood disorders as a direct physiologic result of the seizures.[3] Antiepileptic medications may also increase depression and anxiety in this group as a side effect.[3] Adjustment to illness may be an additional cause of mood disturbances, including depression and anxiety.[3]

Multiple possible etiologies exist for mood disorders in the NES population. The experience of the mood disorder may be a primary problem that contributes to conversion seizures, or a psychological effect of the NES and associated disability. Repression of mood disturbance could contribute to rejecting psychiatric treatment to relieve the mood symptoms. An individualized approach to explore underlying mechanisms that contribute to mood disturbance is required to properly evaluate the need for psychotherapeutic or psychopharmacologic treatment. Our findings suggest that the clinician should not rely on self-report scales to assess mood disturbance in the NES population. Clinician ratings yield more accurate assessments of mood. Reliance on self-report measures could lead to falsely rejecting psychiatric symptoms that would support a psychiatric diagnosis.

References

1. Victoroff JI, Benson F, Grafton ST, et al. Depression in complex partial seizures. Arch Neurol 1994;51:155–163.
2. Devinsky O, Vazquez B. Behavioral changes associated with epilepsy. Behav Neurol 1993;11:127–149.
3. Robertson MM, Trimble MR, Townsend HR. Phenomenology of depression in epilepsy. Epilepsia 1987;28:364–372.
4. Alper K. Nonepileptic seizures. Epilepsy II: Special Issues 1994;12:153–173.
5. Roy A. Pseudoseizures: a psychiatric perspective. J Neuropsychiatry 1989;1:69–71.
6. Cohen RJ. Suggestion as a provocation test for EEG. Ann Neurol 1982;11:391–395.
7. Alper K, Devinsky O, Perrine K, et al. Psychiatric classification of nonconversion nonepileptic seizures. Arch Neurol 1995;52:199–201.
8. Beck AT, Steer RA. Beck Anxiety Inventory Manual. San Antonio, TX: Harcourt Brace, 1993.
9. Beck AT, Epstein N, Brown G, Steer RA. An inventory for measuring clinical anxiety: psychometric properties. J Consult Clin Psychol 1988;56:893–897.
10. Gallagher D, Nies G, Thompson LW. Reliability of the Beck depression inventory with older adults. J Consult Clin Psychol 1982;50:152–153.

11. Maier W, Buller R, Philipp M, Heuser I. The Hamilton anxiety scale: reliability, validity and sensitivity to change in anxiety and depressive disorders. J Affect Dis 1988;14:61–68.
12. Kobak KA, Reynolds WM, Rosenfeld R, Greist JH. Development and validation of a computer administered version of the Hamilton depression rating scale. Psychol Assess J Consult Clin Psych 1990;2:56–63.
13. Wesley AL, Gatchel RJ, Polatin PB, et al. Differentiation between somatic and cognitive/affective components in commonly used measurements of depression in patients with chronic low back pain. Let's not mix apples and oranges. Spine 1991;16:S213–S215.
14. Hamilton M. The assessment of anxiety states by rating. Br J Med Psychol 1959;32:50–55.
15. Beck AT, Steer RA. Relationship between the Beck anxiety inventory and the Hamilton anxiety scale with anxious outpatients. J Anxiety Dis 1991;5: 213–223.

CHAPTER 12

Relationship between Quality of Life Variables and Personality Factors in Patients with Epilepsy and Non-Epileptic Seizures

*David W. Loring, Kimford J. Meador,
Don W. King, and Bruce P. Hermann*

Quality of Life

Quality of life assessment allows for a characterization of disease effects on patient lifestyle and daily functioning, and many quality of life definitions exist. In patients with chronic medical conditions, however, health status is a major determinant of quality of life. Most contemporary conceptualizations of health-related quality of life regard it as "a judgment of one's well-being based on consideration of physical, mental, social, and general health status." In contrast to other approaches to describe diseases and their effects, quality of life emphasizes the patient's perception rather than that of the health care provider.

Two approaches to quality of life assessment in clinical populations exist, although these approaches are not mutually exclusive. In one method, the effects of general health concerns on quality of life are assessed and, in the other, disease-specific effects are investigated. General health-related questions characterize general disease effects and allow for comparisons of quality of life across different diseases and treatments. However, general health measures run the risk of failing to address issues that are *specific* to the disease, and questions that address issues that are relatively unique to the disease but nevertheless exert effects on quality of life may be missed.

Quality of life assessment has been effective in characterizing the effects of cancer and cancer treatment (e.g., chemotherapy effects). Cancer is a chronic condition that, although treatable, is typically not cured and presents with significant treatment side effects. Thus, a significant impact on quality of life should be anticipated.

Quality of life measurement has been proven helpful for evaluating patient treatment. Croog et al.[1] observed that despite the equivalence efficacy of three antihypertensive medications for blood pressure control, medication differences were present for quality of life areas ranging from motor coordination to sexual function. Thus, by describing the interactions between disease and psychosocial factors, quality of life measurement allows for comparison of treatment approaches to a specific disease and can be used as an outcome variable.

Quality of Life in Epilepsy

The paroxysmal nature of epilepsy limits important aspects of independence and sense of well-being, such as one's ability to drive, that are not associated with other chronic medical conditions. In addition, significant effects of medication, cognitive dysfunction, and social isolation may be associated with epilepsy and its treatment.

Patients with epilepsy who are rendered seizure free after epilepsy surgery report a higher quality of life than patients who continue to have seizures postoperatively.[2] In addition, when comparing the generic core of the inventory examining general health concerns, seizure-free patients report a higher quality of life than patients with chronic medical conditions, and epilepsy surgery patients with continued seizures after surgery had poorer scores on emotional well-being, overall quality of life, and social function scales than those with hypertension, diabetes, and heart disease.

Similar effects have been observed by others. Hermann et al.[3] noted significant improvement in personality and psychosocial function in patients who underwent epilepsy surgery, but only in those who were completely seizure free. Patients who continued to have seizures, even auras, did not report improvement in their behavioral status. Among the different measurement scales related to seizure outcome and quality of life after anterior temporal lobectomy, health perceptions and energy/fatigue scales appear the most sensitive to differences in seizure outcome classification (seizure free, auras, continued seizures), with the pain scale being the least sensitive.

Non-Epileptic Seizures

Non-epileptic seizures (NES) are paroxysmal events that are seen in a heterogeneous group of patients. Commonly, they are manifestations of conversion disorders/somatization, although they may also be seen with other psychiatric diagnoses, such as anxiety disorders, psychosis, or even attention deficit disorder.[4] Video-electroencephalographic (EEG) monitoring examining electrographic activity with behavioral presentation remains the definitive technique to diagnose NES. However, rare cases have been reported, typically with frontal lobe seizure onset, in which electrographic seizure activity may not be recorded with scalp electrodes. Psychological assessment is also of benefit in discriminating between NES and epilepsy and has been advocated as a screening method for initial NES evaluation.

Quality of Life in Patients with Non-Epileptic Seizures

Until recently, the only systematic inventory of quality of life behaviors for patients with seizures has been the Washington Psychosocial Seizure Inventory (WPSI; 363). Although the WPSI is not a specific quality of life scale, it does capture a component of quality of life because of its assessment of psychosocial function. NES patients achieve poorer scores than do epilepsy patients on three scales of the WPSI, namely, family background, adjustment to seizures, and medicine and medical management.

Discrimination of Patients with Non-Epileptic Seizures from Patients with Epilepsy

The Minnesota Multiphasic Personality Inventory (MMPI) has been the primary personality test used to discriminate patients with NES from patients with epilepsy. Wilkus et al.[5] reported significant group differences on MMPI scales 1 (hypochondriasis), 3 (hysteria), and 8 (schizophrenia). In addition to the ability of the MMPI to differentiate patients when applied on the group level, the test also can discriminate group membership when applied on an individual patient basis. Decision rules based primarily on the first three scales of the MMPI (hypochondriasis, depression, and hysteria) were able to correctly classify approximately 755 of the patients studied.

Wilkus et al.[5] observed distinct MMPI profiles that distinguished patients with NES from those with epilepsy and, furthermore, developed decision rules using scale 1 (hypochondriasis) and scale 3 (hysteria) elevations that correctly classified 80% of the NES patients and 88% of the epilepsy patients. Other NES/epilepsy patient differences were present on scale 4 (psychopathic deviate) and scale 8 (schizophrenia). Attempts at repeating these findings of Wilkus et al. have been generally positive, with several failures to replicate resulting from possible differences in patient composition. Despite these differences, scale 3 (hysteria) has been able to effectively discriminate groups.

To investigate whether differences between patients with NES and those with epilepsy exist, we administered the Quality of Life in Epilepsy (QOLIE) and MMPI-2 to patients who were admitted to our epilepsy monitoring unit for further characterization of their spells and to patients who were undergoing evaluation for possible surgical intervention. The QOLIE-89 is a quality of life inventory that contains both generic components and scales designed to measure specific epilepsy-related quality of life issues. The MMPI-2 is an objective personality measure that is the most commonly used approach to measure and characterize personality functioning. However, only one published report on the utility of MMPI-2 in discriminating epilepsy from NES presently exists.

Two primary goals of the present investigation were present. The first was to determine if similar differences on formal personality testing between epilepsy and NES groups would exist using the MMPI-2, a more recent revision of the MMPI. Obtaining comparable findings using a similar but somewhat different instrument on a different sample of patients would demonstrate the robustness of the previously reported MMPI scale differences. Furthermore, the QOLIE-89 was administered to examine for possible differences in how the patients perceive the effects of their disorder on quality of life. Because the QOLIE contains both a generic health-related core and scores specifically designed to assess the effects of seizures on quality of life, examination of the pattern can help demonstrate whether differences in quality of life, if present, are caused by general health-related concerns or may be due more to the effects of the patient's paroxysmal disorder on lifestyle.

Methods

Twenty-four patients who were diagnosed with NES and 39 patients with complex partial seizures of temporal lobe origin were our subject sample. There was a greater representation of women in the NES group (19 of 24 patients) than in the epilepsy group (18 of 39 patients; chi-square = 6.7, p = .0097). The patient groups did not differ in age (NES patients = 35.6 years, standard deviation [SD] = 10.4; epilepsy patients = 32.5 years, SD = 10.0) or education (NES patients = 12.9 years, SD = 2.3; epilepsy patients = 12.7 years, SD = 2.5). However, epilepsy patients developed their habitual seizure pattern on average at 13.4 years (SD = 12.5), and NES patients developed their seizures at 28.8 years (SD = 15.3; $p < .05$).

NES diagnosis based on video-EEG monitoring in which typical clinical attacks were not consistent with complex partial seizure symptoms were without EEG correlates for both ictal and postictal recordings. Patients with episodes that involved sensory phenomena only were excluded due to the difficulty of verifying the nature of these episodes. Patients with paroxysmal events such as syncope associated with other physical conditions were not considered as part of the subject pool. The patients with confirmed epilepsy all had complex seizures of temporal lobe origin, and most of the patients were candidates for epilepsy surgery at the time of evaluations. Four patients with NES who had true epileptic seizures were excluded from these analyses. The MMPI-2 and QOLIE-89 were both admitted during the admission for video-EEG monitoring. Patients with an invalid MMPI-2, operationally defined as F scores of at least 100, were excluded (N = 3).

Personality

The MMPI-2 is the most commonly used objective personality test. It consists of 556 questions, although all basic clinical scales are derived from the first 370 questions. The MMPI-2 yields scores on three validity measures and 10 clinical scales. The 10 clinical measures are referred to both by their scale number or the personality constructs that they were originally designed to measure. The 10 clinical scales are scale 1 (hypochondriasis), scale 2 (depression), scale 3 (hysteria), scale 4 (psychopathic deviate), scale 5 (masculinity/femininity), scale 6 (paranoia), scale 7 (psychasthenia), scale 8 (schizophrenia), scale 9 (hypomania), and scale 0 (social introversion).

Scores for each scale are reported as standardized T scores, with a mean of 50 and a standard deviation of 10. For each scale, higher values represent personality factors, which reflect greater abnormality. Clinical elevations are inferred for scale elevations of 65 or greater.

Quality of Life in Epilepsy

The QOLIE-89 consists of both a generic core to address general health concerns and additional epilepsy-specific content areas. Eighty-nine questions are asked and include questions from the RAND 36-Item Health Survey (SF-36) supplemented with questions targeted to measure problems that are frequently associated with epilepsy, attitudes toward epilepsy, and self-esteem in patients with moderately controlled epilepsy. The RAND

36-Item Health Survey includes scales that assess (1) general health perceptions, (2) physical function, (3) role limitation due to physical problems, (4) role limitations due to emotional problems, (5) social function, (6) energy and fatigue, (7) emotional well-being, and (8) physical pain.

In addition to the eight scales from the SF-36, nine new scales that were primarily related to epilepsy are included in the QOLIE-89. These are (1) overall quality of life, (2) work/driving/social function, (3) attention/concentration, (4) health discouragement, (5) seizure worry, (6) memory, (7) language, (8) medication defects, and (9) social isolation. In addition, an overall summary score is obtained. Scores on each scale are transformed into T scores with a mean value of 50 and a SD of 10. In the QOLIE-89, higher scores reflect higher quality of life.

Factor analysis of the QOLIE has revealed four relatively distinct factors: epilepsy-specific concerns, cognitive effects, mental health states, and physical health. These factors are relatively independent, with no individual QOLIE subscale having loadings greater than 0.3 on multiple factors.

Results

Type I versus Type II Errors

A risk associated with performing multiple univariate comparisons is the increased likelihood that, as a function of multiple comparisons, some group comparisons will be statistically significant due to chance alone rather than reflecting genuine differences between the groups (type I error). No universally accepted approach exists to account for the increased type I error rate associated with multiple comparisons. One approach is to use a priori a more conservative level of statistical significance (e.g., $p < .01$ rather than $p < .05$) or to use adjustments in the critical probability level that are based on the number of statistical comparisons made (e.g., Bonferroni). However, this increases the likelihood of failing to detect and report significant differences that are genuine but at lower levels of statistical probability (i.e., type II errors). Because these data represent an early stage of investigation with new instruments in this population (MMPI-2 rather than MMPI, QOLIE-89), we considered type II errors to be as serious as type I errors, chose not to use any experiment-wise alpha adjustment on our results, and considered any statistical results with probability levels of less than .05 to be significant. Results from this early stage of comparisons can then form the basis of more hypothesis-specific studies on different samples, and replication and extension studies can demonstrate the degree that these results capitalize on chance-specific factors.

Minnesota Multiphasic Personality Inventory 2

Results of the two groups on the MMPI-2 are presented in Table 12.1. Significant group effects were present on scale F (infrequency scale; $p = .0054$),

TABLE 12.1
Minnesota Multiphasic Personality Inventory 2 Means (and Standard Deviations) for Patients with Non-Epileptic Seizures and Patients with Epilepsy

Scale	NES	Epilepsy	p Level
Lie scale	57.8 (9.6)	54.4 (10.7)	.2151
Infrequency scale	66.2 (16.1)	58.6 (14.4)	.0054
K scale	44.9 (10.8)	44.8 (15.6)	.9789
Scale 1 (hypochondriasis)	73.3 (12.6)	62.9 (11.4)	.0013
Scale 2 (depression)	72.6 (3.7)	63.9 (11.5)	.0239
Scale 3 (hysteria)	75.8 (14.1)	60.8 (12.3)	.0001
Scale 4 (psychopathic deviate)	59.7 (12.4)	55.6 (10.6)	.1664
Scale 5 (masculine/feminine)	49.9 (10.7)	49.2 (10.5)	.8014
Scale 6 (paranoia)	63.2 (17.2)	58.4 (12.9)	.2149
Scale 7 (psychasthenia)	68.8 (16.2)	61.0 (13.8)	.0473
Scale 8 (schizophrenia)	70.2 (15.8)	64.7 (14.1)	.1526
Scale 9 (hypomania)	55.9 (13.8)	57.6 (10.7)	.5928
Scale 0 (social introversion)	60.4 (10.2)	55.9 (12.1)	.1313

NES = non-epileptic seizure.

scale 1 (hypochondriasis; p = .0013), scale 2 (depression; p = .0239), scale 3 (hysteria; p = .0001), and scale 7 (psychasthenia; p = .0473). No other MMPI-2 scale differed between groups. The mean two-point code type for epilepsy patients was two to eight, and the mean two-point code type for NES patients was one to three.

Quality of Life in Epilepsy 89

Results of the two groups on the QOLIE-89 are presented in Table 12.2. Significant group effects were present on health perceptions (p = .0036), physical function (p = .0014), role limitations–physical (p = .0008), pain (p = .0002), work/driving/social function (p = .0063), health discouragement (p = .0045), seizure worry (p = .0295), and the QOLIE summary score (p = .0022). In each case, patients with NES rated the quality of their life lower than did the patients with epilepsy. Interestingly, four of the seven scales on which the groups differ were from the generic component of the RAND scale, with the remaining three differences present on the epilepsy-targeted scales. Thus, the major differences reported by these cohorts of patients were related more to general health and to specific effects of seizures on quality of life.

To explore the potential utility of these measures in group discrimination, we submitted data obtained from both scales to a stepwise discriminant analysis. The first variable entered into the equation was scale 3 (hysteria) from the MMPI-2. The second variable entered into the equation was health discouragement. No other MMPI-2 or QOLIE-89 scale provided

TABLE 12.2
Quality of Life in Epilepsy 89 Means (and Standard Deviations) for Patients with Non-Epileptic Seizures and Patients with Epilepsy

	NES	Epilepsy	p Level
Epilepsy targeted			
Seizure worry	39.2 (9.3)	45.6 (11.9)	.0295
Medication effects	45.9 (9.2)	49.0 (10.5)	.2384
Health discouragements	37.0 (10.6)	45.2 (10.8)	.0045
Work/driving/social function	36.1 (7.2)	43.1 (10.6)	.0063
Cognitive			
Language	44.6 (13.2)	47.7 (10.6)	.3084
Attention/concentration	41.3 (13.9)	47.2 (12.0)	.0776
Memory	43.6 (11.7)	47.5 (10.2)	.1624
Mental health			
Overall quality of life	40.5 (12.2)	45.8 (11.6)	.0900
Emotional well-being	42.0 (12.2)	48.1 (11.9)	.0564
Role limitations–emotional	45.3 (11.8)	49.1 (10.7)	.1978
Social isolation	36.0 (9.4)	38.5 (7.9)	.2616
Social support	46.3 (10.9)	45.2 (9.0)	.6544
Energy fatigue	42.0 (12.6)	48.1 (11.4)	.0536
Physical health			
Health perceptions	40.1 (9.5)	48.0 (10.5)	.0036
Physical function	35.6 (14.0)	47.1 (12.8)	.0014
Role limitations–physical	38.4 (9.9)	47.8 (10.6)	.0008
Pain	35.7 (12.6)	46.8 (9.7)	.0002
Overall			
Summary score	38.6 (11.4)	48.2 (11.7)	.0022

NES = non-epileptic seizure.

unique information for the discriminant function. The discriminant function based on these two variables correctly classified 76% of the NES patients and 71% of the epilepsy patients. When using a jackknife procedure in which the discriminant function is based on the data for all subjects except the patient being classified, a slight decrease in the classification percentage of NES patients was observed, from 76% to 72%, with no change in the classification of epilepsy patients.

Discussion

These results confirm previous findings that many NES patients can be discriminated from patients with epilepsy based on certain MMPI-2 scales, namely, scales 1 (hypochondriasis) and 3 (hysteria), with the magnitude of difference being greater for scale 3.

Examination of the QOLIE-89 factor groupings is informative. Of the four general factors present in the scale, the most consistent group differences were present on those scales that assessed the role of physical health on quality of life. All four of these scales (health perception, physical function, physical role limitations, and pain) produced significant group differences at a high level of statistical significance (each scale ≤.0014). As suggested by the group MMPI-2 differences and the overall shape of the group MMPI-2 profile, NES patients present as being physically ill, with frequent reports of pain (e.g., back pain, headache). Furthermore, a tendency exists in this group of patients toward development of physical symptoms in response to stress consistent with a somatoform diagnosis. However, in contrast to patients with less depression who are more likely to develop conversion symptomatology, patients with similar MMPI-2 profile types do not present with the "everything is okay" orientation. Thus, findings that NES patients describe overall poor health, poor physical function, limitations imposed on physical function, and pain are consistent with the MMPI-2 results. Interestingly, the four scales that comprise the physical health factor appear in the generic core of the SF-36.

Group differences were present for three of four scales that were epilepsy specific (seizure worry, health discouragement, work/driving/social function), although the magnitude of effect for seizure worry was less ($p = .0295$) than for other significant QOLIE-89 subtest comparisons (all significant at $p = .0063$ or better). No difference in medication effects was seen, a finding that is somewhat surprising because most of the non-NES patients were undergoing evaluation for anterior temporal lobectomy and would be expected to be receiving a greater number of medications at higher dosages.

These findings examining epilepsy-specific quality of life issues may be related to disease chronicity. The mean age of seizure onset differed in these two groups, with the epilepsy patients developing their habitual seizure pattern on average at 13.4 years (SD = 12.5) and NES patients developing their seizures at 28.8 years (SD = 15.3). Thus, although epilepsy patients report significant epilepsy effects on work/driving/social function (second lowest QOLIE scale), these limitations are well known to the patient with chronic epilepsy. In contrast, someone with a recent onset of paroxysmal spells is suddenly faced with the implications that restricted driving can produce on daily functioning and quality of life. Similarly, the more recent diagnosis of "seizures" may make NES patients feel more discouraged.

To investigate this possibility, we performed another series of analyses, but restricted the age of onset to 18 years or younger. Despite the smaller sample size, producing less statistical power, the MMPI-2 differences remained on scale 1 ($p < .04$) and scale 3 ($p < .0001$); no group difference on work/driving/social function, seizure worry, or health discouragement was found. Differences remain on QOLIE scales of physical function, role limitations–physical, pain, and the summary quality of life measure. No other QOLIE scale differences were present.

The lowest QOLIE scale for NES patients was for social isolation (T = 36.0). However, this was also the lowest subtest present in the epilepsy patient group (T = 38.5), and no statistically significant differences were noted between groups.

An important consideration is the realization that perhaps the major thrust of personality testing and assessment of quality of life issues is not likely directly related to the diagnostic efficacy of these tests, which is analogous to the situation in neuropsychology in the 1980s when neuropsychologists played a prominent role in evaluating whether a patient might be considered to have brain damage. Presently, the use of advanced neuroimaging has largely replaced the need for neuropsychological assessment to perform evaluations for the diagnosis of organicity and, rather, in most circumstances current evaluations are designed to assess the cognitive and behavioral correlations of known and documented brain pathology.

Thus, in this context, the success of personality assessment, psychosocial testing, and quality of life testing should not be solely considered based on the ability of these measures to accurately discriminate group membership. Because patients who develop NES earlier in life have fewer quality of life complaints than do patients with NES onset after age 18 years, accurate and early diagnosis can likely contribute significantly to improved quality of life in NES patients and provides one justification for the expense associated with extensive video-EEG monitoring. Early and accurate NES diagnosis, associated with higher reported quality of life, may ultimately translate into the need for fewer medical services, such as emergency room visits and so forth, associated with NES episodes.

References

1. Croog SH, Levine S, Testa MA, et al. The effects of antihypertensive therapy on the quality of life. N Engl J Med 1986;314:1657–1664.
2. Vickrey BG, Hays RD, Rausch R, et al. Qulaity of life of epilepsy surgery patients as compared with outpatients with hypertension, diabetes, heart disease, and/or depressive symptoms. Epilepsia 1994;35:597–607.
3. Hermann BP, Wyler AR, Ackerman B, Rosenthal T. Short-term psychological outcome of anterior temporal lobectomy. J Neurosurg 1989;71:327–334.
4. Devinsky O, Thacker K. Nonepileptic seizures. Neurol Clin 1995;13:299–319 (updated Epilepsia 1989;30:339–347).
5. Wilkus RJ, Dodrill CB. Factors affecting the outcome of MMPI and neuropsychological assessments of psychogenic and epileptic seizure patients. Epilepsia 1989;30:339–347.

CHAPTER 13

Part Summary: Psychological and Neuropsychological Evaluation of the Patient with Non-Epileptic Seizures

Carl B. Dodrill and Mark D. Holmes

The chapters in this section have introduced several issues of importance with respect to the psychological and neuropsychological evaluation of patients with non-epileptic seizures. This overview focuses on two of these: the use of neuropsychological tests to differentiate between patients with epilepsy and patients with non-epileptic seizures, and the use of personality and adjustment inventories to make the same distinction. In addition, new data are presented from the authors' own laboratory, and efforts are made to draw conclusions that will stand the test of time.

Neuropsychological Performance and Non-Epileptic Seizures

Several of the authors in this section have rightfully raised the question about the possible usefulness of tests of mental abilities in differentiating persons with non-epileptic seizures from those with epilepsy. The rationale for this line of thinking is easily understood. Individuals with epilepsy have an organic brain disorder that may have a continuing impact on functioning, even between seizures. Persons with non-epileptic seizures have disorders, which are primarily psychiatric or behavioral in origin, and no compromise in brain functions is therefore necessarily implied. Neuropsychological tests are sensitive to brain damage, and it therefore stands to reason that patients with epilepsy may well perform more poorly on neuropsychological tests than patients with non-epileptic seizures.

Literature Review

Despite the reasonableness of the rationale just offered for finding cognitive differences between non-epileptic and epileptic patients, such differences have not always been discovered. In one early paper,[1] for example, it was noted that patients with non-epileptic seizures were neither more intelligent nor less impaired neuropsychologically than a matched group of patients with epilepsy. A second study[2] found that patients with non-epileptic seizures were less impaired cognitively than persons with epilepsy, but the epileptic seizure group was also less well educated. The critical importance of education was demonstrated in a third study in which it was shown that non-epileptic patients performed better on cognitive tests when they were better educated but that when education was controlled, all or nearly all of the differences disappeared.[3] A fourth paper reported cognitive impairment in 16 of 20 persons with non-epileptic seizures.[4] A fifth investigation showed no cognitive differences between small but intensively studied non-epileptic and epileptic seizure groups.[5] A sixth report noted no differences in intelligence between non-epileptic patients and temporal lobe surgery candidates, but the non-epileptic patients had a superior performance over the surgery candidates on some tests of memory.[6] However, no differences were found between epileptic and non-epileptic patients in an additional investigation of both intelligence and neuropsychological functions.[7] A small number of perceptual tests were reported in an eighth study, with a tendency for non-epileptic patients to make more errors than epileptic patients.[8] Finally, non-epileptic seizure patients performed similarly to surgical patients on the recall but less well on the recognition portion of a verbal memory task, perhaps because of a reluctance to guess or due to denial.[9]

In summary, for these nine studies in the literature, no general neuropsychological superiority of non-epileptic patients to people with epilepsy has been demonstrated when these individuals are matched for critical variables such as age, gender, and education. Small differences on measures of perception and memory have been found that sometimes favored non-epileptic patients over epilepsy surgery candidates[6] and which at other times favored the epilepsy surgery candidates.[7,8]

Why do the non-epileptic patients not consistently outperform matched patients with epilepsy? One explanation, offered in the first of these studies,[1] is that patients with non-epileptic seizures very commonly have positive neurologic histories. In that particular study, 80% of the non-epileptic patients in fact had events in their histories that were likely to have impacted the functioning of the nervous system, including head injuries, brain surgeries, infectious disorders, birth trauma, and combinations of these and similar events. It may be that persons with compromises in brain functions are less able to cope with stressors in everyday life and that they are therefore more likely to develop emotional disorders such as those that often underlie non-epileptic seizures.

Original Investigation

Despite the studies just cited, the data presented by the other authors in this section again raise the possibility that patients with non-epileptic seizures may be distinguishable from those with epilepsy by cognitive measures. Because of this, data were assembled to see if this question could be answered more definitively than has been possible heretofore with a large group of patients. In particular, 100 patients were found who had undergone video-electroencephalographic (EEG) monitoring at the Regional Epilepsy Center of the University of Washington and who had demonstrated multiple non-epileptic attacks that were said to be typical of the spells reported before their hospitalizations. This sample of 100 is intended as an inclusive sample for our center because it includes most of the non-epileptic cases from previous studies.[1,7] Each patient demonstrated behavioral unresponsiveness during the attacks with no EEG changes. The events were usually characterized by motor movements, such as bilateral shaking, body stiffening, out-of-phase bilateral body movements or pelvic thrusting, and/or by affective changes, such as moaning, weeping, affective changes symptomatic of panic, and forcible eye closure during the ictus. In no instances were there EEG changes characteristic of epilepsy, and no interictal EEG discharges occurred with any of these patients. Individuals with subjective spells only (reports of "seizures" but with no EEG or behavioral changes) were excluded.

A group of patients with epilepsy was formed for purposes of comparison. These individuals were all under evaluation for possible epilepsy surgery, and nearly all went to operation. In every instance, these persons demonstrated epileptic seizures accompanied by epileptiform patterns, and in no instance did they demonstrate attacks that appeared likely to represent non-epileptic seizures. A total of 100 cases were selected; they were chosen to match the 100 non-epileptic cases for age, gender, and years of formal education. Of the 100 surgical cases, 56 had epileptiform discharges recorded primarily over the left cerebral hemisphere, and 44 had discharges primarily from the right cerebral hemisphere.

TABLE 13.1
Basic Information on Groups of Non-Epileptic and Epileptic Patients

Variable		Non-Epileptic (n = 100)	Epileptic (n = 100)	Significance
Age	M	32.48	32.54	.962
	SD	9.79	7.74	
Education	M	12.24	12.31	.843
	SD	2.70	2.28	
Gender	Female	72	72	1.00
	Male	28	28	
Onset of attacks	M	22.97	13.54	.001
	SD	12.39	9.42	

M = mean; SD = standard deviation.

Basic information about data on the two groups is provided in Table 13.1. The only statistically significant difference found between the two groups was on the variable of age of onset of attacks and, as has been noted in many of these studies, persons with non-epileptic seizures had much later onsets of attacks than did individuals with epilepsy.

Data from the Wechsler Adult Intelligence Scale-Revised are presented in Table 13.2. Patients with non-epileptic seizures performed

TABLE 13.2
Means (and Standard Deviations) of Non-Epileptic (n = 100) and Epileptic (n = 100) Groups on the Wechsler Adult Intelligence Scale-Revised

Variable	Non-Epileptic	Epileptic	Significance
Verbal IQ	93.91 (14.62)	89.85 (10.53)	.038
Performance IQ	92.37 (14.42)	89.28 (11.37)	.122
Full Scale IQ	92.78 (14.51)	88.62 (10.28)	.031
Information	8.78 (3.05)	8.41 (2.69)	.364
Comprehension	9.81 (3.05)	8.95 (2.78)	.038
Arithmetic	8.17 (2.88)	8.57 (2.63)	.306
Similarities	9.45 (2.89)	8.91 (2.61)	.167
Digit Span	8.94 (3.05)	8.65 (2.91)	.492
Vocabulary	9.70 (3.08)	8.66 (2.66)	.011
Digit Symbol	8.03 (2.56)	7.57 (2.78)	.225
Picture Completion	9.06 (2.72)	8.70 (2.61)	.341
Block Design	8.89 (2.62)	8.99 (2.59)	.785
Picture Arrangement	9.18 (2.84)	8.12 (2.24)	.004
Object Assembly	9.25 (2.96)	8.42 (2.60)	.037

TABLE 13.3
Mean Scores (and Standard Deviations) of Non-Epileptic (n = 100) and Epileptic (n = 100) Groups on the Neuropsychological Battery for Epilepsy

Variable	Non-Epileptic	Epileptic	Significance
Stroop I (secs)	105.18 (42.69)	110.90 (39.10)	.328
Stroop II-I (secs)	166.48 (61.67)	159.44 (56.67)	.405
WMS-I Logical Memory Immediate (total)	18.45 (6.30)	17.61 (6.68)	.360
WMS-I Visual Reproduction Immediate	8.63 (3.24)	8.75 (2.80)	.785
Perception examination, total errors	12.09 (15.00)	13.18 (13.14)	.639
Name writing (letters/secs)	.84 (.29)	.79 (.29)	.238
Category	43.08 (27.17)	47.80 (28.81)	.236
TPT, Total Time (mins)	18.59 (11.70)	22.22 (13.29)	.042
TPT, Memory	7.35 (1.72)	7.01 (1.55)	.149
TPT, Localization	3.77 (2.38)	3.05 (2.09)	.026
Seashore Rhythm	24.38 (4.58)	23.12 (4.28)	.047
Seashore Tonal Memory	21.20 (6.95)	19.05 (6.84)	.029
Finger Tapping, total	89.21 (14.12)	88.40 (13.53)	.679
Trail-Making Test, Part B (secs)	84.46 (48.36)	104.40 (64.16)	.014
Aphasia Screening, total errors	3.78 (4.64)	3.43 (3.40)	.544
Construct dyspraxia, rating*	1.20 (.92)	1.19 (.86)	.937
Percent of 16 scores outside normal limits	48.06 (24.71)	55.12 (26.60)	.053
Halstead Impairment Index	.44 (.27)	.50 (.28)	.113

TPT = Tactual Performance Test; WMS-I = Wechsler Memory Scale-I.
*Rating of constructional dyspraxia: 0 = none; 1 = questionable; 2 = mild; 3 = moderate; 4 = severe.

slightly better on this test than did epilepsy surgery candidates, with statistical significance achieved especially in the verbal area with this large sample. The variable best separating the groups (Picture Arrangement) was able to correctly classify 60% of patients when an optimal cutoff score was established (45% of the non-epileptic group had scores greater than 9, 76% of the epilepsy group had scores less than 10).

Attention is next turned to the results of the Neuropsychological Battery for epilepsy,[10] which is an expanded Halstead-Reitan battery with particular attention to the variables most relevant in epilepsy. Table 13.3

shows that in the 16 brain-sensitive test measures in this battery, patients with non-epileptic seizures performed better than the surgery group on 12, with statistically significant differences found on four, all of which favored the non-epileptic seizure groups. The most noticeable statistically significant difference was on part B of the Trail Making Test, in which a cutoff line between 79 and 80 seconds rendered a correct classification rate of 61% (66 of non-epileptic cases had scores lower than 80, 56 epilepsy cases had scores higher than 79).

In conclusion, for the question of differential neuropsychological abilities across non-epileptic and matched epileptic groups, it is evident that some slight differences exist that favor the non-epileptic patients. These differences are so slight, however, that they are of no practical use in assisting to make a differential diagnosis between these groups. Note is made that even the 60% accuracy rate is likely to shrink at least somewhat on cross-validation. Of likely greater significance is the fact that mental abilities for both the non-epileptic and the epileptic groups are below average and outside normal limits, as would have been readily evident had a normal control group been included. Thus, the key point is not that patients with non-epileptic seizures may have slightly worse scores on tests of abilities than persons with epilepsy. Rather, it is that both groups are on the low side of average intelligence, and both show mild but definite impairment in brain functions. This impairment is likely due to both the positive neurologic histories[1] frequently found in these cases and to maladaptive response styles.[8,9]

Emotional Adjustment and Non-Epileptic Seizures

The second part of this chapter deals with the use of personality and adjustment inventories to help in the differential diagnosis of epileptic and non-epileptic patients. There has been some dispute in the literature with respect to the value of tests such as the Minnesota Multiphasic Personality Inventory (MMPI) to differentiate between epileptic and non-epileptic patients. In fact, one review of the area is especially critical, saying that "no psychological profile appeared to be of help in the differentiation" of patients in epileptic and non-epileptic groups.[11] Such a conclusion is surprising in view of the fact that the authors have found that the MMPI is of definite value in daily clinical work with patients who have non-epileptic seizures. Clearly, a review of the literature is needed to determine whether or not personality inventories are of value in differentiating epileptic from non-epileptic cases and, if so, to what degree they can be relied on to make this differentiation. In this literature review, we focus on the MMPI exclusively because it is only rarely that other tests have been studied in attempting to differentiate between epileptic and non-epileptic patients.

Literature Review

All of the known literature on the MMPI and non-epileptic seizures is summarized in Table 13.4 except for those cases in which the same data set was presented on two or more occasions, whereupon, with a single exception due to new information presented,[3] it was cited only once. A total of 15 investigations appear here, and due to diversity in defining non-epileptic seizures and in establishing contrasting groups, a summary of all of these papers is somewhat challenging. Nevertheless, the conclusions were fundamentally positive from 11 studies[1,3,4,10,12–18] relative to the use of the MMPI to differentiate non-epileptic from epileptic patients. In contrast to the negative review of the area,[11] the investigators from these studies concluded that the MMPI was helpful even though imperfect in differentiating between non-epileptic and epileptic groups. Many of these investigators pointed out that their patients with non-epileptic seizures represented a heterogeneous sample, with various causes of their non-epileptic seizures likely, which no doubt relates to the fact that multiple elevations were commonly noted on the various MMPI scales even though the greatest elevations were typically observed on hysteria and schizophrenia. In general, the authors concluded that although the differential diagnosis problem is difficult, the MMPI was at least of some help in making this diagnosis.

The question should be raised about the four studies in which the investigators concluded that the MMPI had limited value.[5,19–21] Reasons are evident to the current authors why the MMPI may not have performed as well as anticipated in each of these studies. In the first of these,[5] the primary sample was a group of 12 patients who represented especially difficult diagnostic problems and for whom invasive electrodes had to be placed to determine if the attacks were epileptic or non-epileptic. This sample was thus highly atypical. A secondary sample in the same paper of surgical patients produced a "hit" rate of 71%, which other investigators considered to be of value but which these investigators thought to be poor. In the second study,[19] the non-epileptic patients selected had primarily motor manifestations to their attacks rather than affective components, and this restriction in subject selection no doubt resulted in reduced effectiveness of the MMPI, as was later shown.[3] The third investigation included a variety of patients with syncope, sleep disorders, migraine, and so forth, which were said to manifest non-epileptic "events" that other investigators would not include in a non-epileptic seizure group.[20] Finally, investigators in the fourth study[21] could not effectively differentiate non-epileptic and mixed (epileptic plus non-epileptic) patients with the MMPI, but because both of their groups had the same non-epileptic disorder, the differentiation between those groups using the MMPI would appear to be difficult. In short, all four studies used samples that were atypical in one respect or another, and results were not considered to be satisfactory.

TABLE 13.4
Summary of Studies of Patients with Non-Epileptic Seizures Using the Minnesota Multiphasic Personality Inventory (MMPI)

Investigator(s)	Subjects	Results and Rule Classification
Shaw (1996)	15 patients with non-epileptic attacks (13 also had epilepsy), 15 with epilepsy only, 15 "pseudoneurologic" patients; EEG monitoring not used.	Pseudoneurologic scale separated epileptic and mixed epileptic/non-epileptic groups with an uncross-validated hit rate of 83% overall; mixed group had somewhat poorer adjustment.
Finlayson and Lucas (1979)	13 adolescents with non-epileptic attacks from files indexed "seizure with conversion reaction"; EEG monitoring not used.	MMPI findings not presented in detail; unusual thought patterns most in evidence in combination with hysteroid tendencies; depression was variable.
Wilkus et al. (1984)	25 patients (84% women) with solely non-epileptic attacks, 25 patients (84% women) with solely epileptic attacks.	Configural rules set up that correctly classified 84% of all cases (80% of non-epileptic, 88% of epileptic).
Vanderzant et al. (1986)	19 patients (68% women) with non-epileptic attacks consisting only of loss of consciousness or bilateral motor activity; 20 patients (50% women) with generalized seizures selected from the clinic population; groups not matched for age or education.	Rules of Wilkus et al. (1984) correctly classified 61% of all cases (37% of non-epileptic, 88% of epileptic); diverse personalities emphasized with sampling differences across groups likely.
Henrichs et al. (1988)	31 with solely non-epileptic attacks (61% women), 113 with focal or generalized discharges (a consecutive series of cases with unequivocal findings).	Rules of Wilkus et al. (1984) correctly classified 72% of all cases (68% of non-epileptic, 73% of epileptic); concluded patients are heterogenous.
Barrash et al. (1989)	44 with solely non-epileptic attacks, 43 with epileptic and non-epileptic (83% women for both groups); non-epileptic events included physical problems with episodic behavioral manifestations, such as syncope, sleep disorders, migraine, etc.	Rules of Wilkus et al. (1984) correctly classified 70% of all cases (53% of non-epileptic, 79% of epileptic); found seven subtypes of MMPI profiles by cluster analysis; concluded patients are heterogenous.

Wilkus and Dodrill (1989)	Same patients as Wilkus et al. (1984); all patients classified according to extent of motor and affectual expression during typical attacks.	Non-epileptic patients with major affectual/minimal motor features to their spells were more disturbed on the MMPI than were patients with partial seizures; non-epileptic patients with minimal affectual/major motor features could not be distinguished on the MMPI from patients with generalized seizures.
Drake et al. (1992)	20 patients (95% women), 16 with some previous suggestion of epilepsy but with currently negative EEGs; most showed back arching and pelvic thrusting.	MMPIs available on 16 patients were elevated in 15 "conversion V" profiles (hypochodria and hysteria up, depression down) common, although no scores were given and no configural rules were applied.
Hermann (1993)	12 patients (83% women) with especially difficult diagnostic questions (non-epileptic seizures vs. epilepsy) that remained even after scalp monitoring; strip electrode implantation resulted in six diagnosed as having epilepsy and six as having non-epileptic seizures.	Rules of Wilkus et al. (1984) correctly classified approximately 50% of all cases (60% of non-epileptic, 39% of epileptic).
	92 patients (60% women) with intractable seizures of temporal origin; all had EEG monitoring, and none had suspected non-epileptic seizures.	Rules of Wilkus et al. (1984) correctly classified 71% of patients as epileptic (29% were classified as non-epileptic).
Dodrill et al. (1993)	23 patients (87% women) with non-epileptic seizures and 22 epilepsy surgery candidates (36% women); these patients had not been studied previously.	Rules of Wilkus et al. (1984) correctly classified 76% of all cases (70% of non-epileptic, 82% of epileptic).
Derry and McLachlan (1996)	24 patients (54% women) with non-epileptic seizures of which 13 were also said to have epilepsy; 115 patients (53% women) had epilepsy only.	The authors devised their own set of decision rules based on the new form of the MMPI (MMPI-2) with a 94% classification accuracy overall (92% for mixed, 94% for epilepsy).

(continued)

TABLE 13.4
Summary of Studies of Patients with Non-Epileptic Seizures Using the Minnesota Multiphasic Personality Inventory (MMPI) (Continued)

Investigator(s)	Subjects	Results and Rule Classification
Mason et al. (1996)	27 patients (78% women) with non-epileptic seizures and 27 patients (59% women) with epilepsy.	Rules of Wilkus et al. (1984) with adjustments for MMPI-2 rather than the MMPI correctly classified 65% of all cases (60% of non-epileptic, 70% of epileptic).
Connell and Wilner (1996)	21 patients (86% women) with non-epileptic seizures and 24 patients (63% women) with epileptic seizures.	MMPI-2 used along with biographic variables in a multivariate context; age at onset of attacks and the hysteria scale together best predicted group classification ($p < .0001$).
Warner et al. (1996)	58 patients (78% women) with non-epileptic seizures and 89 patients (63% women) with epilepsy.	Rules of Wilkus et al. (1984) were applied to MMPI-2 profiles with an accuracy rate of 74% overall (74% of non-epileptic, 74% of epileptic); Derry and McLachlan rules correctly classified 69% of all cases (71% of non-epileptic, 67% of epileptic).
Kalogjera-Sackellares and Sackellares (1997)	55 patients (84% female) had either non-epileptic seizures alone (N = 40) or non-epileptic seizures plus epilepsy (N = 15) as determined by records review; 43 cases had EEG monitoring.	Rules of Wilkus et al. (1984) applied to the "pure" group showed a 60% correct classification (rules do not apply to a mixed sample); basic MMPI scales did not differ across the two groups.

An objective evaluation of the results from the studies can be done with a configural rule approach. Although investigators occasionally developed their own unique MMPI scales or configural rules,[12,17] when configural rules were used, they were typically those of Wilkus et al.[1] These rules state that, among monitored patients, an MMPI profile is characteristic of non-epileptic seizures when one or more of the following apply: (1) Hysteria or hypochondriasis is 70 or higher and one of the two highest points, disregarding masculinity-femininity and social introversion; (2) hysteria or hypochondriasis is 80 or higher even though not among the two highest points; and (3) both hysteria and hypochondriasis are higher than 59, and both are at least 10 points higher than depression.

In nine studies the Wilkus et al. rules were applied to the patient groups evaluated.[1,5,14,16–21] It is important to note that this group includes all four negative studies, and thus it does not appear to be biased in the direction of finding unrepresentative positive findings. Of a total of 272 patients with non-epileptic seizures included in the nine studies, 174 (64%) were correctly classified using the Wilkus et al. (1984) rules. Of the 469 patients with epilepsy to whom the rules were applied, 352 (75%) were correctly classified by the rules. Overall, the correct classification rate for epileptic and non-epileptic subjects was 71% (Fisher's exact, $p = .0018$). This figure includes all negative studies in the literature and also some groups of patients for whom the diagnosis of non-epileptic seizures could be questioned, as well as some persons classified as "epileptic" based on histories rather than EEG monitoring. A reasonable statement about the configural rules (and the MMPI) is that it is able to classify approximately seven of 10 patients with either epileptic or non-epileptic attacks, or possibly slightly better when patients are carefully defined.

Summary and Recommendations for Future Work

The findings from the literature and an original investigation showed that patients with non-epileptic seizures only are very slightly more capable cognitively than matched persons with epilepsy. The difference is on the order of four IQ points, not a great enough difference on any variable to be of practical use in differentiating epileptic from non-epileptic patients. In the area of adjustment, the MMPI has been by far the most commonly used measure to distinguish between patients having epileptic and non-epileptic attacks. Such a test is imperfect and has a correct classification rate of 70%, or slightly better with careful definition of subject groups. It is nevertheless useful in day-to-day work with people with non-epileptic seizures.

For future work in this area, several areas are evident. Application of gender-specific rules to MMPI profiles has not been explored, but it might result in better classification rates. Such inventories also have not been applied prognostically in terms of relief from seizures, but they might be very useful in that context. The combination of personality variables with biodata variables such as age at onset of attacks is especially promising,[9] and it may in fact be one of the best ways to improve accuracy in differential diagnosis. Finally, there are now indications that what patients do during the non-epileptic attacks is related to their personality profiles,[3] and considering these behaviors could significantly improve correct classification rates or at least identify those cases in which a correct classification is unlikely.

References

1. Wilkus RJ, Dodrill CB, Thompson PM. Intensive EEG monitoring and psychological studies of patients with pseudoepileptic seizures. Epilepsia 1984;25:100–107.
2. Sackellares JC, Giordani B, Berent S, et al. Patients with pseudoseizure: intellectual and cognitive performance. Neurology 1985;35:116–119.
3. Wilkus RJ, Dodrill CB. Factors affecting the outcome of MMPI and neuropsychological assessments of psychogenic and epileptic seizure patients. Epilepsia 1989;30:339–347.
4. Drake ME, Pakalnis A, Phillips BB. Neuropsychological and psychiatric correlates of intractable pseudoseizures. Seizure 1992;1:11–13.
5. Hermann BP. Neuropsychological Assessment in the Diagnosis of Non-Epileptic Seizures. In AJ Rowan, JR Gates (eds), Non-Epileptic Seizures. Boston: Butterworth–Heinemann, 1993;221–232.
6. Novelly RA. Cerebral Dysfunction Non-Epileptic Seizure Disorders. In AJ Rowan, JR Gates (eds), Non-Epileptic Seizures. Boston: Butterworth–Heinemann, 1993;233–242.
7. Dodrill CB, Wilkus RJ, Batzel LW. The MMPI as a Diagnostic Tool in Non-Epileptic Seizures. In AJ Rowan, JR Gates (eds), Non-Epileptic Seizures. Boston: Butterworth–Heinemann, 1993;211–219.
8. Binder LM, Salinsky MC, Smith SP. Psychological correlates of psychogenic seizures. J Clin Exp Neuropsychol 1994;16:524–530.
9. Bortz JJ, Prigatano GP, Blum D, Fisher RS. Differential response characteristics in nonepileptic and epileptic seizure patients on a test of verbal learning and memory. Neurology 1995;45:2029–2034.
10. Dodrill CB. A neuropsychological battery for epilepsy. Epilepsia 1978; 19:611–623.
11. Kuyk J, Leijten F, Meinardi H, et al. The diagnosis of psychogenic non-epileptic seizures: a review. Seizure 1997;6:243–253.
12. Shaw DJ. Differential MMPI performance in pseudo-seizure epileptic and pseudo-neurologic groups. J Clin Psychol 1966;22:271–275.
13. Finlayson RE, Lucas AL. Pseudoepileptic seizures in children and adolescents. Mayo Clin Proc 1979;54:83.

14. Henrichs TF, Tucker DM, Farha J, et al. MMPI indices in the identification of patients evidencing pseudoseizures. Epilepsia 1988;29:184–187.
15. Derry PA, McLachlan RS. The MMPI-2 as an adjunct to the diagnosis of pseudoseizures. Seizure 1996;5: 35–40.
16. Mason SL, Mercer K, Risse GL, Gates JR. Clinical utility of the MMPI-II in the diagnosis of non-epileptic seizures (NES). Epilepsia 1996;37(Suppl 5):18.
17. Connell BE, Wilner AN. MMPI-2 distinguishes intractable epilepsy from pseudoseizures: a replication. Epilepsia 1996;37(Suppl 5):19.
18. Warner MH, Wilkus RJ, Vossler DG, et al. MMPI-2 profiles in differential diagnosis of epilepsy vs. psychogenic seizures. Epilepsia 1996;37(Suppl 5):19.
19. Vanderzant CW, Giordani B, Berent S, et al. Personality of patients with pseudoseizures. Neurology 1986;36:664–668.
20. Barrash J, Gates JR, Heck DG, et al. MMPI subtypes among patients with nonepileptic events. Epilepsia 1989;30:730–731.
21. Kalogjera-Sackellares D, Sackellares JC. Personality profiles of patients with pseudoseizures. Seizure 1997;6:1–7.

PART III

Cognitive and Psychological Functioning and Treatment of the Pediatric Patient with Non-Epileptic Seizures

CHAPTER 14

Cognitive Features and Predisposing Factors in Children with Psychogenic Seizures

Ann Hempel

The psychosocial and cognitive characteristics of children and adolescents who manifest psychogenic non-epileptic seizures have not been studied extensively. Available research suggests that, as in the adult patient population, psychogenic seizures (PS) are more common among females than males.[1] Intellectual functioning is often satisfactory,[2,3] and outcome in terms of reduction or cessation of PS appears more favorable in children and adolescents than in adult-onset patients.[4]

In both children and adults, PS are often believed to represent one manifestation of conversion disorder and, as such, are assumed to be unintentionally produced.[5] In theory, a conversion reaction represents either repression of unacceptable emotions or dissociation from distressing experiences,[5,6] and for this reason somatic symptoms are presumed more likely to occur at times of stress.[7] Although a history of sexual abuse often is reported in adults who manifest PS,[6] more commonly cited stressors in children have included family conflict, academic difficulties, and poor peer relationships.[1,5]

In early studies, a number of other variables were considered associated features of conversion disorder. These included secondary gain, presence of a model for the symptom, and lack of concern about the symptom (*la belle indifférence*).[7] There is general agreement that, although not uncommon, these features do not occur with sufficient regularity in these patients to be considered diagnostic of conversion disorder.[8,9]

The degree to which the adult or child PS patient is aware of the association between stressors and symptom production, or might be consciously producing the symptoms, is difficult, if not impossible at times, to ascertain (R. Martin, personal communication, 1996). Nevertheless, even if a child or adolescent patient's symptoms are suspected of being under voluntary control, the individual is given the benefit of the doubt to maintain a therapeutic alliance between the medical staff and patient and to provide a face-saving opportunity for the patient to relinquish the symptom.[10] Besides conversion disorder, some authors propose that PS might also represent a manifestation of other conditions, such as dissociative disorder, factitious disorder, malingering, or an anxiety disorder, or reinforced behavior patterns.[8,11]

The aim of this chapter is to review previous studies on PS and conversion disorder in children and adolescents to identify common features of this group and to present new data on the cognitive functioning and psychosocial background of a sample of PS patients.

Literature Review

Of the 14 studies that examined psychosocial variables in children and adolescents (Table 14.1), only three[3,12,13] focused specifically on PS. The majority of patients in all three studies had a history of significant stress. Stressors were most commonly related to family or parental situations,

TABLE 14.1
Studies on Psychosocial Variables in Conversion Disorder/Psychogenic Seizures in Children

Psychogenic seizures
Gross and Huerta (1980)[14]
Lancman et al. (1994)[4]
Wyllie et al. (1990)[13]
Conversion disorder
Goodyer (1981)[15]
Grattan-Smith et al. (1988)[10]
Jensen and West (1945)[16]
Kotsopoulos and Snow (1986)[17]
Lehmkuhl et al. (1989)[18]
Leslie (1988)[19]
Maisami and Freeman (1987)[20]
Maloney (1980)[21]
Siegel and Barthel (1986)[22]
Steinhausen et al. (1989)[23]
Volkmar et al. (1984)[24]

TABLE 14.2
Demographic Variables

Variable	Range	Mean	Number of Studies	Aggregate n
Percent female	53–81	69	13	491
Mean age of onset	10.5–13.8 yrs	12.4 yrs	3	79
Mean age at evaluation	10–15 yrs	12.7 yrs	12	476
Mean duration of symptoms at time of evaluation	7–9 mos	8.6 mos	4	145
Percent of conversion disorder patients evidencing PS	0–68	27	12	436

PS = psychogenic seizures.

such as divorce, parental medical problems, parental alcohol dependence, and parent-child conflict. Other stressors included peer relationship problems, sexual abuse, and grief. Psychiatric diagnosis of the patient was presented in two studies.[4,14] In these studies, the diagnosis of conversion disorder was most common, although other disorders, such as depression, obsessive-compulsive disorder, and psychosis, were sometimes seen. One study[4] reported that the majority of patients evidenced "normal" intelligence (IQ = 80–120).

For this chapter, the results of all 14 studies were aggregated to provide overall estimates of psychosocial and demographic features of pediatric patients who evidence conversion disorder or PS. As indicated in Table 14.2, the majority of patients were female and, on average, symptoms first appeared and patients were seen for an evaluation during early adolescence. The earliest reported age of onset ranged from 5 to 8 years, suggesting that the presentation of psychogenic symptoms is not restricted to older children and adolescents. In the 11 studies on conversion disorder, 27% of the aggregate sample manifested PS as their principal symptom. In the three studies that reported specifically on children who presented with PS, several of the more common symptom manifestations included unresponsiveness or fainting, tremor, and thrashing of all extremities. A small minority of patients displayed lateralized movements.

Table 14.3 presents combined results of the studies with respect to variables that historically have been considered characteristic of conver-

TABLE 14.3
Prevalence of Associated Features of Conversion Disorder

Feature	Range (%)	Percent of Patients	Number of Studies	Aggregate n
Any stressor present	46–97	77	5	221
Model for symptom	15–66	36	6	242
Somatic symptom preceded by illness or injury	40–55	50	2	82
La belle indifférence	19–55	34	4	129
Secondary gain	—	41	1	27

sion disorder. The majority of patients across studies had a history of a significant stressor. In a large proportion of patients, the somatic symptoms were preceded by illness or injury, or there was a model for the symptom. Secondary gain and indifference toward the symptoms were often noted, but not in the majority of patients.

Some of the more common stressors that appeared to be associated with symptom onset and maintenance are presented in Table 14.4. Surprisingly, parental psychopathology emerges as one of the most common stressors among the studies that included this variable in their investigations, whereas sexual abuse was reported in only 17% of the total aggregate sample. The prevalence of a history of sexual abuse in pediatric conversion disorder/PS patients appears no greater than in the general population; approximately 27% of women and 16% of men who were questioned in a large national survey reported a history of some form of sexual abuse.[25] The combined results of the studies suggest that family

TABLE 14.4
Prevalence of Stressors Associated with Conversion Disorder or Psychogenic Seizures

Stressor	Range (%)	Percent of Patients	Number of Studies	Aggregate n
Psychopathology in family	25–85	64	6	289
School problems	5–90	36	5	176
Family discord	20–56	34	5	181
Peer relationship problems	10–47	30	4	149
Family structure not intact	19–38	28	4	112
Sexual stressor	2–70	17	6	184
Parental alcohol dependence	5–25	16	3	55

TABLE 14.5
Prevalence of Comorbid Psychiatric Disorders

Disorder	Range (%)	Percent of Patients	Number of Studies	Aggregate n
Any comorbid diagnosis	20–80	38	3	76
Disruptive behavior disorder	5–53	35	3	65
Psychosis	—	16	1	19
Depression	7–25	10	4	108
Anxiety	2–30	10	5	128
Personality disorder	2–11	5	2	61

discord, peer relationship problems, and school problems appear to occur more frequently than sexual abuse in pediatric conversion disorder/PS patients.

Table 14.5 presents the prevalence of comorbid psychiatric diagnoses. Psychosis was reported in only a single study,[13] and in that study three of 19 patients evidenced that disorder. Anxiety disorders and depression were each observed in 10% of the aggregate patient sample, which does not exceed the population estimates in this age group.[26,27] This finding suggests that child or adolescent patients with conversion disorder or PS are not disproportionately affected by affective or anxiety disorders.

Minnesota Epilepsy Group Study Methods

Records of 20 patients with non-epileptic seizures were reviewed retrospectively. The patients had been admitted to the epilepsy unit for long-term video-electroencephalographic (EEG) monitoring to clarify the nature of possible seizure episodes. Patients were included in the present study if their typical events were recorded, the events did not have an EEG correlate, and the episodes were not due to non-epileptic physiologic events. Patients whose paroxysmal events represented a manifestation of a disruptive behavior disorder (e.g., tantrums, aggression, difficulty in sustaining attention) were excluded. Of the 20 PS patients, six also had a history of epileptic seizures.

The records of 27 epilepsy patients, who served as a comparison group, were reviewed. These individuals had undergone long-term video-EEG monitoring and neuropsychological testing to evaluate their candidacy for epilepsy surgery. All patients were found to have a clearly lateralized left or right seizure focus.

As indicated in Table 14.6, the majority of PS patients were female, which is consistent with previous studies. In contrast, an equal number of

TABLE 14.6
Minnesota Epilepsy Group Demographic and Background Variables

Variable	Psychogenic Seizures (n = 20)	Epileptic Seizures Only (n = 27)	p
Female (%)	70	52	NS
Mean age of onset	12.2 yrs	5.3 yrs	<.001
Mean age at evaluation	13.6 yrs	11.4 yrs	.04
Mean duration of symptoms at time of evaluation	15.8 mos	74.3 mos	<.001

NS = not significant.

males and females was present in the epilepsy patient sample. On average, PS patients were significantly older at the time of symptom onset, were slightly older at the time of inpatient evaluation, and had experienced symptoms for a shorter duration than patients evaluated for epileptic seizures. This sample of PS patients is similar to those described in previous studies with respect to age of onset and age at evaluation, both of which were commonly observed during early adolescence.

As in previous studies, it was common for PS patients to have experienced a stressor in some form (Table 14.7). The majority of patients appeared to receive secondary gain, such as avoidance of stressful situations (e.g., school), increased attention from parents, and increased caring and concern from peers and teachers. Indifference toward the symptoms was not commonly observed, although few patients expressed a high level of distress or concern about their symptoms. Many patients had a model for the symptoms, such as a family member or acquaintance at school. For some patients, their symptoms did not appear to mimic the symptoms of someone known to them; however, not uncommonly, a patient had family members whose health complaints of another nature were prominent. In approximately one-third of the patients, onset of the symptoms was preceded by illness or injury. From the standpoint of behavior learning theory,

TABLE 14.7
Minnesota Epilepsy Group Prevalence of Associated Features of Conversion Disorder

Feature	Percent of Psychogenic Seizure Patients
Any stressor present	100
Secondary gain	70
Model for symptoms	60
Preceded by illness or injury	35
La belle indifférence	30

TABLE 14.8
Minnesota Epilepsy Group Percentage of Psychogenic (n = 20) and Epileptic (n = 27) Seizure Patients Experiencing Each Stressor

Stressor	Psychogenic (%)	Epileptic (%)	p
Parent/child conflict	45	11	.02
Parental psychopathology	10	0	NS
Parental alcohol dependence	10	11	NS
Marital discord	30	0	NS
School problems	70	67	NS
Peer relationship problems	45	37	NS
Sexual stressor	10	4	NS
History of parental divorce/separation	35	26	NS
High parental or child expectations	25	4	NS
Below-average IQ	40	44	NS

NS = not significant.

it is possible that secondary gain (e.g., avoidance of aversive situations, increased social support) resulting from an initial illness or injury might have served to reinforce the patient's expression of psychological distress through physical symptoms.

The incidence of various possible stressors was reviewed for both epilepsy and PS patients (Table 14.8). A number of stressors were common to both groups, including school problems, peer relationship problems, and below-average IQ. Parent-child conflict (e.g., lack of support from an emotionally unavailable parent, frequent disagreements with a step-parent) was more commonly noted in families of PS patients than epilepsy patients; however, because family relationship issues were not always explored at length during evaluations of epilepsy patients, the incidence of family discord in the comparison group may have been underestimated. Sexual abuse and parental alcohol dependence were infrequently reported in both the PS and epilepsy groups, consistent with previous studies on patients with PS or conversion disorder. Parental psychopathology also was infrequently observed in the psychosocial backgrounds of PS patients in this study, contrary to findings reported in six previous studies.

Several PS patients who displayed satisfactory (average to high average) intellectual functioning and academic performance denied experiencing significant interpersonal or scholastic difficulties. Some of these individuals were described as exceptionally good students by the parents when, in fact, on formal testing they displayed average skills. Others were described as gifted in other ways, such as in music or drama, but the extent of their talent could not be verified by objective evidence (e.g., awards, being offered prestigious opportunities in the arts), raising the possibility that parents exaggerated their children's abilities and may have unintentionally communicated unrealistically high expectations to them. Two patients had a history of

TABLE 14.9
Minnesota Epilepsy Group Percentage of Psychogenic (n = 20) and Epileptic Seizure (n = 27) Patients Evidencing a Comorbid Psychiatric Diagnosis

Diagnosis	Psychogenic (%)	Epileptic (%)
Any comorbid diagnosis	60	52
Disruptive behavior disorder	45	48
Anxiety disorder	15	0
Depression	15	4

accomplishment and were unable to continue their previously high level of performance despite holding themselves to very high standards. High expectations by the parent or child were more often evident in the PS than in the epilepsy group, but this difference was not statistically significant.

Although the incidence of individual stressors was often comparable for PS and epilepsy patients, PS patients were found to experience a significantly greater number of stressors on average. The mean number of reported stressors was 1.3 for epilepsy patients and 2.5 for PS patients.

As indicated in Table 14.9, the majority of both PS and epilepsy patients received a comorbid psychiatric diagnosis. However, the diagnosis was more likely to reflect a form of disruptive behavior disorder (e.g., attention deficit hyperactivity disorder, oppositional defiant disorder) than an "internalizing" disorder such as anxiety or depression. Consistent with results of previous studies, incidence of anxiety and depression in the PS patient group did not appear to exceed population base rates.

Measures of intellectual functioning and academic achievement were administered to the majority of PS and epilepsy patients. Mean verbal, performance, and full-scale IQ scores for all groups fell in the lower end of the average range, suggesting that PS patients are not necessarily more likely than epilepsy patients to evidence satisfactory cognitive functioning (Table 14.10). As indicated in Table 14.8, a large proportion of both epilepsy and PS patients obtained IQ scores that were low average or below.

TABLE 14.10
Minnesota Epilepsy Group Intellectual Functioning of Psychogenic (n = 13), Epileptic and Psychogenic (n = 5), and Epileptic (n = 27) Seizure Patients

Scale	Psychogenic	Psychogenic + Epileptic	Epileptic
VIQ	93	93	90
PIQ	96	95	94
FSIQ	94	94	91

FSIQ = full-scale intelligence quotient; PIQ = performance intelligence quotient; VIQ = verbal intelligence quotient.

TABLE 14.11
Minnesota Epilepsy Group Number of Grade Levels below Grade Placement for Psychogenic (n = 16) and Epileptic (n = 26) Seizure Patients

Subject	Psychogenic	Epileptic	p
Reading	1.49	.89	NS
Mathematics	1.75	.86	.07
Written language	2.3	1.4	.10
Average underperformance	1.8	1.0	.09

NS = not significant.

In addition to an increased number of stressors, PS patients displayed a greater severity of academic underachievement, on average, than those in the epilepsy sample. That is, PS patients performed below grade placement by more grade levels than did epilepsy patients, although this group difference fell short of statistical significance (Table 14.11). Only a minority of both PS and epilepsy patients (31%) demonstrated skills that were commensurate with grade placement in all academic areas. Psychogenic seizure patients (56%) were only slightly more likely than epilepsy patients (38%) to underachieve by two grade levels in at least one subject area.

Discussion

Results of the Minnesota Epilepsy Group study are consistent with the foregoing research on conversion disorder and PS in children in a number of respects. The PS patient is usually female and often experiences nonepileptic seizures during early adolescence. Stressful experiences are common and sometimes numerous and may serve to precipitate unexplained physical symptoms in children and adolescents who do not have the means to cope with stressors in more adaptive ways. As in previous studies, we found that a history of sexual abuse was the exception rather than the rule. Patients who evidenced PS were more likely to have a history of family discord, school problems, or inadequate peer support than to report traumatic events. The commonly held belief that PS patients are usually cognitively intact is not supported by our data. Rather, it is a minority of patients who do not evidence academic underachievement or slightly below-average intellectual functioning. Not infrequently, their academic struggles are associated with an attention deficit or other disruptive behavior disorder rather than an internalizing disorder such as anxiety or depression.

Results of this study are also consistent with previous research with respect to associated features of conversion disorder. We found that PS patients often received secondary gain in some form for their symptoms, had a model for their symptoms, and showed a general lack of concern about their health or its impact on their life circumstances. However, as in previous research, these characteristics did not occur with sufficient consistency to support their use as diagnostic criteria.

These data and those of other investigators have a number of clinical implications. One is that children who present with PS should be evaluated not only for psychological disorders but also for learning or other cognitive problems. Given the high rate of psychosocial stressors in the lives of PS children and adolescents, the clinician should be prepared to inquire not only about a history of abuse, but also about family relationships, peer relationships, and academic functioning. When patients and their families respond to interview questions with a cursory reassurance that everything is fine, a more extensive psychological assessment consisting of objective and projective personality measures may still be warranted. A family interview by a skilled psychotherapist to assess family dynamics should also be considered in the event that dysfunctional patterns of interaction may be contributing to the maintenance of the symptom(s).[28]

References

1. Goodyer IM. Epileptic and pseudoepileptic seizures in childhood and adolescence. J Am Acad Child Psychiatry 1985;24:3–9.
2. Lowman RL, Richardson LM. Pseudoepileptic seizures of psychogenic origin: a review of the literature. Clin Psychol Rev 1987;7:363–389.
3. Metrick ME, Ritter FJ, Gates JR, et al. Nonepileptic events in childhood. Epilepsia 1991;322–328.
4. Lancman ME, Asconape JJ, Graves S, Gibson P. Psychogenic seizures in children: long term analysis of 43 cases. J Child Neurol 1994;9:404–407.
5. Wyllie E, Friedman D, Lüders H, et al. Outcome of psychogenic seizures in children and adolescents compared with adults. Neurology 1991;742–744.
6. Brunquell PJ. Psychogenic seizures in children. Int Pediatr 1995;10:47–54.
7. Bowman ES. Etiology and clinical course of pseudoseizures. Psychosomatics 1993;34:333–342.
8. Friedman SB. Conversion symptoms in adolescents. Pediatr Clin North Am 1973;20:873–882.
9. Ford CV, Folks DG. Conversion disorders: an overview. Psychosomatics 1985;26:371–386.
10. Grattan-Smith P, Fairley M, Procopis P. Clinical features of conversion disorder. Arch Dis Child 1988;63:408–414.
11. Williams DT, Mostofsky DI. Psychogenic Seizures in Childhood and Adolescence. In TL Riley, A Roy (eds), Pseudoseizures. Baltimore: Williams & Wilkins, 1982;169–184.
12. Gates JR, Mercer K. Nonepileptic events. Semin Neurol 1995;15:167–174.

13. Wyllie E, Friedman D, Rothner D, et al. Psychogenic seizures in children and adolescents: outcome after diagnosis by ictal video and electroencephalographic recording. Pediatrics 1990;85:480–484.
14. Gross M, Huerta E. Functional convulsions masked as epileptic disorders. J Pediatr Psychol 1980;5:71–79.
15. Goodyer I. Hysterical conversion reactions in childhood. J Child Psychol Psychiatry 1981;22:179–188.
16. Jensen RA, West AD. Conversion hysteria in children. Lancet 1945;65:172–175.
17. Kotsopoulos S, Snow B. Conversion disorders in children: a study of clinical outcome. Psychiatr J Univ Ottawa 1986;11:134–139.
18. Lehmkuhl G, Blanz B, Lemkuhl U, et al. Conversion disorder (DSM-III 300.11): symptomatology and course in childhood and adolescence. Eur Arch Psychiatry Neurol Sci 1989;238:155–160.
19. Leslie SA. Diagnosis and treatment of hysterical conversion reactions. Arch Dis Child 1988;63:506–511.
20. Maisami M, Freeman JM. Conversion reaction in children as body language: a combined child psychiatry/neurology team approach to the management of functional neurological disorders in children. Pediatrics 1987;80:46–52.
21. Maloney MJ. Diagnosis hysterical conversion reactions in children. J Pediatr 1980;97:1016–1020.
22. Siegel M, Barthel R. Conversion disorders on a child psychiatry consultation service. Psychosomatics 1986;27:201–204.
23. Steinhausen H, Aster M, Pfeiffer E, Gobel D. Comparative studies of conversion disorders in childhood and adolescence. J Child Psychol Psychiatry 1989;30:615–621.
24. Volkmar FR, Poli J, Lewis M. Conversion reaction in childhood and adolescence. J Am Acad Child Psychiatry 1984;23:424–430.
25. Finkelhor D, Hotaling G, Lewis IA, Smith C. Sexual abuse in a national survey of adult men and women: prevalence, characteristics, and risk factors. Child Abuse Neglect 1990;14:19–28.
26. Reynolds WM. Depression. In VB Van Hasselt, M Hersen (eds), Handbook of Adolescent Psychopathology. New York: Lexington Books, 1995;297–348.
27. Kearney CA, Silverman WK. Anxiety Disorders. In VB Van Hasselt, M Hersen (eds), Handbook of Adolescent Psychopathology. New York: Lexington Books, 1995;435–464.
28. Minuchin S, Baker L, Rosman BL, et al. A conceptual model of psychosomatic illness in children. Arch Gen Psychiatry 1975;32:1031–1038.

CHAPTER 15

Characteristics of Pediatric Non-Epileptic Seizure Patients: A Retrospective Study

Jane Williams and Mitzie L. Grant

The advent of video-electroencephalographic (EEG) monitoring has dramatically improved the ability to diagnose non-epileptic seizures (NES) in pediatric patients. Increased identification of these children has raised unanswered questions concerning the prevalence and etiology of non-epileptic events during childhood.

Several potential risk factors for the development of NES have been identified from pediatric studies. The occurrence of a high rate of family or personal stress,[1,2] a predominance of females diagnosed with the disorder,[1,2] and a family history of epilepsy[1] have all been reported. Research with children diagnosed with conversion disorder, whose symptoms frequently involve NES, suggests other possible risk factors, including academic failure,[3] psychiatric impairment of a parent,[3,4] exposure to a personal model for conversion symptoms,[5,6] associated symptoms involving pain,[5,6] abnormal familial situation or family dysfunction,[5] and secondary gain.[5] In two interesting pediatric case studies, Silver[7] attributes conversion disorder involving NES to a stress reaction resulting from unrecognized and untreated learning disabilities.

Studies with adults diagnosed with NES suggest additional risk factors that may be applicable to a pediatric population. These include a history of sexual abuse,[8,9] associated neurologic dysfunction such as traumatic head injury or neurologic disease,[9,10] and epileptic seizures co-occurring with non-epileptic events.[10]

Comparison of risk factors in children and adults indicates that developmental differences may exist in the etiology and course of NES. Children with NES may not demonstrate the severity of psychopathology and personality disorder that are frequently reported in the adult literature, because childhood causes may be more related to an anxiety reaction to stress or to externalizing (acting out) behaviors in the child.[1,2,8,11]

Age-based differences in occurrence may be present, although prevalence rates in childhood are unknown. Wyllie et al.[12] indicate that NES are rare in a pediatric population younger than 10 years of age because these children are more likely to have movement disorders, syncope, hyperventilation, parasomnias, and breath-holding spells. Goodyer[11] states that NES become more common in adolescence. However, Duchowny et al.[13] report a high incidence of NES presenting as rhythmic movements or staring in children younger than 10 years of age who were believed to have epileptic seizures before video-EEG monitoring.

Developmental differences in occurrence may also exist based on gender. Wyllie et al.[12] report that the preponderance of females may become more prevalent in adulthood.

At present, information is limited concerning the psychological and biological characteristics of children who experience non-epileptic events. Identification of risk factors associated with NES in childhood may contribute to increased understanding of the pathogenesis of this disorder. Knowledge of psychosocial and biological factors that contribute to the evolution and maintenance of NES symptoms may result in a more effective treatment approach as well as preventive practices for children at risk for development of this disorder.

Research Study Subjects and Procedures

A retrospective study was conducted to examine possible risk factors associated with NES in a pediatric population. All patients had been hospitalized between 1990 and 1995 at Arkansas Children's Hospital for video-EEG monitoring due to possible seizures. To be included in the study, the child had to experience typical clinical episodes that occurred without concomitant electrographic changes during monitoring. These behavioral events and EEG recordings were reviewed by one of five pediatric neurologists and were diagnosed as being NES.

Charts were reviewed for 97 patients. Of the initial reviews, 17 patients were excluded because no typical events were recorded, seven were excluded due to an inability to clearly determine a diagnosis, and eight were excluded because their events were the direct result of a physical precipitant; the latter group included five children with movement disorders, one child with a true tremor, one child with autistic blinking, and one child with syncope from orthostatic hypertension. Both inpatient and

TABLE 15.1
Demographic Characteristics

Characteristic	Number	Percent
Gender (n = 65)		
Female	42	65
Male	23	35
Ethnicity (n = 65)		
White	54	83
Black	11	17
Payment source (n = 65)		
Commercial insurance	31	48
Medicaid	20	31
Self-pay	14	21
Parental educational level (n = 74)		
Maternal (n = 40)		
Less than twelfth grade	5	12
GED or high school graduate	21	53
Vocational training or college	14	35
Paternal (n = 34)		
Less than twelfth grade	8	24
GED or high school graduate	15	44
Vocational training or college	11	32
Family structure (n = 65)		
Intact family	32	49
Reconstituted family	10	15
Single-parent family	15	23
Lives with extended family members	5	8
Institutional care	3	5

GED = General Education Development.

outpatient records were examined for the remaining 65 children and adolescents, who ranged in age from 7 to 17 years (mean = 13 years, 3 months; standard deviation = 30 months).

The chart reviews were conducted by two clinical psychologists. If information was not directly written in the medical record for an individual subject on any psychosocial or medical factor, then the variable was coded as "unknown."

Results

Demographic Characteristics

There was a female predominance of patients (65%), and ethnicity was reflective of the population within the region (Table 15.1). Financially, the reported payment source indicated that the majority of children (79%) were medically covered. After the diagnosis of NES, the parents of at least 20 patients (31%) applied for Social Security disability payments.

The majority of parents were high school graduates or had additional education beyond a high school diploma. The children generally lived with immediate or extended family members, with few requiring institutional care. Twenty-six of the children (40%) were first-born offspring in the family.

Developmental History

Developmental history was ascertained for 54 children. Within this group, 40 children (74%) reached developmental milestones within the normal range or at an advanced rate, seven children (13%) had normal motor development with delays in speech and language skills, and seven children (13%) had delayed development.

School Performance and Placement

Of the 50 children and adolescents whose school placement was determined, 24 of the patients (48%) were in regular education classes. For the remaining subjects, a high rate of learning problems was reported, with 20 children (40%) diagnosed with learning disabilities and six children (12%) diagnosed with mental retardation. Speech and language services were provided for six children.

After the onset of the NES, changes in school attendance were reported for 22 children (34%). These changes consisted of decreased attendance for 13 children and nine children who no longer attended school or were being home-schooled due to the episodes.

School performance was reported to have declined for 20 children (31%) before or after the onset of the non-epileptic events. Continuing school difficulties that were long-standing in nature were reported for nine additional children. At least 20 of all the children and adolescents (31%) diagnosed with NES had repeated one or more grades.

Psychosocial Stressors

Psychosocial stressors were defined as life-changing events, including death of a family member, sexual or physical abuse, forced separation from family members, physical disability or illness of a parent, major illnesses, financial stressors, moving, relational difficulties, and significant family conflict. No significant stressors were reported for 14 children (22%). Twenty-two children (34%) had experienced one significant stressor, 12 children (18%) had experienced two stressors, 10 children (15%) had experienced three stressors, five children (8%) had experienced four stressors, and two children (3%) had experienced five stressors.

Only 39 of the total sample of children and adolescents were queried concerning sexual or physical abuse. Of the respondents, 21 patients (54%) denied any abuse, 12 patients (31%) had been sexually abused, and six patients (15%) had been physically abused. None of the patients reported both sexual and physical abuse.

Psychiatric History

Psychiatric status before the present hospitalization was determined for 53 children. Of these, 26 children (49%) had received no previous psychiatric diagnosis; 10 children (19%) had been diagnosed with externalizing disorders, including attention deficit hyperactivity disorder, oppositional defiant disorder, or conduct disorder; 10 children (19%) had been diagnosed with affective disorders, including anxiety and depression; five children (9%) had been diagnosed with both externalizing and internalizing disorders; one child (2%) had been diagnosed with an adjustment disorder; and one child (2%) had been diagnosed with an affective disorder with psychotic features. None of the children or adolescents had been diagnosed with major psychosis or personality disorders. At least one previous hospitalization for psychiatric care was reported for eight children, and six patients had a history of suicidal ideation or attempted suicide.

Family psychiatric history was elicited for 44 patients. Ten of the families denied any psychiatric difficulties. Of the remaining families, eight had members with mood disorders; 13 had members with externalizing behaviors, including problems with impulse control, addictions, and antisocial behavior; seven had members with mood disturbance and externalizing behaviors; one had members with psychosis; four had members with mood disturbance, addictions, and psychosis; and one had members with addictions and psychosis. A history of substance abuse was reported in 16 families (36%).

Medical and Neurologic History

Non-neurologic medical history indicated that 16 children (25%) had no reported health problems; 39 children (60%) had a history of minor health difficulties, such as chronic otitis media requiring pressure equalization tubes, pneumonia, appendicitis, heart murmur, or urinary tract infections; and 10 children (15%) had major physical conditions that altered their lifestyle or were life threatening, such as multiple sclerosis, leukemia, juvenile arthritis, cardiomyopathy, or severe physical trauma. Within the total sample, 14 children (22%) had physical conditions that are known to be reactive to stress, such as asthma, ulcers, gastrointestinal disorders or pain, and chronic fatigue.

Of the total population, 34 children (52%) had no known neurologic disorder. A history of epileptic seizures was reported for 14 children (22%), mild to severe head injuries were noted for 10 children (15%), static or degenerative encephalopathy was indicated for five children (8%), and movement disorders not related to their non-epileptic events were noted

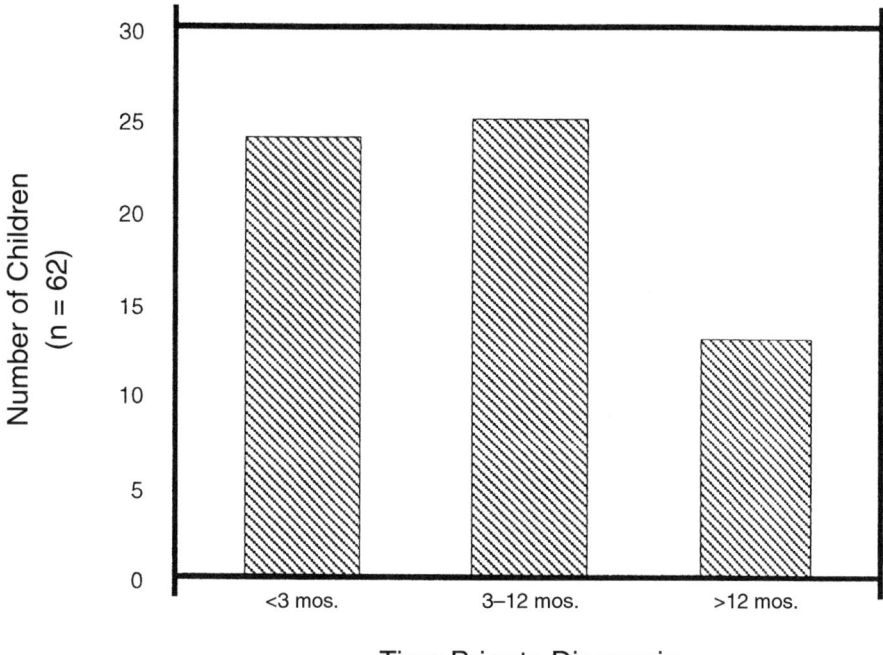

FIGURE 15.1. The majority of children experienced the onset of non-epileptic seizure symptoms within the year before diagnosis.

for two children (3%). Twenty-four children reported experiencing significant headaches. A familial history of seizure disorder was indicated for immediate or extended family members for 35 patients (54%).

Non-Epileptic Seizure Diagnostic and Treatment Course

The occurrence of NES in the identified population was characterized by a recent onset and high rate of frequency before diagnosis. The majority of children and adolescents (79%) had experienced initial events less than 1 year before hospitalization (Figure 15.1), and most of the patients (84%) were reporting daily to weekly episodes (Figure 15.2). A dramatic increase in frequency was described for 21 children immediately before video-EEG monitoring. On hospital admission, 41 children (63%) were taking anticonvulsants.

During the hospitalization, completed psychiatric consultations were recorded for 39 patients. Of the patients seen in consultation, 11 received a primary diagnosis of a somatoform disorder, including nine with conversion disorder and two with somatization disorder; 11 children received a primary diagnosis of an affective disorder, including anxiety or depression, or both;

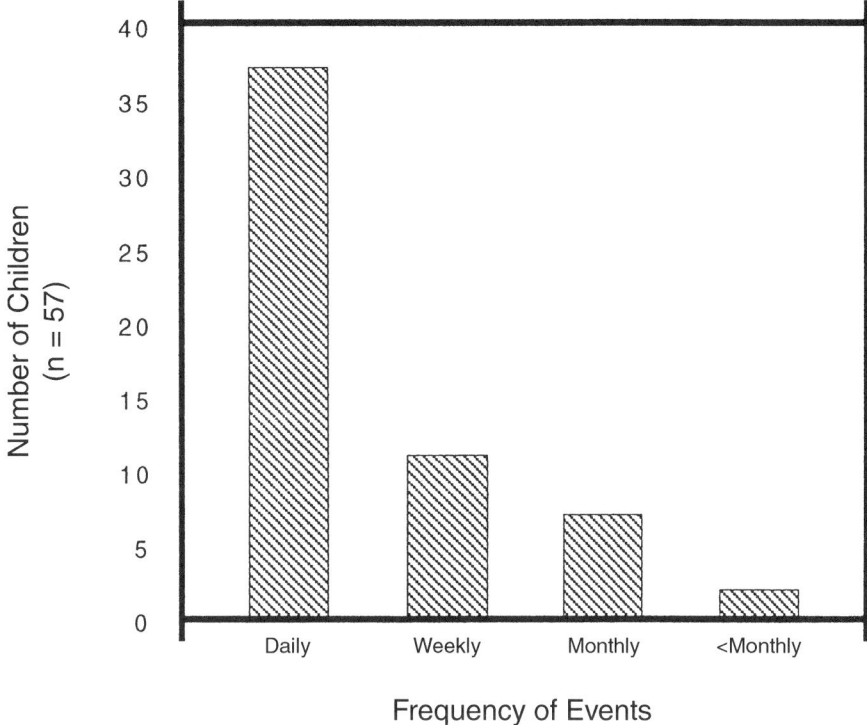

FIGURE 15.2. The majority of children were experiencing a high rate of episodes before diagnosis of non-epileptic seizure.

six children received a primary diagnosis of psychological factors affecting physical condition; two children received a primary diagnosis of oppositional defiant disorder; one child received a primary diagnosis of impulse control disorder; and one child received a primary diagnosis of psychosis. In addition to the primary diagnosis, numerous children received either a secondary diagnosis or several rule-out diagnoses. The psychiatrists were unable to make a definitive diagnosis for seven children who received from three to five rule-out diagnoses each.

Outpatient psychiatric care was recommended by the neurologist or psychiatrist for 48 children (74%), and eight children (12%) were referred for inpatient psychiatric care. Referrals back to the neurologist or primary care physician were made for five patients (8%), two patients (3%) returned to institutional care, and two patients (3%) did not receive a referral.

In contrast to the 41 children who were taking anticonvulsants on admission, only 11 children (17%) with co-occurring epileptic seizures continued on anticonvulsants at discharge. Psychotropic medications were prescribed for 17 children after hospitalization.

Discussion

Results from this retrospective study would suggest a high level of heterogeneity concerning social, psychological, and biological characteristics of pediatric NES patients. The distribution of socioeconomic status would indicate that these children come from a wide range of backgrounds and that NES patients are not confined to any particular socioeconomic level. Because nearly two-thirds of the children came from two-parent families, the occurrence of NES did not appear to be more prevalent in single-parent homes.

The age range of children with NES was broad. Almost one-half of the children (46%) were between 7 and 12 years of age, and the remainder were adolescents (54%). This finding contrasts with the belief that NES rarely occurs in younger children and suggests the need for establishing prevalence rates in the pediatric population.

Similar to other pediatric studies, a preponderance of females was diagnosed with NES, although the percentage was relatively smaller than that reported for adults.[12]

One of the most striking findings was the high rate of learning disorders and educational difficulties experienced by these children. More than 50% had been diagnosed with learning disabilities or mental retardation and were receiving special education services. For more than one-third of the children, school attendance had dropped or the child was no longer attending school because of NES symptoms. A substantial number of children reported increased difficulty in school functioning that appeared to be associated with NES, occurring either before the onset of the events or with the advent of NES.

In agreement with other studies concerning the occurrence of NES, a high rate (78%) of psychosocial stressors was found. There was also evidence to support a positive history for sexual or physical abuse in some of these children. The recentness of the psychosocial stressors could not always be ascertained, and some stressors, such as unresolved grief or sexual abuse, were more remote. However, anecdotal information in the medical charts suggested that the reported stressors were having a continued effect on family and personal functioning.

Psychiatric history for the children was diverse. Although psychiatric hospitalization and suicidal ideation were reported for some children and adolescents, one-half of the population had no previous diagnosis of psychiatric disorder. For the children who had a psychiatric diagnosis before the onset of NES, an equal number were diagnosed with externalizing versus internalizing disorders. In agreement with previous findings, these children and adolescents did not have a high rate of psychosis or personality disorders.[1,2,8,11] However, psychiatric difficulties for immediate and extended family members, including both externalizing behaviors and mood disorders, were noted. More than one-third of the families had members with substance abuse problems.

Health status in the children diagnosed with NES varied from an absence of physical conditions to major health problems. The children had not experienced an excessive number of physical problems involving pain or conditions reactive to stress, as noted in studies of children with conversion disorder, although headaches were a common complaint. Documented neurologic conditions were frequent among the children. More than one-fifth of the children had been diagnosed with epileptic seizures, and one-fourth had documented neurologic conditions. More than one-half of the children had an immediate or extended family member diagnosed with a seizure disorder.

Outcome findings would suggest that the pathogenesis of NES is likely multifactoral and may involve a complex interaction of social, biological, and psychological factors. The recentness of onset, high frequency of events, and significant number of stressors found in this population would support the hypothesis that NES may be a maladaptive coping mechanism that develops in reaction to stressful life events or untreated affective disorders. This coping style may be reinforced by avoidance of painful or frustrating situations. On the other hand, some children develop NES from a more behavioral paradigm in which the child models symptoms from observation in the environment and receives secondary gain from increased attention for physical symptoms or avoidance of activities that he or she finds aversive, such as school attendance or interacting with peers. An unexpected finding suggests possible reinforcement for parents in the form of anticipated financial gain. From a cognitive perspective, some children with learning and language disorders who have difficulty expressing affect through a verbal modality may develop NES symptoms as a means of expressing emotional distress in a nonverbal manner. Additionally, a genetic predisposition or physiologic factors may play a role in the expression of this disorder, as noted in the prevalence of neurologic symptoms and family occurrence of epilepsy.

Although the high percentage of children who receive anticonvulsants before video-EEG monitoring would indicate that NES is difficult to diagnose, the characteristics identified in this study may be useful for the physician to consider when NES is suspected. The heterogeneity of this population suggests the need for further research concerning the influence and interaction of psychosocial and biological variables. Most information reported to this point has been obtained from retrospective chart reviews. Prospective studies involving a multifactorial model would provide more insight concerning the direct and indirect influence of variables in the development of this disorder.

Acknowledgments

Appreciation is expressed to the Departments of Neurology, Psychiatry, and Social Work at Arkansas Children's Hospital for their assistance with this study.

References

1. Lancman ME, Asconape JJ, Graves S, Gibson PA. Psychogenic seizures in children: long-term analysis of 43 cases. J Child Neurol 1994;9:404–407.
2. Wyllie E, Friedman D, Rothner AD, et al. Psychogenic seizures in children and adolescents: outcome after diagnosis by ictal video and electroencephalographic recording. Pediatrics 1990;85:480–484.
3. Lehmkuhl G, Blanz B, Lehmkuhl U, Braun-Scharm H. Conversion disorder (DSM-III 300.11): symptomatology and course in childhood and adolescence. Eur Arch Psychiatr Neurol Sci 1989;238:155–160.
4. Steinhausen HC, Aster M, Pfeifter E, Gobel D. Comparative studies of conversion disorders in childhood and adolescence. J Child Psychol Psychiatry 1989;30:615–621.
5. Siegel M, Barthel RP. Conversion disorders on a child psychiatry consultation service. Psychosomatics 1986;27:201–208.
6. Graftan-Smith P, Fairiey M, Procopis P. Clinical features of conversion disorder. Arch Dis Child 1988;63:408–414.
7. Silver L. Conversion disorder with pseudoseizures in adolescence: a stress reaction to unrecognized and untreated learning disabilities. Am Acad Child Psychiatry 1982;21:508–512.
8. Bowman ES. Etiology and clinical course of pseudoseizures. Psychosomatics 1993;34:333–342.
9. Alper K, Devinsky O, Perrine K, et al. Nonepileptic seizures and childhood sexual and physical abuse. Neurology 1993;43:1950–1953.
10. Krumholz A, Niedermeyer E. Psychogenic seizures: a clinical study with follow-up data. Neurology 1983;33:498–502.
11. Goodyer IM. Epileptic and pseudoepileptic seizures in childhood and adolescence. J Am Acad Child Psychiatry 1985;24:3–9.
12. Wyllie E, Friedman D, Lüders H, et al. Outcome of psychogenic seizures in children and adolescents compared with adults. Neurology 1991;41:742–744.
13. Duchowny MS, Resnick TJ, Deray MJ, Alvarez LA. Video EEG diagnosis of repetitive behavior in early childhood and its relationship to seizures. Pediatr Neurol 1988;4:162–164.

CHAPTER 16

Psychological Assessment and Treatment of Non-Epileptic Seizures and Related Symptoms in Children and Adolescents

Audrey M. W. Ho, Marilyn J. Ransby, Kevin Farrell, Mary Connolly, and Nancy Thornton

Although children and adolescents with psychogenic non-epileptic seizures (NES) represent a relatively small proportion of referrals to psychological services, they present with complex medical, psychological, and social needs that make disproportionate demands on professional time and hospital resources. Thus, several investigators have attempted to address questions about the differential diagnosis and nosology in this population.[1-4] In contrast, relatively few investigations have described or evaluated treatment programs for children and adolescents with NES.

Limited follow-up data are available on pediatric patients with conversion disorder, including those with NES. Some investigators report that many such patients emerge from psychiatric treatment free of the presenting symptom.[5,6] In other studies, however, no significant improvement was observed in treated patients,[7] or the interventions were so heterogeneous that the relative advantage of one treatment over another could not be systematically evaluated.[8] The research literature on treatment outcome is difficult to interpret because few investigators describe their treatment programs or assessment tools in sufficient detail to allow replication. Furthermore, measurement of treatment outcome is often limited to an easily quantified behavioral criterion such as symptom relief, which may not be the best indicator of long-term psychological health or of subsequent use of medical resources.

A report by Turgay[6] offers a relatively detailed treatment program description and evaluation. He studied 89 conversion disorder patients aged 5–17 years who received both family and individual therapy. Treatment was aimed at (1) reducing anxiety, (2) increasing "insight into the meaning of the symptoms," and (3) changing other troublesome behavioral patterns. Turgay used several theoretical approaches and addressed patient/family denial of the psychological aspects of the symptoms, provided education about conversion disorders, and facilitated identification of strengths and weaknesses in family functioning. Turgay did not find a significant correlation between initial symptom severity and treatment outcome but concluded that several child characteristics, including younger age, greater ego strength, and a capacity for insight, appeared to be associated with a more favorable treatment response. Other variables that seemed to be related to better outcome included cooperation of the child and family with the treatment team and an absence of serious family dysfunction.

Symptom Management Program at a Children's Hospital

The treatment approach at British Columbia Children's Hospital is holistic and eclectic. Multiple modalities are used in the assessment and treatment of NES, with the central focus being the child.

The symptom management program follows several theoretical models, including the general systems theory of Bertalanffy,[9] in which people are seen as members of a family system that is a subsystem of a larger social system. This view is consistent with Minuchin and Fishman's[10] approach to family therapy in that the child is a member of a nuclear and extended family system in which each family member plays a role in maintaining the homeostasis of the system and, in a dysfunctional family system, in maintaining the presenting problem.

Theoretical constructs from the psychodynamic approach serve as a framework for understanding the psychological underpinnings of NES. When homeostasis is threatened, such as by a significant life event, symptoms serve as communication to both the internal child and members of the child's system. A symptom also functions as a mechanism for resolving internal conflict between instinctual drives and social demands. The symptom may relieve anxiety by permitting a channel for expression, which elicits a caring response from the social system and gratifies the child's dependence needs. Helping the child to gain insight into the psychological dimensions of the symptoms is a central therapeutic aim.

The psychodynamic component of the assessment helps the patient or parents, or both, retrieve information related to relevant life events and stressors that may be obvious to the therapist but not to the family. Using the peeling of an onion as an analogy, we view the patient's symptoms as the outer layers of the onion and the most available. The recovery of memories of stressful experiences leads the assessment into the middle layers of the onion. If the child and family feel supported and are given license to emotionally experience traumatic events as stressful, then they will journey into their past and present emotional life, which is the core of the onion—the conflict.

The cognitive behavioral approach serves primarily as a treatment approach to help the child and parents cope with and change the illness condition. This approach might involve teaching a vocabulary for emotional expression, teaching them how to match body language with the emotional vocabulary terms, and practicing the use of emotional vocabulary while expressing their feelings and experiences.

The A-B-C triplet change model provides a framework for defining treatment gains. It defines improvement in affect (A), behavior (B), and cognition (C) as three goals of therapy. In the NES patient, awareness of psychological distress may be limited, and one goal is to increase the patient's and family's awareness of *affect* that is channeled through physical symptoms. Improvement in *behavior*, both in terms of a reduction in physical symptoms and an increase in use of coping skills (e.g., relaxation exercises), is another goal of treatment. Finally, treatment is aimed at increasing patients' and families' *cognitive* awareness of the underlying sources of distress and helping them to cognitively appraise events in more adaptive ways.

Table 16.1 illustrates the continuum of improvement in affect, behavior, and cognition that is observed over the course of treatment. At the beginning of treatment, the child and parents focus only on the symptoms but, as treatment proceeds, past memories come to the surface. This recognition of life events as being stressful leads to awareness of the connection between emotional and physical symptoms, followed by an appreciation of the importance of emotional life.

Preliminary Report on the Symptom Management Program

A retrospective chart review of 50 consecutive neurology referrals to the symptom management program from October 1993 to October 1995 served as the basis of this study. Four of the 50 patients were eliminated from the study due to treatment dropout (two patients), development of a psychotic disorder (one patient), or referral to mental health services elsewhere (one

TABLE 16.1
A-B-C Triplet Availability and Eventual Homeostasis

Level	Initial Presentation	Initial Intervention	Psychological Formulation and Treatment	Termination/Follow-Up
Affective	No matching emotions for traumatic experiences, ignoring the presence of emotion or lack of vocabulary for emotions	Aware of some emotions; realize emotion is being misplaced and acquire license to express emotions through assessment and treatment	Acknowledge the role of emotions under stressful circumstances; willingness to express oneself	Acknowledge the importance of emotional life, express emotions appropriately, experience a wide range of emotion
Behavioral	Focusing on symptoms and difficulty of functioning	Physiotherapy and relaxation exercise to relieve symptoms	Respect but de-emphasize symptoms	Symptoms serve as alarm to communicate stress
Cognitive	Little/no report of related life stressors	Recalling facts; a safe contained environment facilitates the recovery of painful experiences	Aware of the association between stress and physical symptoms	Be aware and attend to life stress; stress need not manifest via physical mode Homeostasis

patient). The symptoms of the remaining 46 children were divided into four categories: (1) NES; (2) gait problems, paralysis, and falls; (3) muscle weakness with severe pain; and (4) hysterical blindness and hand cramps. Some patients evidenced more than one type of symptom. The distribution of patients by symptoms, age, and gender is summarized in Table 16.2.

Description of the Assessment and Treatment Program

The psychological assessment serves four purposes: (1) to provide information to assist in the differential diagnosis; (2) to offer the patient opportuni-

TABLE 16.2
Distribution of Patients by Symptom, Age, and Gender

Symptoms	7–9 yrs		10–12 yrs		13–15 yrs		16–17 yrs	
	Male	Female	Male	Female	Male	Female	Male	Female
Seizures or convulsions	1	2	1	4	2	4	0	1
Motor symptoms (gait problems, paralysis)	0	3	1	5	1	3	0	1
Sensory symptoms (pain, weakness, numbness)	2	0	1	3	0	9	0	0
Mixed presentation (blindness, hand cramps)	0	0	0	0	0	2	0	0
Subtotal	3	5	3	12	3	18	0	2
Total	8 (17%)		15 (33%)		21 (47%)		2 (4%)	

ties to experience self-expression in a relaxed and nonthreatening environment and to feel the connection between the symptom presentations, associated emotions, and stressful events; (3) to assess the child's psychological coping skills; and (4) to prepare the child and family gradually for the possibility that a psychological intervention may be an essential component of the treatment plan.

A firm diagnosis of NES or conversion disorder is not required for referral to the symptom management program. We acknowledge that many investigators have concluded that a substantial proportion of children and adolescents referred for seizure assessments have comorbid epileptic and psychogenic seizure disorders.[3,7,11] However, the question of whether psychological conflicts or significant life stressors are antecedents or consequences of seizure behavior is often difficult to answer in the initial stages of the neurologic assessment. The concurrent investigation of organic and psychological factors can reduce the shock when the final diagnosis of NES is given; it also reduces the risk of commencing with psychological assessment of a child who has an organic basis for his or her symptoms.

An introduction to the mind-body connection is presented early in the program, emphasizing to the family that, even in conditions in which an organic etiology has been confirmed, psychological factors can exacerbate physical symptoms. It is also emphasized that even though the medical evaluations suggest that the condition is unlikely to have a neurologic origin, the medical team does not dismiss the importance or seriousness of the symptoms.

At each stage of the assessment-treatment process, resistance is anticipated in both children and their family members. Because significant resistance has been noted by several other groups of clinicians who have treated this population,[5,12] we deliberately plan for its inevitable interference with treatment progress. At significant milestones the psychologist takes a detour in the treatment plan to deal with the specific forms of resistance. The responses of parents may vary from watchful suspicion to overt anger and confrontational accusation. The child may become withdrawn or express anger and skepticism toward the psychological approach. At these junctures the therapist might try to reduce resistance by empathetically listening to their concerns and providing reassurance. Alternatively, other team members, particularly neurologists, can be enlisted as allies.

The first meeting usually is attended by both the child and family members as a unit. At that time, the rationale for a psychological approach is explained and the concept of the mind-body connection is reviewed. Stories about jungle animals and the fright-flight response often are told to demonstrate the physiologic aspects of stress. These are pediatric analogies for Maisami and Freeman's[5] peptic ulcer example for parents. During this initial meeting, the therapist acknowledges the seriousness of the symptoms and assesses the extent to which the patient and family are willing to accept a psychological intervention as an adjunct to the medical program. When parental resistance is encountered in the first or subsequent meetings, the therapist empathizes with their frustration and reassures them that the team is not overlooking the organic-physiologic aspect of the problem. If the parent does not readily offer consent for a psychological intervention, the therapist asks to see the parents alone for two reasons: (1) The child is not placed in the awkward position of facing mixed loyalties, and (2) the therapist can explore the parents' resistance and respond to their concerns. If parents are insistent on symptom relief yet denounce a psychological approach, an intervention that is not highly emotionally laden, such as assertiveness training for a child who is bullied at school, could be considered as a starting point to provide some symptom relief and to increase the parents' confidence in psychological approaches to treatment.

After consent to proceed is given by the parents, the therapist sees the child alone. During the first session with the child or adolescent, the therapist invites the patient to become a collaborator in the search for a solution that can lead to healing and symptom relief. After the child and therapist agree to work toward solving the mystery of the symptom and its origins, the symptom can be externalized to help relieve some of the anxiety associated with it and to aid the child in focusing on its symbolic meaning. One method of externalizing the symptom is to have the child

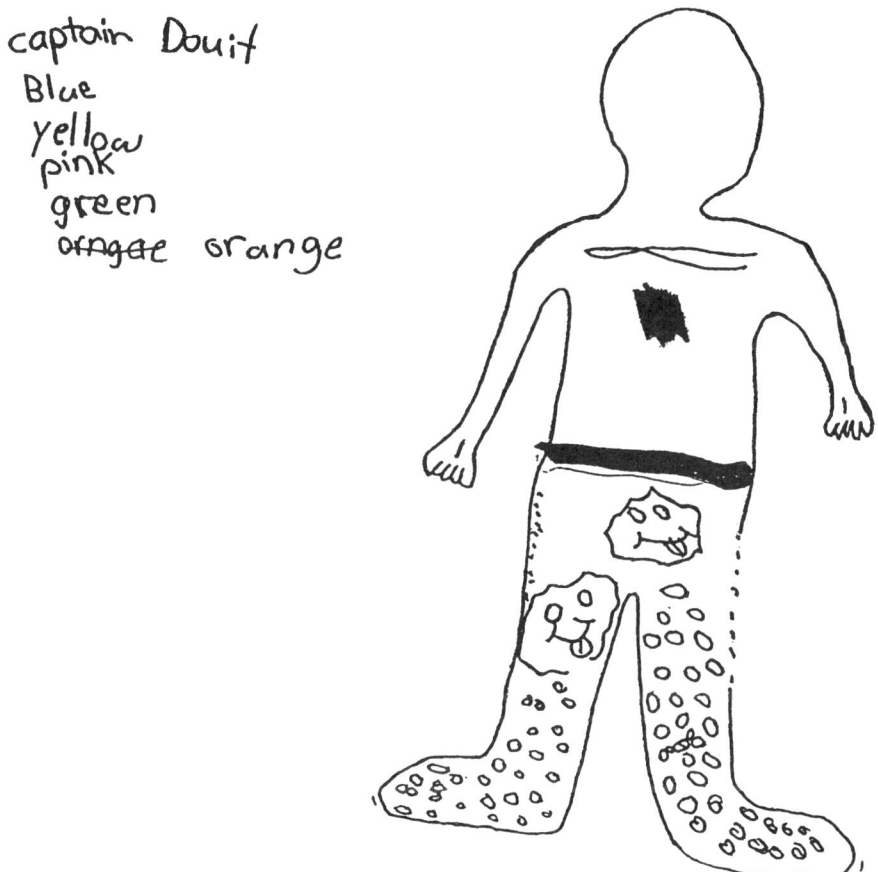

FIGURE 16.1. Externalizing control.

draw how he or she visualizes it. For example, one child who experienced leg weakness drew a picture of a hero, "Captain Douit" (Figure 16.1), who was appointed to capture the culprit, "Jelly Bean" (Figure 16.2), who caused her weakness. Another method of externalizing the symptom, which also serves as a gauge of symptom severity, involves a Likert scale analogue in which one hand of the child and one hand of the therapist are traced on paper and each finger is assigned a number from 1 to 10, with 10 representing the worst symptom severity and 1 representing the least severity (Figure 16.3). The child then rates the severity of his or her symptoms on the scale. The initial session can also be used to begin teaching the child symptom management techniques, such as muscle relaxation, to convey that the symptom is taken seriously and to help establish in the patient a sense of confidence and control over the symptom.

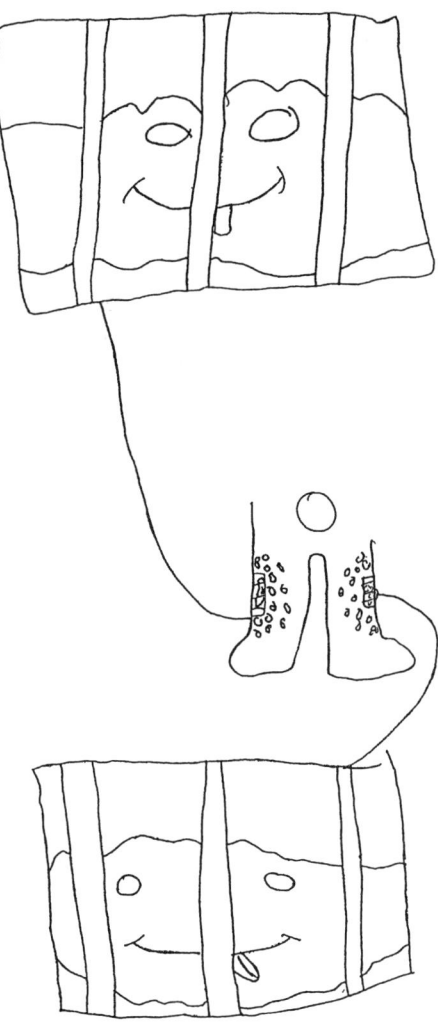

FIGURE 16.2. Externalizing heal-

Projective assessment can be used to obtain information about the child's psychological functioning that may not be apparent to the family or therapist. Projective testing can also facilitate emotional expression and help the child to become comfortable in discussing issues of an emotional nature. Examples of projective techniques include the following:

1. In the *button game*,[13–15] a large cookie tin filled with hundreds of buttons of various shapes and sizes is presented to the child. Initially, the child is asked to select one button representing himself or herself and each member of the family. The family constellation is defined by the child and may include pets, extended family members, or significant others. Then the child is asked to arrange the but-

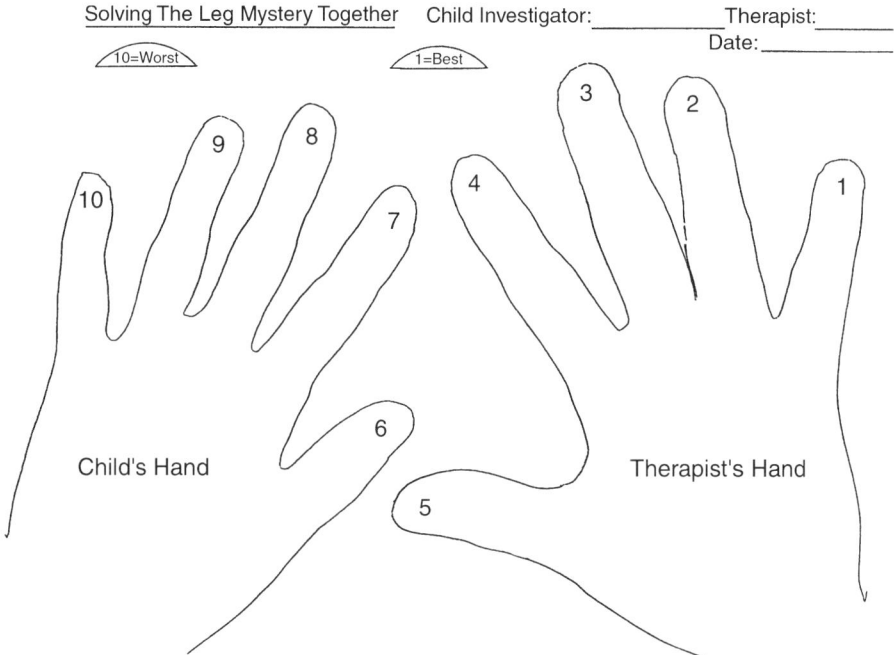

FIGURE 16.3. Symptoms severity scale.

tons in a pattern to show the relationships between and among family members. Some people in a family, the therapist explains, are very close to each other, and others may be far apart; some people seem to go together and some people don't. The child then arranges the buttons on a large sheet of white paper to show the family constellation from his/her perspective. The therapist next asks the child to explain the representation. Among the cases we have seen was a 10-year-old girl with NES who had an intense grief reaction. The girl arranged the buttons representing immediate family members, a deceased twin cat A, and the surviving but aging twin cat B in close proximity to each other (Figure 16.4). A button representing a lost dog was positioned away from the cluster of buttons. The patient began to grieve the loss of the dog and the deceased cat A with her mother and began to discuss her fear of the death of the remaining cat B (see Figure 16.4). The button game, which can also review a child's inability to conceptualize a nuclear family unit, included distant relatives, pets, and friends (Figure 16.5).

2. The *house-tree-person technique*[14] involves having the child draw a house, a tree, and a person. The drawing process itself, its content, and the postdrawing questioning supply data on the child's self-perception and significant background information. The following case of a 10-year-old girl provides an example of this technique: The

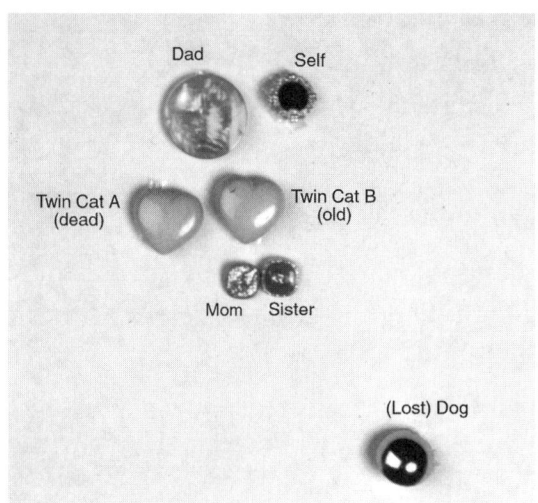

FIGURE 16.4. A grieving family.

girl developed epileptic seizures after a fall on the school playground when she was 6 years of age, and she began to evidence NES at 10 years of age. Her parents focused their efforts on the epilepsy and never validated the trauma of the fall. The girl initially drew a picture of a house with smoke coming from the chimney and a for-sale sign on the lawn, a tree with a hole in it, and a person with a fearful expression on her face (Figure 16.6). After 9 months of psychological treatment, the child drew a picture in which the for-sale sign was gone, the tree was healed, and the person was depicted as socially engaging (saying "Hi!") (Figure 16.7).

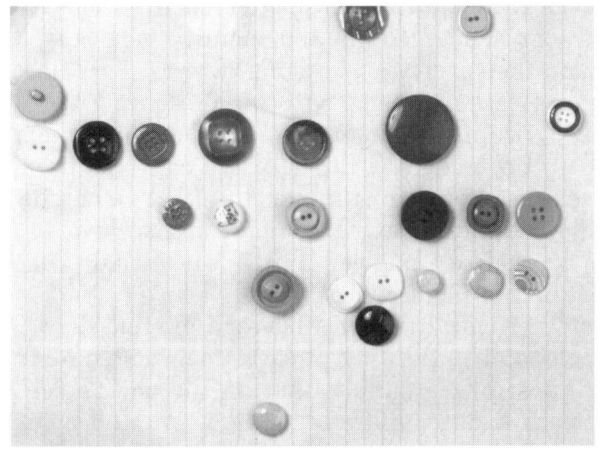

FIGURE 16.5. An ill-defined and over-inclusive family.

Psychological Assessment and Treatment of Non-Epileptic Seizures 217

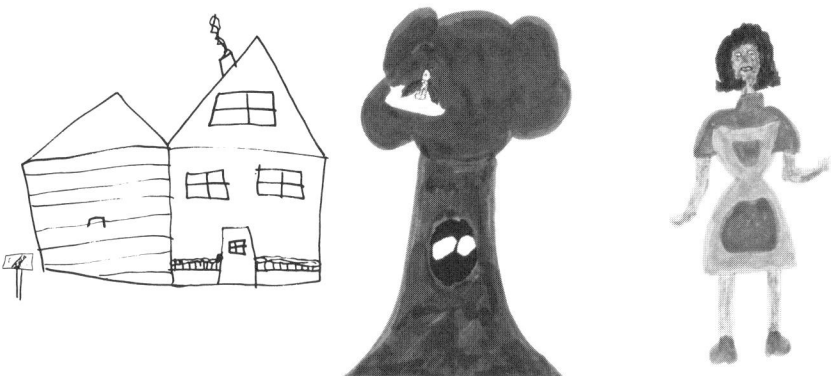

FIGURE 16.6. Pretreatment house-tree-person drawings.

3. The *child/person in the rain technique* was adapted from the Children's Self-Report Inventory.[17] It involves asking the child to draw a picture of himself or herself in the rain. The resulting drawing gives the therapist some idea about the patient's coping skills and behaviors. For example, a child who appears to deny difficulties may draw a sun in the rain, and a child who feels vulnerable may either omit the umbrella or rain hat or include broken or defective protective devices (Figure 16.8).

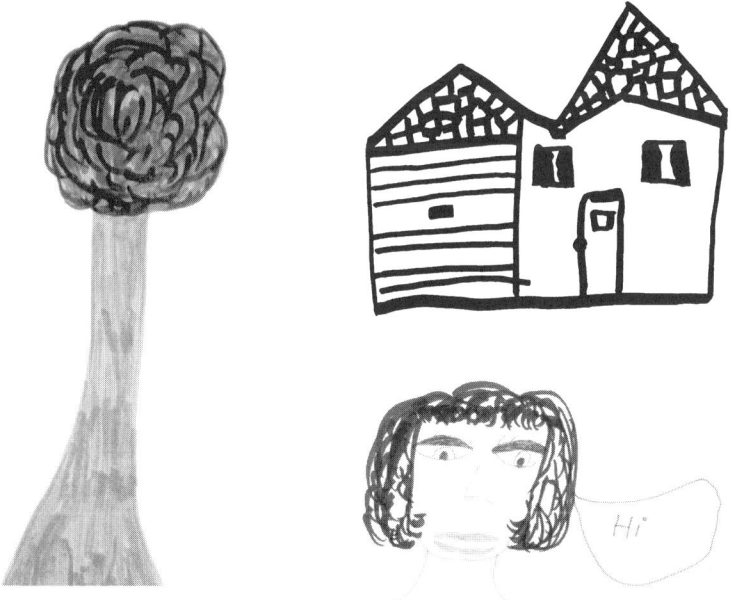

FIGURE 16.7. Post-treatment house-tree-person drawings.

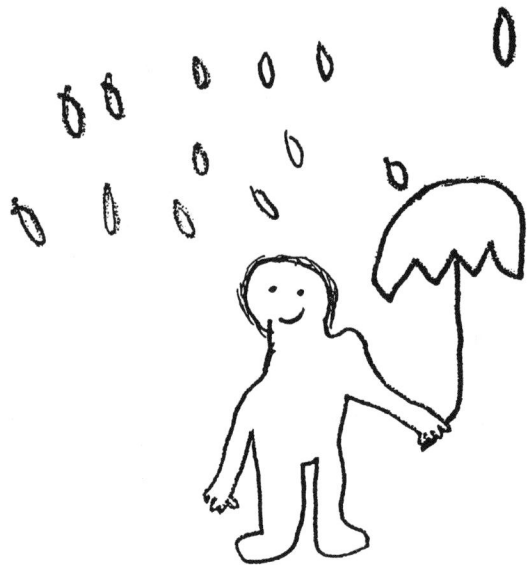

FIGURE 16.8. A child in the rain.

4. The *rosebush technique*[18] begins as a relaxation and visualization exercise in which the child is asked to imagine himself or herself as a rosebush. The patient is to visualize the stems, flowers, leaves, and branches. After relaxation, the child is given a sheet of paper and a pencil and is asked to draw himself or herself as the rosebush that emerged during the guided visualization. After the drawing exercise, the child is asked to respond verbally to a series of 12 questions about the rosebush, such as, "What do you look like? Tell me about your thorns. Who takes care of you?" This technique has been found to discriminate between well-adjusted, resilient sexually abused children and their nonresilient sexually abused peers.[19] In the case described in the example of the house-tree-person technique, the girl drew a sad-faced rosebush that was continuously being cut by mean people under the hot sun and rain (Figure 16.9A). During psychological treatment, a traumatic event from her earlier childhood was successfully retrieved and effectively dealt with. After treatment she drew a happy rosebush that was well supported (Figure 16.9B).
5. The *squiggle game*[20] can best be described as a nonverbal conversation between the therapist and child using doodle-type drawings as the communication vehicle. The therapist starts by making a simple mark, for example, a half circle. The child is then invited to use the curve to "make something" of his or her choice. The game proceeds with the child and therapist taking turns completing one another's squiggles. As the game proceeds, sensitive material often evolves. For

Psychological Assessment and Treatment of Non-Epileptic Seizures   219

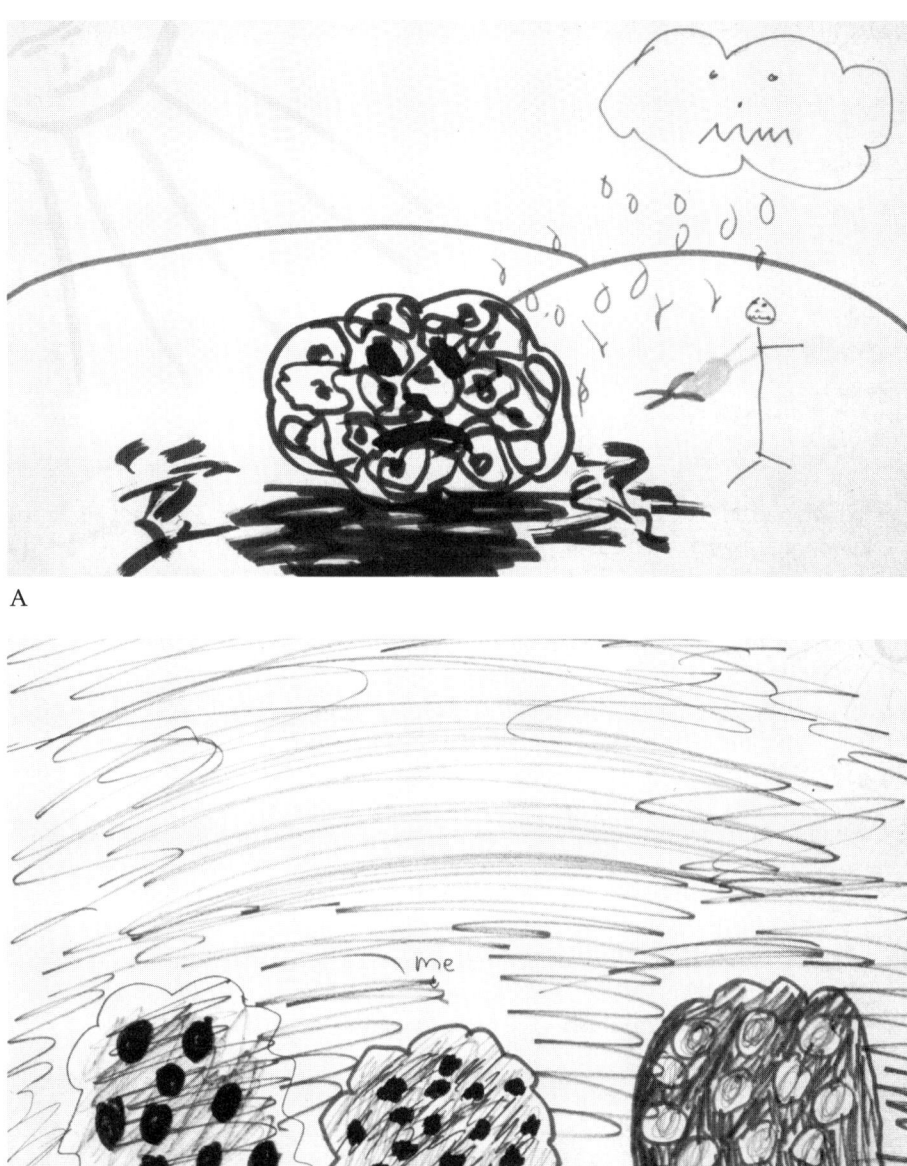

FIGURE 16.9.   The pretreatment (**A**) and post-treatment (**B**) rosebush drawings.

instance, themes of loneliness, sadness, fear, or anger may emerge. The therapist can then respond to the child's drawings of emotional expression by providing support, by helping the child to contain strong feelings, and by seeking additional information.

Feedback in Preparation for a Psychological Formulation: A Recapitulation

Children usually respond positively to the projective assessment, and rapport is quickly established. As children feel comfortable in this therapeutic climate, memories of traumatic events may surface. If the recollections that surface take the form of both emotional expression and a cognitive awareness, we proceed to the next step. If both the child and the parents appear to be ready to come to an understanding of the problem and we have sufficient evidence, we check our hypothesis or tentative formulation with them, first with the child and then with the family. If the formulation is incomplete, the parents are engaged as partners in solving the mystery, and objective assessments are conducted. Objective assessments might involve self- or parent-report measures of the child's symptoms of anxiety, depression, and disruptive behaviors. Intellectual and educational testing is often conducted concurrently with other assessment procedures to determine if academic problems or a specific learning disability may be contributing to school-related stress. If there is support for the tentative hypothesis, a full team meeting is convened. A formulation session with the family is also conducted to develop a treatment plan. At that point, resistance usually is diminished and the patient and family are able to engage in open inquiry if there are doubts about the formulation.

If resistance exists at the end of the projective assessment, the sources of resistance are explored. The parents may feel neglected by previous medical or psychological professionals, or they may feel that their parenting skills are being questioned. There may be severe psychopathology or illness in the family that interferes with their coping. Whatever the source of resistance, the parents and child are helped to deal with unresolved issues, fears, or frustrations *before* the formulation of the psychological problem is formally addressed. After the formulation meeting, children's awareness may be at any level of the A-B-C triplet (see Table 16-1). Some children may be at the emotional level, whereas others may be at the cognitive or behavioral level, or at varying combinations of the three.

Psychological Treatment

Psychological intervention starts with anxiety and symptom relief. The psychodynamic approach to assessment and treatment helps to identify issues and relieve symptoms. For example, drawing and storytelling can reduce children's anxiety, aid their memory recall, enhance their emotional expression, and help them gain insight into the meaning of the symptom. Psychotherapy takes place within the assessment sessions as the child's problems emerge.

The second level of therapy targets emotional expression and affect availability. Behavioral and cognitive approaches can help the child and parents cope more adaptively with stress and change the illness conditions. Children can be taught a vocabulary for emotional expression, practice new skills using role playing, and learn that certain emotions can elicit certain physical reactions.

Challenging resistance is both a goal and a process that requires tactful management. When resistance by the child is encountered, humor and other familiar coping strategies can be helpful. For example, if a child says "I forgot" or "I don't know" when asked to tell about his or her experiences, the therapist could introduce a character named "Mr. Forgot" who needs some help from "Mr. Memory." This paradoxical approach seems to appeal to children and helps them save face. The parents are reassured that the therapist has expertise in handling these issues and are encouraged to "hang in" and be patient with the seemingly slow therapeutic process.

Therapy for children who are unaware of the conflict should avoid direct confrontation or interpretation of their defenses. Nonverbal play therapy can help the child deal with anxiety at a manageable level while allowing his or her defense mechanisms to remain unbroken.

Therapy for parents and family members puts the child's symptoms back into the family context. Dysfunctional family patterns are common in this population,[4,8,21,22] and parents may have unresolved emotional conflicts that prevent them from attending to their children's distress. Parents may repress, deny, or discount the impact of trauma on their children, particularly if the parents themselves have a history of multiple traumas. Treatment can be aimed at assisting family members to become aware of differences in perception between themselves and the child. For example, parents are not always aware of sibling rivalry or teasing by a sibling and may not be aware of the distress this causes the child. Once the child's perceptions are made known to the parents, they often facilitate alternative ways of coping with and managing life stressors.

Termination and Follow-Up

Termination is never abrupt because the child needs help to deal with separation from the therapist and the hospital. To ease the transition to the home environment, follow-up appointments or community services are planned before discharge. During the termination sessions, the treatment process is summarized to the child. A session also is held to prepare parents, because their readiness to adjust to the new situation may lag behind that of their child. Often the child has become more mature and positive in expressing his or her needs, and the parents' anxiety levels may be higher. It should be noted that it is very important during the termination sessions to respect the confidential nature of the content shared in the sessions and to protect the confidentiality of information provided by both the child and parents during sessions with the other party. The child is congratulated in front of the family for solving the mystery and making progress on the 10-point finger scale. The family also is encouraged to continue this open approach to solving problems.

TABLE 16.3
Summary of Stressors and Number of Treatment Modalities by Patient Group

Patient Group	Number	Mean Traumatic Life Events	Teased in School	Bullied at Home/School	Needed 5+ Types of Treatment
NES	23	3.78	52%	26%	87%
NES + organic	19	3.84	83%	5%	74%
Organic	4	1.6	50%	0%	75%

NES = non-epileptic seizures.

Summary of Treatment Outcome

As previously noted, patients were referred for psychological assessment when psychogenic causes of their symptoms were suspected but an NES diagnosis was not yet confirmed. At the conclusion of the diagnostic process, it was found that, of the 46 patients who underwent the evaluation, 23 evidenced NES, 19 evidenced both NES and an organic condition (mixed group), and four had an organic basis for their symptoms but had psychological complications. Patients with an organic basis for their symptoms appeared to have experienced fewer traumatic life events, although at least one-half of the patients in all groups experienced bullying and teasing at school and needed help to deal with such experiences. Bullying and teasing at home and by peers outside of school occurred with greater frequency in the NES group and appeared to be associated with other factors, such as family functioning and neighborhood security. The patient sample was too small to permit statistical analyses of group differences. However, descriptive data suggest that the NES and mixed group were similar with respect to severity and complexity of psychological issues and treatment needs (Table 16.3).

All three groups required more than one modality of treatment. Table 16.3 indicates the percentage of patients who required a combination of five or more forms of treatment. The types of treatments that were used and the percentage of patients who received each form of treatment are presented in Table 16.4. Most patients and families received more than three types of treatments, and some received treatment in all seven modalities.

The assessment time and treatment duration ranged from 7 days to 1 year. Most patients were admitted as inpatients for 1–2 weeks. On termination of treatment, all 46 patients indicated that they had regained functioning and were relieved of their chief complaints.

Therapists rated the child's functioning with respect to the A-B-C triplet on a five-point Likert scale, with one representing the best adjustment and five representing the worst. Mean pre- and post-treatment A-B-C

TABLE 16.4.
Number of Patients by Treatment Method (n = 46)

Type of Treatment	Number	Percent
Family education on mind-body connection	45	97.8
Child education on mind-body connection	45	97.8
Relaxation behavior training	44	95.7
Emotional change training	40	87.0
Post-traumatic stress disorder education and management	34	73.9
Stop teasing training	27	58.7
Cognitive change training	23	50.0

ratings are presented in Table 16.5. Because multiple matched t tests were conducted, Bonferroni critical values were used when determining significance level. The statistical significance of pre- to post-treatment changes in behavior could not be determined because all patients received a rating of five at pretreatment, violating the homogeneity of variance criterion for the statistical test. However, an inspection of mean scores suggests that symptom severity was reduced. Results also indicate that children experienced a significant improvement in affect availability and cognitive awareness.

Twenty-six variables relating to child and family functioning were rated by the therapist on a five-point Likert scale, as described previously. These variables were combined to form seven child and family coping factors. Table 16.6 indicates correlation coefficients between five-point therapist ratings and therapist ratings of need for treatment at discharge. All factors were significantly correlated with need for treatment, particularly factors relating to family functioning and parental awareness of affect, behavior, and cognition.

TABLE 16.5
Child Pre- and Post-Treatment Rating

Factor	Measure	Pretreatment	Post-Treatment	t Value	p Value
Affect	Mean	3.978	1.9348	11.45	<.0001
	SD	1.1252	1.036		
Behavior	Mean	5.000	2.1304	15.26	—
	SD	0.0000	1.2756		
Cognition	Mean	4.2391	2.1957	11.63	<.0001
	SD	0.6389	0.9802		

SD = standard deviation.

TABLE 16.6
Correlations between Coping Scores and Family Factors with Need for Outpatient Care after Hospitalization

Factor	Correlation Coefficient
Family dysfunctioning	0.8151[a]
Parental pretreatment affect	0.6692[a]
Parental pretreatment behavior	0.6434[a]
Parental pretreatment cognition	0.5123[b]
Existence of trauma	0.4126[b]
Parental resistance	0.4391[b]
Child pretreatment affect	0.4160[b]

[a] $p \leq .01$.
[b] $p \leq .001$.

Discussion and Future Directions

These preliminary data suggest that a psychodynamic approach to assessment and a multimodal approach to psychological treatment can be of benefit to NES patients and patients with other forms of psychogenic symptoms. Therapist ratings suggest that patients experienced improvement in awareness of affect, behavior, and cognition over the course of treatment, although multiple treatment modalities were often needed. Because the interpretation of projective testing relies heavily on the subjective judgments of the therapist and cannot be easily quantified, and because the nature of the problem evolves as the assessment process proceeds, it can be difficult to evaluate the effectiveness of a psychological treatment program that uses these strategies. To address this problem, we have adopted a two-stage assessment process so that we first gather data by administering objective scales (for example, ratings of life events, emotional expressiveness, family functioning, self-esteem, and coping style) and then use projective techniques to let the child lead us to the meaning of his or her symptoms. Future research could investigate the role of parental variables, such as parental life events, coping, and emotional expression, on the development, persistence, or cessation of NES in children. Future research might also be aimed at developing objective scoring systems for projective tests and establishing standard assessment and treatment protocols to facilitate program evaluation and replication of treatment programs at other centers.

Several recommendations and conclusions can be drawn from the experience at the symptom management program at the British Columbia Children's Hospital:

1. NES is a complex syndrome, and its differential diagnosis is a challenge to clinicians. For this reason, medical and psychological investigations should take place concurrently.

2. Psychological assessment can be perceived as invasive and threatening, particularly in patients and families who have limited awareness of psychological issues. Projective techniques can be helpful in assessing psychological functioning while minimizing the patient's feelings of anxiety and defensiveness.
3. Behavioral and cognitive approaches are essential to offer skills for change at any stage of the assessment and treatment process. They can help to reduce the patient's and family's anxiety about psychological services by demonstrating that, rather than being mysterious or threatening, therapy can involve the teaching of very practical and intuitively logical skills, such as relaxation training. These approaches can also bolster parent confidence in the value of psychological treatment while increasing the child's sense of control over his or her symptoms and stressful experiences.
4. Psychological support should be made available to families because the process of assessment and treatment may uncover emotionally charged material, such as painful recollections or realizations, both in the child and in the family.
5. A systematic investigation into transgenerational trauma and coping may help the therapist, the child, and the family to understand the dynamics of the symptom.
6. A holistic approach, which addresses peer, family, and school functioning, in addition to the internal emotional experience of the child, is important.
7. The assessment and treatment team can serve as a model, both to the child and the family, of an effectively functioning system characterized by openness in communication and supportiveness and respect toward others.

References

1. Goodyer IM. Epileptic and pseudoepileptic seizures in childhood and adolescence. J Am Acad Child Psychiatry 1998;24:3–9.
2. Shapiro EG, Rosenfeld AA. The Somatizing Child: Diagnosis and Treatment of Conversion and Somatization Disorders. New York: Springer-Verlag, 1997.
3. Metrick ME, Ritter FJ, Gates JR, et al. Nonepileptic events in childhood. Epilepsia 1991;32:322–328.
4. Sassower K, Duchowny M. Psychogenic Seizures and Nonepileptic Phenomena in Childhood 1991. In O Devinsky (ed), Epilepsy and Behavior. New York: Wiley-Liss, 1991;223–235.
5. Maisami M, Freeman JM. Conversion reactions in children as body language: a combined child psychiatry/neurology team approach to the management of functional neurologic disorders in children. Pediatrics 1987;80:46–52.
6. Turgay A. Treatment outcome of children and adolescents with conversion disorder. Can J Psychiatry 1990;35:585–588.

7. Wyllie E, Friedman D, Rother AD, et al. Psychogenic seizures in children and adolescents: outcome after diagnosis by ictal video and electroencephalographic recording. Pediatrics 1990;85:480–484.
8. Lancman ME, Asconape JJ, Graves S, Gibson PA. Psychogenic seizures in children: long-term analysis of 43 cases. J Child Neurol 1994;9:404–407.
9. Bertalanffy L. General Systems Theory. In PA LaViolette (ed), A Systems View of Man. Boulder, CO: Westerview Press, 1981.
10. Minuchin S, Fishman HC. Family Therapy Techniques. Cambridge, MA: Harvard University, 1981.
11. Williams DT, Spiegel H, Mostofsky DI. Neurogenic and hysterical seizures in children and adolescents: differential diagnostic and therapeutic considerations. Am J Psychiatry 1978;135:82–86.
12. Shen W, Bowman ES, Markand ON. Presenting the diagnosis of pseudoseizure. Neurology 1990;40:756–759.
13. Yau CWD. The Button Game: Towards the Validation of a Projective Technique. Master's Thesis. Department of Psychology, Hong Kong University Library, 1990.
14. Ho AMW. Projective Techniques: Tools for Assessment and Treatment in Children. Paper presented at the British Columbia Play Therapy Association Workshop, 1995.
15. Ransby M, Carter MA, Piper E, Ho AMW. The Family Relations Button Sort: A Paediatric Interview Technique. Paper presented at the British Columbia Children's Hospital Clinical Rounds, 1998.
16. Buck JN. House, Tree, Person Technique Revised Manual. Los Angeles: Western Psychology Services, 1998.
17. Ziffer RL, Shapiro LE. Children's Self-Report and Projective Inventory Manual. Narberth, PA: Psychological Assessment Services, 1992.
18. Allan JAB. Inscapes of the Child's World: Jungian Counseling in Schools and Clinics. Dallas: Spring, 1992.
19. Carter MA, Allan JAB, Boldt WB. Projective assessment of child sexual abuse. Br J Projective Psychol 1992;37:37–44.
20. Claman L. The squiggle-drawing game in child psychotherapy. Am J Psychother 1980;34:414–425.
21. Mims J, Antonello JL. Treatment of non-epileptic psychogenic events in adolescent patients using the systems model for intervention. Am J Neurosci Nurs 1994;10:298–305.
22. Leslie SA. Diagnosis and treatment of hysterical conversion reactions. Arch Dis Child 1988;63:506–511.

CHAPTER 17

Adolescents' and Parents' Perception of Non-Epileptic Seizures: A Retrospective and Qualitative Glance

Lucyna M. Lach and Louis Peltz

Researchers and clinicians can approach the study of non-epileptic seizures (NES) from various epistemologic and methodologic frameworks. Their approach partly depends on what the state-of-the-art knowledge development is in a substantive area and on the research question that is being asked.[1] This study begins with the following question: What is the lived experience of the pediatric patient with NES or the parent(s) of that patient, or both, regarding the diagnosis of NES? Several assumptions are embedded in this question: (1) The patient or the parent(s), or both, have something to tell us about their lived experience; (2) they are able to intelligibly articulate their encounter; and (3) what they have to tell us is useful, informative, and helpful in some way.

Most psychological research is conducted using a postpositivist epistemologic framework. This means that hypotheses to be tested and variables to be studied are specified a priori by the examiner. The methods used are often guided by previous research or theories and conceptual frameworks. There is an established "gold standard" for sampling strategies, the selection and administration of measures, and the conducting of analyses, which represent the benchmark against which "good" research is evaluated.[2] In essence, the structure of a study or experiment is shaped primarily by the investigator rather than by the natural manifestation of the phenomenon of interest.[3] In a qualitative paradigm, the investigator's aim is to become thoroughly familiar with the experience of an individual subject by minimizing constraints on how the individual reports on his or her experience. The goal of the qualitative paradigm is not necessarily to derive general principles (although deriving general principles can be achieved with this method), but to understand a phenomenon within the individual's own, often dynamic, personal and social context. This permits greater richness and depth in understanding how the individual experiences and makes sense of his or her world.[4]

Qualitative research is the art of asking simple questions and getting complex answers. The challenge lies in managing the simultaneous simplicity and complexity of the data. Two types of qualitative methodologies were used to analyze the transcripts from in-depth interviews: discourse analysis and thematic analysis. They are integrated and involve studying the narrative of an individual's construction of his or her experience in the context of dialogue. The individual's communication is analyzed for themes that reflect beliefs, attitudes, values, or sentiments.[5,6] Meaning in the individual's communication can be conveyed by subtleties in speech at the word, clause, or story levels.[7] For example, hesitations such as pauses or "ummm" can convey that the individual is struggling to express what he or she wants to say. Words such as "so" and "because" often connote that a person is drawing a conclusion or is expressing an attitude about a subject. Therefore, a relationship exists between the way the story is told and the personal meaning of the story. How individuals talk about their experience of NES and the meaning that that experience has for them are, therefore, related. It is important to note that the analysis represents only preliminary findings from a pilot study.

The sample included three adolescent patients whose NES have since resolved and their parent(s). The first patient is an 18-year-old female who received a diagnosis of NES 2 years before participating in this study and had received a diagnosis of complex partial seizures at 9 years of age. Her father is an unskilled laborer with a history of alcohol dependence, and her mother is a homemaker. The second patient is a 13-year-old girl who received a diagnosis of NES approximately 2 years before entering the study but subsequently was also found to be experiencing complex partial seizures and underwent a temporal lobectomy. She is an only child from a single-parent family, and her mother works as a secretary. The third patient is a 13-year-old boy who received a diagnosis of NES 1 year before entering the study. He presents as a bright, articulate, and outgoing individual. He is an only child, and his parents are divorced. Both of his parents are well educated.

Each family was offered the opportunity to be interviewed as part of a study aimed at improving our understanding of NES. Because the interviewer had seen the respondents in counseling sessions during the time of diagnosis, the nature of interviews was both clinical and ethnographic. During the interview the families were asked the following questions:

1. What was your initial response to hearing that you/your son/your daughter was diagnosed with NES? How did you initially understand or make sense of that conclusion? What did you think your mother's/father's/son's/daughter's understanding of the diagnosis was?
2. After you were told of the diagnosis, what difference did it make to you? How did you feel? What did you do differently? How did it change the way you perceive things?
3. How many more episodes did you/your son/your daughter have?
4. What do you think ultimately made a difference in resolving the symptoms? What factors were involved in the resolution of the symptoms? What suggestions or recommendations did you find most helpful from health care professionals? If you or your family received counseling, was it helpful? What was helpful? Through the entire process, what was most helpful?
5. Having gone through that experience with your son or daughter, and knowing that it is resolved, how does it impact you today?

The families' responses were audiotaped and transcribed. The responses were coded into categories using an inductive and interactive process. First, the transcripts were read, and initial themes were identified on a line-by-line basis. The transcripts were then reread until all themes were categorized, and the frequency with which a theme recurred in a transcript was counted. For example, in the first reading of a transcript, the adolescent's expression of frustration and confusion is coded. In the second reading, the adolescent's expressions of frustration, confusion, relief, and hopefulness for the future are grouped and categorized as "emotional reaction." In the next reading, the adolescent's reporting of emotional reaction is recategorized based on the positive and negative aspects of the emotional reaction. The following is a summary of the findings according to themes relevant to the adolescent.

Adolescents' Emotional Response

The adolescents connoted the experience of being diagnosed with NES both positively and negatively. They described themselves as feeling relieved not to have epileptic seizures, pleased not to have to take medication anymore, and hopeful for the future. For example, one adolescent said, "I felt happy because, first of all, I get weak, I got taken off the medication, I didn't have to take that anymore. I think that was the main thing, I didn't like taking medication, but I also felt happy because the doctors have told me over the whole time I've been at the hospital that they thought it was epileptic seizures, so once I found out it was not epileptic and got it explained, that I was, I felt happy about it."

The NES diagnosis also elicited negative emotion, such as confusion, frustration, uncertainty, and anger. The following is an excerpt from the interview with the girl who experienced the diagnosis of NES as an additional burden to her existing diagnosis of epilepsy:

> Interviewer: "Did being told that you had non-epileptic seizures actually change anything for you?"
> Adolescent: "Yeah, I think my attitude changed a bit."
> Interviewer: "Really? In what way?"
> Adolescent: "It was another thing to handle, it's like I already had enough."

Another aspect to the emotional experience was that of loss of identity. It appeared that finding out that they had non-epileptic rather than epileptic seizures affected how the adolescents felt about themselves and who they were. For example, one patient said, "Well, I guess it would have been like a relief in one way, but upsetting on the other hand, that I had been through that. They told me I had epilepsy, that I was epileptic, that I had to wear the necklace and stuff like that to show that I was epileptic. So I guess I really didn't want them to tell me that I don't have seizures and that it's all over."

Adolescents' Behavioral Response

The adolescents' responses to the NES diagnosis could be categorized not only by emotional reaction but also behavioral response—that is, how they cope with it. It is interesting to note that each of the three adolescents seems to have made the decision to accept and cope with the diagnosis. Other strategies identified include staying as calm as possible, seeking out parental support, and keeping up with schoolwork in spite of the intrusiveness of the episodes. The following excerpt is from an interview with a girl who had non-epileptic events when she became angry with her mother. The behavior would escalate and continue for hours because the mother would attempt to restrain her or try other ineffective measures to stop the agitation. The girl's remarks suggest that she made a conscious decision to attempt to cope with her feelings in an alternative way.

> Interviewer: "When you found out that these weren't the kind of seizures that you could treat with medication, did it change anything for you?"
> Adolescent: "Well, I thought like, um, if you think that they're not real and that they are, so, maybe I kind of, after a while, had myself convinced that they weren't real, I said like now I just tried not to get nervous and stuff and I tried not to get angry or anything because I thought that I would have a pseudoseizure or something because every time I got angry . . ."

Adolescents' Cognitive Response

Overall, the adolescents' remarks suggested a feeling that NES are a mystery and that there is nothing they can take for them. The adolescents understood that NES are related to stress, and they could articulate what the stressors might be, such as something related to school, friends, family, or the seizures themselves. They also acknowledged an understanding that NES were not caused by a brain abnormality, that there is no electroencephalographic correlate for the events, and that NES can look like epileptic seizures. They could not describe what the events look like, what they are doing during the episodes, or why they started.

The adolescents' thoughts and feelings about NES appeared to reflect, or were impacted by, what they heard from their parents and the health care team. The adolescents seemed preoccupied with others' perceptions of the NES. Their comments reflected concern that others thought they were faking the events, that the events were under their control, that they were behaving this way for attention, and that the events were a form of a temper tantrum. Essentially, the adolescents were concerned about whether they were believed or not believed and perceived others as either validating or invalidating. The following is an exemplar of this theme:

> Interviewer: "What do you think her reaction was to finding out that she had non-epileptic seizures?"
> Parent: "I don't think [patient] wanted to believe it."
> Adolescent: "Because you thought I was faking it."
> Interviewer: "Because of what?"
> Adolescent: "Because I thought that meant they were made up."
> Interviewer: "Do you remember how you got that idea that maybe they were made up?"
> Adolescent: "I don't know. I guess it was just because of the word 'pseudo,' I don't know."

The word *pseudo* was very salient, even upsetting, to the parents and adolescents. It seemed that somehow the events were being construed as false or not real when from the family's perspective they felt very real. From the adolescents' viewpoint, NES are outside of their control, come without warning, and can occur at inconvenient times. The events can feel violent and intense, and patients can hear people around them. The following is a representative excerpt from the transcribed interviews:

> Adolescent: "The majority of my seizures happen out of the blue, so there was nothing to cause it really, it would just happen in the middle of the day or in the evening or at night, and like, there would be no cause for it."
> Parent: "And often, too, there would be the consequence of having one. It would take away things that he really couldn't do."
> Adolescent: "Yeah, if I was faking it, then, like, wouldn't I stop faking it for the period that I was going skiing, or wouldn't I stop?"

Adolescents' Perception of What Helped

The adolescents were able to talk about things that they believed helped them. They found it helpful when their parents were present during and immediately after the episode. Receiving an adequate explanation directly from the physician was important to them. They appreciated knowing that the symptoms and the possibility of organicity were being taken seriously. Other things that they perceived as helpful included making a connection between stressors and symptoms, decreasing their anxiety about having the episodes, decreasing their anxiety about major stressors in their lives, breathing/relaxation exercises, and hopefulness.

Parents' Emotional Response

Transcripts were reviewed to obtain an understanding of the parents' experiences. The remarks suggest that parents also felt a combination of negative and positive emotions. They experienced shame because of their perceived inability to discuss the diagnosis with close friends and family members. Parents explained that they did not think others would understand and that it was not the kind of diagnosis that would conjure up the same level of empathy and support that a medical diagnosis would elicit from others. It was therefore difficult for them to seek out support among those in whom they would typically confide. Parents also felt guilt and embarrassment because of their failure to identify or prevent the psychological distress that their children experienced. The following excerpt conveys these ideas:

> Parent: "Why don't you contact Barbara Walters?" (laughter) "No, I'm serious, they would probably love to do a piece on it. You would be so good on it. We really think there is an educating thing that would be wonderful to let people know that these exist. They really impact on people's lives very much. In a similar way, there is a dark ages connotation attached to it."
> Interviewer: "What do you think that is all about?"
> Parent: "It's the shame."
> Interviewer: "What's the shame about?"
> Parent: "Because it kind of means because there is still an attitude that if there isn't anything physically happening in the brain, then you should have been able to pick up on it. You should have been able to make sure it wasn't happening to your child, um, your child was going through something and you didn't recognize it, um, it's that kind of, that you find that . . ."

Later in the interview:

> Parent: "What it means is if this child had epileptic seizures, if he had cancer, if he had kidney problems, then [I] could go and talk to other people about it and receive empathy. But in going to explain to somebody that my child has

non-epileptic seizures and these are psychiatrically based or psychologically based . . . it's harder to do."

The parents conveyed frustration with themselves because they felt powerless to change the situation or control the symptoms. They also expressed feelings of frustration with their children for having the symptoms. They still experienced residual worry that the symptoms might have an organic cause, although this concern was not as great as when the diagnosis was first made.

> Mother: "I think you feel such relief that he doesn't have epileptic seizures and it probably goes back to what H. [father] said . . . that kind of vagueness . . . there is something very definitive about epileptic seizures—the brain waves go, the pattern goes skewy, the seizures happen, you totally have no control. There's . . . anything to do with the consciousness has that kind of feeling of . . . it's like when you hear that someone's suffering from clinical depression. How many times do you hear 'well, just get on with your life' kind of thing, you know, that sort of thing. It's very hard to grasp that concept that this might be something that you can't control necessarily . . . um . . . but it is a harder thing to . . . uh . . . and sometimes when he had the seizures, I would feel . . . I felt after I found out they were NES, sometimes I felt angrier toward you [son] sometimes for having them simply because it was like, come on, stop it and control this. Um. And I didn't want him to have NES. I felt a lot of relief that he didn't have epileptic seizures but a lot of frustration that they were NES at the same time."

Parents' Behavioral Response

When asked about what they do during an episode, parents offered the following types of remarks:

> "I try to figure it out. Is this epileptic or non-epileptic?"
> "I assure them of their safety."
> "I walk away."
> "I don't stay with my child, but I keep an eye on [him/her], and I may try to distract them by calling them, asking them to count."
> "I suggest for them to stop and I encourage them to use deep breathing and relaxation."

The parents talked about managing their own anxiety about their child's episodes. They also stated what a parent should not do during an episode, such as get frustrated, tell the adolescent to snap out of it, tell the adolescent to stop, try to physically restrain them, or hold his or her hand.

Parents' Cognitive Response

In analyzing parents' responses, it became clear that understanding NES is a lengthy process that does not end when they are informed of the diagnosis. They need a number of opportunities to ask the question, "What is this?" and need to have numerous conversations with the physician, social worker, psychiatrist, and psychologist about this question. The following is an exemplar of this theme:

> Parent: "Even at this point after the non-epileptic seizures have resolved, I still don't fully understand it because I know I couldn't really tell the difference. Sometimes I thought I could, but I was maybe catching the end of a true seizure or she was just coming out of it. Most of the time I went by the eye, that look, you know, they get with a seizure, but being very honest, I still to this day don't understand."

Parents' remarks suggested that assimilating new information is an ongoing process and that there is a need to match their own experience to the information that they are given before they can follow treatment recommendations. For example, parents could not make a sincere effort in counseling until they felt confident about the medical workup. Parents appreciated when the health care professionals took the time to give thorough explanations and when they validated the parents' feelings that it was a difficult and stressful process.

Parents often asked the following types of questions:

> "What is a non-epileptic seizure anyway?"
> "What proportion of the seizures are epileptic and non-epileptic?"
> "Does he or she have epilepsy?"
> "Is this an epileptic or non-epileptic seizure?"
> "Why should we even call these seizures?"

Parents wondered whether, because the symptoms were so bizarre and severe, the emotional problems were severe. Ultimately, the parents achieved an understanding of their children's physical symptoms as a manifestation of emotional stress and were able to be empathic toward their children. They also were able to understand that their children's level of awareness or consciousness, both of the physical symptoms and their emotional underpinnings, was incomplete or altered during the episodes. The parents were able to make connections between critical psychological events and NES. They often connected the NES to such stressors as anxiety about peers or school performance, some aspect of family relationship, a recent loss, experiencing anger or other form of affect, or just having epilepsy.

Discussion

These preliminary data provide a glimpse into the thoughts and feelings of adolescents diagnosed with NES and their parents. Symptoms are usually a signal that something is wrong in the body. They are a sign of an ailment, illness, or disease. The diagnosis of NES challenges patients and families to view the symptom differently, as a signal of distress. The usual role of the health care professional is to diagnose and treat physical conditions, and the psychological factors may be peripheral to the provider's primary objective. What the interviews discussed in this chapter suggest is that the provider's sensitivity to psychological issues may be essential to the patients' and families' willingness to accept the NES diagnosis and pursue psychological treatment options. A number of factors may be critical to achieving a positive patient outcome, such as the availability of health care providers to have unhurried and often multiple discussions to address families' questions and concerns, providers' ability to express an appreciation of the validity of the symptoms and the stress that families are going through, and the use of nonpejorative terminology during the diagnostic process. Physicians' respect for the patient and family, conveyed by their willingness to speak directly to the patient, and their thoroughness in ruling out physical causes of NES were perceived as an important element in the families' ability to come to terms with the diagnosis.

Factors outside the medical setting can also have a significant bearing on adolescents' and parents' ability to cope with the diagnosis, such as community members' attitudes toward NES and the willingness of educators and other influential people in adolescents' lives to make adjustments toward minimizing stressors. Similarly, internal variables may affect the ability of patients and their parents to deal successfully with NES. Adolescents' sense of identity may be threatened if epilepsy has become a part of how they see themselves as individuals. Parents may feel guilt related to their failure to identify their children's emotional distress, while at the same time feeling frustration with their children's symptoms. Addressing these issues during and immediately after the diagnostic evaluation may help to facilitate the adjustment process.

Because this study consisted of data from only three families, it is unclear to what extent their views are shared by other NES adolescents and their families. One aim of future research would be to obtain a larger sample, including those whose episodes resolved and those whose episodes continued, and to apply the above paradigm to identify commonalities in feelings and attitudes about the diagnostic process. Once these common dimensions are identified, a quantitative approach could be used to determine which factors, such as the patients' ability to acknowledge stressors or parents' awareness of their own feelings, might best predict cessation of NES.

References

1. Miller WJ, Crabtree BF. Clinical Research. In NK Denzin, YS Lincoln (eds), Handbook of Qualitative Research. Thousand Oaks, CA: Sage, 1994;340–352.

2. Bryman A. Quantity and Quality in Social Research. London: Routledge, 1992.
3. Guba EG, Lincoln YS. Competing Paradigms in Qualitative Research. In NK Denzin, YS Lincoln (eds), Handbook of Qualitative Research. Thousand Oaks, CA: Sage, 1994;105–137.
4. Denzin NK, Lincoln YS. Introduction: Entering the Field of Qualitative Research. In NK Denzin, YS Lincoln (eds), Handbook of Qualitative Research. Thousand Oaks, CA: Sage, 1994;1–22.
5. Morse JM, Field PA. Qualitative Research Methods for Health Professionals. Thousand Oaks, CA: Sage, 1995.
6. Reissman CK. Narrative Analysis: Qualitative Research Methods Series, vol 30. Newbury Park, CA: Sage, 1993.
7. Chambon A. The Dialogical Analysis of Case Materials. In E Sherman, WJ Reid (eds), Qualitative Research in Social Work. New York: Columbia University, 1994;205–215.

CHAPTER 18

Munchausen Syndrome by Proxy and Svengali Syndrome

Fritz E. Dreifuss and John R. Gates

Munchausen Syndrome by Proxy

Baron Karl Friedrich Hieronymous Freiherr von Muenchhausen fought with the Russians against the Turks in the eighteenth century and thereafter became known for the tall tales he spun concerning his adventures. These tales were subsequently further fictionalized and presented in popular form.[1]

The adventures of the Baron were farfetched and amusing. In 1951, Asher[2] popularized a syndrome characterized by tales, also farfetched but far from amusing, of patients who allow themselves to be medically mutilated to mislead physicians with tales of fictitious symptoms. Our experience includes a man who purported to have a war-related head wound, had recurrent episodes of fictitious cerebrospinal fluid rhinorrhea, and underwent at least four craniotomies for the treatment thereof, using a series of lies and a number of hospitals to achieve these ends. Patients with fictitious intestinal obstruction leading to abdominal distention and recurrent laparotomies have been seen on at least three occasions, and fictitious episodes of epilepsy and status epilepticus, the latter leading to recurrent intubations and intravenous administrations of diazepam, have become an almost common occurrence in a busy epilepsy center.

Epileptic Munchausen syndrome is a rather rare condition.[3,4] A physician's 21-year-old stepdaughter was referred to us because of recurrent episodes of status epilepticus. No one in the immediate family had epilepsy, but her past history included several febrile convulsions in infancy for which she was treated transiently with phenobarbital; she had been without medication since the age of 4 years, however. She claimed that for almost a year she had had intermittent, recurrent episodes of generalized tonic-clonic status epilepticus that required emergency room management and many hospitalizations. She came to the emergency room as often as twice a week and was frequently intubated and treated with intravenous benzodiazepines and an interim phenytoin management. Ultimately, she could no longer be intubated because of laryngeal stenosis.

It was determined that this patient had never, in fact, had an epileptic seizure after the febrile seizures of infancy, and what seizures were observed were patently malingered. Psychotherapy was successful in purging this symptom from the nervous system; when last heard from she had undergone laparotomy for a putative diagnosis of intestinal obstruction that was not borne out. She has visited several hospitals in the Mississippi Delta for recurrent episodes of abdominal pain.

A similar patient was subsequently seen by us with a rather transparent motivation, but the denouement took several weeks to achieve despite a low diagnostic threshold. We are unaware of any cases of epileptic Munchausen syndrome in which true epilepsy existed, and it appears to be one of the few conditions in which non-epileptic seizures are seen in pure culture.

A variant of the Munchausen syndrome was first described by Meadow in 1977[5] as "the hinterland of child abuse" in which the deceit was practiced by adults and the victims were their children. Several patients with this condition were described by Dreifuss in 1993,[2] and *Munchausen syndrome by proxy* (MSBP), as it has become known, has been copiously written about since 1977. It is likely that most pediatric epileptologists see several cases each year in which epileptic seizures are alleged to afflict a child and have never been observed by anyone other than a parent but which lead to copious examinations including invasive procedures.

Clinical Characteristics

In all of our cases, the mother was the historian, although on occasion the father would participate in the deception. The phenotype of the child's family has been well described, particularly in Rosenberg's report on 117 cases.[7] The perpetrators were the biological mothers in 98% of the cases; one-fourth of these had training in nursing. Ten percent themselves had Munchausen syndrome, and a history of child abuse experienced by the mother occasionally was elicited. (The affected offspring of Munchausen parents have been described as having Polle syndrome after the baron's son who died early in life.) Broken families were common and, in our experience, this syndrome has been frequently seen in military families, especially when there is prolonged paternal absence and paternal neglect. This is also true of those children in the literature who died of nonaccidental poisoning, when the mothers presumably killed the offspring of the men who had spurned them.

All reports reflect what has been our experience also—namely, that the mothers are extremely attentive to their children in the hospital, like to become members of the health care team, acquaint themselves with hospital routine and procedures, and are solicitous of nurses and physicians in their frequent misguided treatment of the child. Often, the mothers will resort to active intervention to prove a point, such as the mother who was apprehended putting a pillow over the child's face to produce an apneic episode so that she could then confront the nurse with proof. (This sequence of events was observed with a video camera.) It has been stated that such mothers feel secure and at home in a hospital setting.

It appears that many surviving children themselves develop Munchausen syndrome,[7] and there is an excess of unexplained deaths in siblings of children who had been recognized as experiencing this form of child abuse.[8,9]

In a typical presentation of the allegedly epileptic child, the mother brings the child to the physician with a complaint of recurrent seizures that may or may not be associated with fever. The child may be drowsy and postictal by description, but evaluation reveals no specific abnormalities. If the child is sent home, he or she will soon be brought back with a recurrence. Sooner or later the child may be hospitalized or subjected to anti-epileptic drug therapy on the basis of the history, only to have more seizures, after which more medication is prescribed. Frequently, the child is taken from physician to physician or from emergency department to emergency department. One such child in our clinic was subsequently admitted in barbiturate-induced stupor. Occasionally, these children are taken from place to place attached to an apnea monitor. The mother of one of our patients, when critically questioned and confronted with the fact that no one but her had ever seen a seizure, began to solicit affidavits from rescue squad crews and emergency department personnel, all of whom had always seen the child just after a seizure had finished. She carried this "documentation" with her as evidence of her "veracity," although she never proved this. Once such mother, in the hope of denying weekend privileges to an estranged husband, solicited an affidavit that she was the only person fit to care for her child by virtue of her experience in the care of the child's seizures.

These children do well when they are separated from their mothers. When the mothers accompany them to the epilepsy unit, seizures occur under bizarre circumstances and are reported by the mother, usually just after the monitoring electrodes are removed. On one occasion, a prolonged electroencephalogram (EEG) recording had an unexplained gap, as if the machine had been turned off, and a seizure was reported to have occurred during this time. As was mentioned by Meadow, such children tended to be referred to centers of excellence, "where many have been included in carefully conducted trials of therapeutic drugs and diets for epilepsy."[10] Thus, the physician is unwittingly co-opted as the perpetrator's instrument.

Management

Patients suspected of having MSBP who are characterized by a fictitious history of epileptic seizures present a special problem in management. In those cases of MSBP in which physical evidence of abuse can be obtained, the course of action is relatively straightforward, including involvement of a social services department, a psychiatric evaluation, the involvement of child abuse personnel, and measures aimed at protecting the child from further damage. In the case of suspected falsification of a seizure history, no physical evidence is available and, unless the patient is in the hospital, a hint of disbelief usually results in failure to honor follow-up visit appointments. The situation is not helped by the present medicolegal climate, in which physicians are afraid to record their suspicions in writing, and in which potentially pejorative comments on hospital charts may lead to the physician being hoisted on his or her own petard. When the suspicion is sufficiently strong that a child is a victim of MSBP, and when the child is not under the protection of a hospital setting, the primary care physician must be included in the gathering of evidence that may ultimately lead to the protection of the child from further medical depredation.

The practical management of the problem of MSBP is difficult, and each case must be treated individually. If physical harm to the child calls attention to the situation, considerable urgency exists to terminate the child's exposure. Proof must be assiduously gathered, and once this evidence is available, the child must be safeguarded. The actual confrontation must occur in such a way that the mother does not pick up the child and leave the hospital. The mother's safety against a threat of suicide must also be ensured, insofar as possible, by the mobilization of social workers, psychologists, hospital administrative personnel, security personnel, a chaplain, an experienced child abuse pediatrician, the attending physician, and nurses.

The usual course of events is that the child is placed in protective foster care while the parent receives psychotherapy or other counseling. In all but the most egregious cases, the child is usually returned to the family.

When no overt physical harm befalls the child in whom a factitious seizure disorder is the presenting symptom, there is a strong likelihood that nothing can be proved beyond a reasonable doubt. It is our usual practice to confront the parents with the suspicion that the child's symptoms are being consciously or unconsciously exaggerated, and strongly recommend psychotherapy. Strange as it may seem, many parents avail themselves of this avenue, and some of these children do well in their home environment. At other times, the parents remove the child from the care of the physician making the diagnosis. The family physician and, in the case of mobile families, physicians at known points of contact should be alerted so that they do not participate in further deception. It is toward the education of the unwitting participant in this process that programs aimed at the detection of the syndrome are addressed. The salient features of this tragic condition are the presentation of illness in a child who has been repeatedly presented for illnesses that are either simulated or produced by parents or caretakers who deny knowledge of the cause.

The most common presenting symptoms include bleeding, seizures, depression of central nervous system function, apnea, diarrhea or vomiting, fever, or rash. According to Meadow, diagnostic clues include unexplained recurrent or persistent illness with symptoms and signs that do not correspond, and patients who carry a diagnosis of an "uncommon disorder" or in whom an experienced physician has "never seen a case like this."[5,11,12] The illness usually abates in the mother's absence.

It has been noted that the mothers frequently are extremely solicitous of the child in the hospital, although they are relatively unconcerned in light of the apparent gravity of the situation. The mothers frequently have nursing experience and may themselves have a history of factitious illness.

Social factors frequently include medical abuse of other siblings and a history of marital dysfunction, frequently with an absent father or paternal drug or alcohol abuse. The mothers sometimes have a history of experiencing abuse.

The legacy of the illness is likewise tragic in that there is frequently persistence of feigned illness and long-term morbidity, including failure to thrive. There is an approximately 10% death rate in the abused children, and approximately 10% of their siblings may die from unexplained causes. Early recognition of this condition is therefore essential.

Apart from the immediate unpleasantness, such a child is often deprived of a normal childhood, missing much school and many recreational pleasures. It is interesting that a referring physician, when confronted with the suspicion, often becomes defensive and extols the parent's virtues.

Svengali Syndrome

Ozkara and Dreifuss[3] touched on a further variant of MSBP that is distinguished by the intermediation of a member of the opposite sex who uses the occurrence of seizures in the victims to exert control over them. This condition is referred to as the *Svengali syndrome* in the present publication.

Franz Anton Mesmer (1734–1815) introduced hypnosis to the practice of his time and titled it "animal magnetism," which he applied as a cure for a number of conditions. Although he apparently believed that he was producing a physical effect, the principal modality used was suggestion, preceding the dawn of psychology by 100 years. Benjamin Franklin, Lavoisier, and Guillotin were members of a French scientific commission that investigated the practice. According to Orne and Dinges (1989), the practice of mesmerism resulted in a strong, erotic attraction by many female patients toward the "magnetizer." In the induction of a sleep-like state, later called *hypnotism*, subjects performed in a somnambulistic manner. It was Charcot who dignified hypnosis in the practice of neurologic medicine.

In 1894, George duMaurier wrote the novel *Trilby*, which told the story of Trilby O'Ferral, an English artist's model in Paris. The girl had ambitions as a singer, although she was virtually tone deaf. Under the tutelage of a Polish-German musician, Svengali, she was transformed into a leading prima donna. During a protracted period, she was under his hypnotic sway. So long as Svengali conducted, she was the toast of musical Europe. During this time, she became oblivious of her previous friends and acquaintances and remained under Svengali's mesmeric spell until he fell ill and subsequently died, whereupon her talent evaporated. She returned to her previous nonmusical state until she, too, sickened and faded away.

The Svengali syndrome is closely related to the Munchausen complex or syndromes. It more strongly resembles psychogenically precipitated or exacerbated epileptic seizures, however.

A 19-year-old woman had dropped out of school at the age of 15. She had developed juvenile absence at the age of 13 in association with her introduction to hallucinogenic drugs. Occasionally she experienced an early-morning generalized tonic-clonic convulsion, particularly if she had been sleep deprived. Her seizures came under reasonable control with valproate. At the age of 16, she had an induced miscarriage. At the age of 18, she was working as a waitress and developed a romantic attachment with a man who was an emergency medical technician. At about this time, her seizures, which had been in abeyance for several years, recurred in the form of frequent, generalized tonic-clonic seizures. She was unaware of these seizures, but her friend informed her that they occurred approximately two to three times a week. Allegedly these seizures occurred predominantly during sleep. A sleep-deprived electroencephalogram revealed a single, short burst of irregular fast spike and wave activity that was fragmentary and unassociated with clinical accompaniments. She was in the hospital for a number of days, and it became clear that, although she had a history of primary generalized epilepsy, the seizures for which she was admitted had only been observed by her boyfriend. While she was under investigation, her friend insisted on reading her chart, interviewing the physicians, and assuming the role of "protector." When these privileges were denied him and he was challenged on ethical grounds, he prevailed on the patient to discharge herself against medical advice. With this demand, he lost his hold over her, and shortly after she left the hospital she left her "protector" and again became seizure free. She undertook training as a nurse's aide and, when last seen, she continued to do well while still taking valproate for her primary generalized epilepsy.

Another patient, a 53-year-old woman, has been repeatedly studied for a complaint of blackout spells preceded by a smell of burning rubber. For a period of 15 years, she has had episodes of diminished sensation and weakness of the limbs on the right. She has had multiple, repetitive thallium tests for a complaint of substernal pain with exertion. All studies have repeatedly been unrevealing, including repeated neurologic examinations, which have shown a nonorganic-type sensory disturbance that splits the midline; there has always been a finding of weakness unassociated with tone or reflex alteration. She has had repeatedly normal EEGs and scans.

For many years her seizures did not significantly trouble her, but then recurred just as before. Prolonged EEG monitoring on many occasions was performed with negative results. She has recently become enamored of a house guest who is considerably younger than she and who apparently inserts an airway into her pharynx; when she wakes up she is told she has had a seizure. She has never had a seizure witnessed by a medical professional. She has a strong family history of abuse by a parent and later by one of her husbands.

A third patient has a rather similar story. She is 38 years old and has a 2-year history of recurrent seizures that had been predominantly observed by her husband, who is an emergency medical technician and who practices resuscitation when she has an attack. When the rescue team arrives, she is postictal and receives benzodiazepines intravenously and is then taken to the hospital. However, it appears that her seizures have not actually been observed by anyone but the husband who resuscitates her. She also has had complaints of dizziness and chest pain and has been repeatedly evaluated for a cardiac problem that has not been identified. She has been seen by numerous physicians, including three neurologists.

Although it has been noted that Munchausen syndrome presenting as epileptic seizures is relatively uncommon, one suspects the reason for this is that the repertoire of potential epileptic seizure phenomena is sufficiently large that even the most cynical epileptologist tends to allow a certain latitude before invoking the diagnosis of malingering, particularly having regard for the potential medicolegal implications of error. It is just this latitude permitted by the variability of epileptic seizures, as well as a memory of errors in the diagnosis of hysterical seizures, that was later discovered to represent frontal lobe epilepsy. This latitude has allowed Munchausen syndrome to escape serious consideration in many patients who, in fact, have experienced severe medical depradations because Munchausen syndrome has not been considered in the diagnosis.

The variant that one might call the *Svengali syndrome* is of interest because it represents not only a *folie-à-deux*, in which the active participant is a health care professional and the patient is relatively passive and easily manipulated. It would appear that the principal motivation is the display of dominance and ego enhancement thus enjoyed. The author has seen a true *folie-à-deux*, in which a husband-and-wife team, both emergency medical technicians, were involved—she with intractable migraine, he with intractable "post-traumatic" seizures, neither with any objective findings and both of many years' duration.

References

1. Raspe RE. The Surprising Adventures of Baron Munchausen. New York: Peter Pauper, 1944.
2. Asher R. Munchausen's syndrome. Lancet 1951;1:339–341.
3. Ozkara C, Dreifuss FE. Differential diagnosis in pseudoepileptic seizures. Epilepsia 1993;34:294–298.
4. Savard G, Andermann F, Teitelbaum J, Lehmann H. Epileptic Munchausen syndrome: a form of pseudo-seizures distinct from hysteria and malingering. Neurology 1988;38:1628–1629.
5. Meadow R. Munchausen Syndrome by Proxy: the hinterland of child abuse. Lancet 1977;2:343–354.
6. Dreifuss FE. Munchausen Syndrome by Proxy. In AJ Rowan, JR Gates (eds), Non-Epileptic Seizures. Boston: Butterworth–Heinemann, 1993;202–207.
7. Rosenberg DA. Web of deceit: a literature review of Munchausen syndrome by proxy. Child Abuse Neglect 1987;11:547–563.
8. White ST. Surreptitious warfarin ingestion. Child Abuse Neglect 1985;9: 349–352.
9. Roberts IF, West RJ, Ogilvie D, Dillon MJ. Malnutrition in infants receiving cult diets: a form of child abuse. BMJ 1979;1:296–298.
10. Pickel S, Anderson C, Holliday MA. Thirsting and hypernatremic dehydration: a form of child abuse. Pediatrics 1970;45:54–59.
11. Meadow R. Management of Munchausen syndrome by proxy. Arch Dis Child 1985;60:385–393.
12. Meadow R. Fictitious epilepsy. Lancet 1984;2:25–28.

CHAPTER 19

Part Summary: Cognitive and Psychological Functioning and Treatment of the Pediatric Patient with Non-Epileptic Seizures

Ann Hempel

The chapters in this section provide varied perspectives on the psychosocial aspects of non-epileptic seizures (NES) in children. In some ways, the data that are presented may appear to be at variance with conventional wisdom. For example, conventional wisdom would suggest that children with NES often have a history of sexual abuse or experience a mood disorder, whereas the present data indicate that such conditions are seen in a relative minority of pediatric NES patients. These and other data discussed below suggest that the psychological underpinnings of NES in children may be very different from those in adults.

The idea that NES in children and adults represent different psychological phenomena is supported by research on conversion disorder in children and adolescents. In Chapter 14, for example, in the summary of previous studies, Hempel reports that the incidence of sexual abuse and affective disorders in children and adolescents with conversion disorder does not exceed the base rate in the general population. Family discord, peer relationship problems, and school problems were, on average, more common than sexual abuse. Similar types of stressors were found among

NES patients in the Minnesota Epilepsy Group study (see Chapter 14). Although a substantial number of patients in the study by Williams and Grant (see Chapter 15) had a history of sexual abuse, an even larger proportion required special education services for learning disabilities or other learning problems, and many patients experienced a decline in school performance in close temporal proximity to the onset of NES. In addition to a high incidence of school problems, it was found that a large proportion of pediatric NES patients evidenced below-normal IQ, disruptive behavior disorders, or both. In both Chapters 14 and 15, multiple stressors are reported to be common among pediatric NES patients, suggesting that a single factor, such as an isolated traumatic event (e.g., sexual abuse) or a single psychological condition (e.g., mood disorder), is unlikely to represent the sole cause of NES in many of these individuals.

Similarities with earlier conceptualizations of conversion disorder are reported in Chapters 14, 15, and 16. Pediatric NES patients were more often female than male and were commonly of preadolescent or early-adolescent age. It is reported both in Chapters 14 and 15 that pediatric NES patients often had a history of health problems or had a model for the symptoms, and that, as Siegel and Barthel[1] found, they often received secondary gain. These findings suggest that a patient's previous direct or indirect experience with health problems may set the stage for a pattern of maladaptive coping in which physical symptoms become the means by which the patient obtains relief from stress and emotional support from others.

Chapter 18 serves to remind the reader that NES may originate with the parent as a form of Munchausen syndrome by proxy. However, Dr. Dreifuss also presents cases that, like many of the other data reported in this section, are outside the bounds of conventional clinical lore. He reports several cases in which a man, usually a medical technician, persuades an adult female partner to believe that she is experiencing seizures and provides or seeks unnecessary medical treatment for her. Dr. Dreifuss terms the phenomenon the *Svengali syndrome*, a variant of Munchausen by proxy, in which vulnerable women, either through willful or passive acceptance of manipulation by their male partners, report and seek treatment for conditions that have no medical basis. Hence, a condition that heretofore has been considered a disorder restricted to childhood can also be experienced by susceptible adults.

Chapter 16 provides a worthwhile overview of the issues that confront psychosocial providers in dealing with pediatric NES patients and their families. Ho et al. describe procedures for assessment and treatment that convey respect for the child's symptoms and allow the family to achieve an understanding of underlying psychological issues in a gradual and minimally anxiety-provoking manner. An important component of their assessment and treatment approach rests on psychodynamic theory. The tenets of this theory do not readily lend themselves to empirical validation. One assumption is that memories of traumatic events can be repressed and cause psychological disturbance. The second is that the symptoms resolve when the patient achieves a conscious awareness of the event and its accompanying emotions. The concept of repressed memories has been challenged by some investigators, who contend that traumatic events can be forgotten and sometimes recovered years later when prompted by an effective retrieval cue, in the same way as ordinary events, not because memories of traumatic events are pushed out of consciousness by intrapsychic conflict.[2] The therapist's emphasis on uncovering repressed memories increases his or her risk of overlooking other potential sources of stress, such as learning problems, peer relationship difficulties, and family discord, which may be best addressed by alternative, or additional, methods to those described by Ho et al.

The hypothesis that a forgotten traumatic event is the cause of a young patient's psychogenic symptoms can never actually be tested or proved. Nonetheless, the assessment and treatment practices described in Chapter 16, which rest, in part, on this hypothesis, can have merit even if they benefit the patient for reasons other than the uncovering of repressed memories. Projective testing and discussion of test results with parents may serve not only to increase the patient's and family's awareness of the emotional aspects of events in their lives but may also allow a gradual desensitization to discussing issues of an emotional nature. The procedures may also provide a means of validating the child's emotional experience and communicating to parents that the child's emotional distress is no less deserving of compassion and support than a physical health problem.

There are a number of assumptions regarding the psychological functioning of pediatric NES patients that have, as yet, little empirical support but seem intuitively feasible if only because they are compatible with the anecdotal experiences of many clinicians. In Chapter 16, Ho et al. state that NES patients and their families often ignore the presence of emotions, do not have a vocabulary for emotions, and may not be aware of life stressors that contribute to the child's symptoms. In fact, the pilot data presented in Chapter 17 suggest that adolescent NES patients and their parents found it helpful to become aware of the link between NES symptoms and stressors, although one still cannot be sure that the NES adolescent is necessarily any worse at identifying emotions than the typical adolescent. One also cannot know if NES patients and parents might minimize psychological distress as a means of bolstering their assertion to health care providers that the symptoms have a physical basis, particularly when their defensiveness has been raised by the comments of others who might have suggested, perhaps undiplomatically, that the symptoms are "all in their head." Increasing one's access to the NES patient's emotions through therapy may indeed be beneficial, just as it may be in treating other psychological disorders. In fact, the effectiveness of cognitive behavior therapy for treating depression, which has as one component increasing the patient's awareness of the relationship between thoughts and feelings, is well documented.[3]

Chapter 17 provides much-needed insight into the internal experiences of NES adolescents and their parents. Lach's interview data suggest that patients grapple with thoughts and emotions of which many providers may be unaware. For example, adolescents may be keenly attuned to whether others perceive their symptoms as real, which may make it difficult for them to move on in the therapeutic process until their concerns about others' reactions are addressed. It may be difficult for some adolescents to relinquish their symptoms, because having seizures may represent an important aspect of their identity. The interview data also suggest that parents experience a range of sometimes conflicting emotions, including feelings of both frustration and compassion toward their children, feelings of guilt and inadequacy toward themselves, and impatience with those in the community whose intolerance of psychological problems increases their sense of shame. These internal forces, as well as situational factors, may impede the patient's and family's acceptance of the NES diagnosis and their willingness to seek appropriate services. Helping the family to become aware of these issues, even at the beginning of the diagnostic process, may help to lessen possible resistance.

There are a number of points on which there is general agreement among presenters in this section:

1. Because the incidence of learning and behavior problems is quite high in this patient group, the psychological assessment should include not only measures of emotional and personality functioning, but also an evaluation of cognitive variables, such as intelligence, academic achievement, and attention, even when concerns about school performance or behavior have not been raised by the family.
2. Because pediatric NES patients often experience multiple stressors, assessment and therapy aimed at identifying subconscious processes, in and of itself, would likely be insufficient for successful treatment of most patients. Other interventions, which in many instances may be more appropriate than insight-oriented therapy, might include the following:
    a. In a cognitive-behavioral paradigm, the patient could be taught skills to deal with stress, such as relaxation and cognitive coping strategies, or how to relate more effectively to peers (e.g., deal with bullies).
    b. In a behavioral paradigm, positive consequences that appear to be maintaining the symptoms (such as being sent home from school after NES episodes) could be eliminated. Conversely, other positive consequences (such as parental attention) could be made contingent on positive, non-illness behaviors, such as the child's use of appropriate coping behaviors or improved school performance.

c. The patient's environment could be modified to minimize stressors. This might involve making adjustments to the patient's school program to address learning problems, obtaining assistance for the parents in dealing with their own psychological issues, and changing the nature of family dynamics through family therapy.
   d. If mood, anxiety, or attention problems are suspected of contributing to the patient's maladjustment, treatment with psychotropic medications could be considered.
3. The patient's symptoms should be taken seriously by the treatment team, not only to ensure that medical problems are carefully ruled out but also to maintain trust and rapport with the family while the diagnostic process proceeds.
4. During hospitalization for long-term video-electroencephalographic recording, the possibility that the events are psychogenic should be communicated early to the family (and, when appropriate, also to the child or adolescent) to allow the family to begin the process of assimilating new information that may be inconsistent with their belief that the symptoms have a physical origin. Early discussion of a possible psychogenic basis can also allow more time for education of the family and development of a treatment plan.
5. The psychosocial provider should work in a collaborative manner with the family to sort out problems in a nonjudgmental, nonthreatening way. The patient and parents may feel patronized and become defensive if the therapist takes the role of an "expert" who sees it as his or her responsibility to tell the family what they do not already know. Working with NES patients and their families requires a willingness on the provider's part to work with the family in a sensitive and unhurried manner, taking the time necessary to carefully assess all possible psychosocial stressors and respond to the family's concerns over, at times, lengthy and multiple conversations.

Several additional points are worth mentioning. Data from two published studies, by Turgay[4] and Walczak et al.,[5] suggest that shorter duration of NES is associated with better outcome. Previous data also indicate that acceptance of the NES diagnosis is associated with better outcome in adult patients.[6] It is possible that these two variables are related such that the longer patients expend effort and resources toward seeking medical services for their symptoms, and recruit social support from others for what they consider "legitimate" health problems, the more invested they become in maintaining belief in a physical cause of the condition, because to abandon this belief would create an uncomfortable level of cognitive dissonance. Patients may feel that they have wasted their own and others' time and money in seeking assistance for something as seemingly frivolous as a psychological or emotional problem. They may also find it too threatening, particularly after months or years of dismissing others' insensitive remarks about "faking" the symptoms, to admit that there is an emotional element to the NES episodes or that the NES diagnosis somehow implies that they are "crazy." For this reason, it is important that patients be seen for a caring, thorough, and comprehensive diagnostic assessment as early as possible in the course of their symptoms to minimize resistance to the diagnosis and to decrease the risk of a protracted course of NES. These considerations may help to maximize the effectiveness of the diagnostic process.

References

1. Siegel M, Barthel R. Conversion disorders on a child psychiatry consultation service. Psychosomatics 1986;27:201–204.
2. Hyman IE, Loftus EF. Some People Recover Memories of Childhood Trauma That Never Really Happened. In PS Appelbaum, LA Uyehara, MR Elm (eds), Trauma and Memory: Clinical and Legal Controversies. Oxford: Oxford University, 1997;3–24.
3. Craighead WE, Craighead LW, Ilardi SS. Psychosocial Treatments for Major Depressive Disorder. In PE Nathan, JM Gorman (eds), Treatments That Work. Oxford: Oxford University Press, 1998;226–239.
4. Turgay A. Treatment outcome for children and adolescents with conversion disorder. Can J Psychiatry 1990;35:585–588.
5. Walczak TS, Papacostas S, Williams DT, et al. Outcome after diagnosis of psychogenic nonepileptic seizures. Epilepsia 1995;36:1131–1137.
6. Mercer K, Gates J, Risse G, Mason S. Nonepileptic seizures: treatment and outcome. Paper presented at the annual meeting of the American Epilepsy Society, San Francisco, December 1996.

PART IV

Psychiatric Aspects of the Patient with Non-Epileptic Seizures

CHAPTER 20

Nosology, Classification, and Differential Diagnosis of Non-Epileptic Seizures: An Alternative Proposal

Ronald L. Martin and John R. Gates

> "When I use a word," Humpty Dumpty said, in a rather scornful tone, "it means just what I choose it to mean—neither more nor less."
> "The question is," said Alice, "whether you can make words mean so many different things."
>
> Lewis Carroll, *Through the Looking Glass*[1]

Problems in the Nosology and Classification of Seizure-Like Events

A great deal of time and effort can be spent debating definitions and terminology. Yet, although semantic arguments can be trying and seemingly fruitless, productive study of a medical condition demands a clear, precise, logically coherent, universally applicable, and consistently interpreted descriptive nosology. Such a nosology allows unambiguous communication and fosters meaningful classification,[2] which in turn facilitates differential diagnosis. On the other hand, if everyone, in a prideful "Humpty Dumpty" fashion, uses words to mean whatever they choose them to mean, the result is chaos. It must be remembered that Humpty's pride preceded his fall.

Unfortunately, the study of "seizure-like events"—that is, events that either are or are prone to be misidentified as seizures—has been marred by the lack of such a nosology and classification. Of particular difficulty are nonseizure "seizure-like events," which are better understood as associated with psychological processes. Traditionally, such events have been designated variously (to include a few) as hysteroepilepsy, pseudoseizures, or hysterical pseudoseizures, as well as hysterical, psychogenic, functional, or nonphysiologic seizures. The histories, rationales, and disadvantages of such terms have been well described many times.[3-6] More recently, the term *non-epileptic seizures*, often abbreviated as NES, has been endorsed, at least by some.[6,7] This term was adopted after a long process of considering traditional terms, including those listed previously, each of which is objectionable in one way or another. Of particular concern was the pejorative connotation of terms with the prefixes *hystero-*, *psycho-*, and even *pseudo-*. *Hystero-* and *psycho-* may impart "it's all in your head," and *pseudo-* might indicate that something is not "real" and perhaps is even deliberately falsified, that is, feigned.[8] Such concerns are understandable because there is often a need to inform patients and their families of a diagnosis in this increasingly medically sophisticated society. What clinicians want to convey is, "Yes, you (or your family member) have a *real* problem," but, "No, you do not have epilepsy." The term *non-epileptic seizures* facilitates this communication.

Thus, a major motivation for the adoption of "non-epileptic seizures" was its euphemistic value. In psychiatry, similar motivation contributed to the adoption, by some, of the eponymic *Briquet's syndrome* to replace the diagnosis of "hysteria."[9] *DSM-III* (*Diagnostic and Statistical Manual of Mental Disorders*, Third Edition)[10] substituted the descriptive term *somatization disorder* for the same entity, which was placed in the grouping of "somatoform disorders." Both *somatization disorder* and *somatoform disorders* were retained in *DSM-III-R* (Revised)[11] and *DSM-IV*.[12] Thus, euphemisms are an accepted approach. But does such an advantage of the term *non-epileptic seizures* outweigh the disadvantages?

In many ways, the current use of the term *non-epileptic seizures* is unsatisfactory. Etymologically, the term is misleading. The most widely accepted definitions among neurologists, psychiatrists, and other health professionals of the term *seizure* include designations of some combination of such adjectives as *paroxysmal*, *spontaneous*, and *transient excessive discharge of cortical neurons*. "Epilepsy" designates a chronic pattern of recurrent, spontaneous, or unprovoked seizures. To an individual who is familiar with such commonly accepted definitions of *seizure* and *epilepsy*, but not informed of the "special" meanings of *non-epileptic seizures*, the most apparent connotation of the term would be in reference to "symptomatic" seizures, that is, seizures provoked by various identifiable precipitants, such as metabolic disturbances (electrolyte disturbances such as hyponatremia, hypoglycemia), high fever, and external causes such as acute head trauma and electric shock. Such events would be seizures yet would not be epileptic seizures.

As additional evidence of problems in the current use of the term *non-epileptic seizures*, in most articles the justification for its use is reiterated, followed by a delineation of its specific meaning in the article's context. Thus, in some instances the term is applied to any event that is or resembles a seizure but is not a manifestation of epilepsy.[6,7] Included under the rubric of "non-epileptic seizures" are such disparate entities as febrile or metabolically provoked seizures, syncope, transient ischemic attacks, panic attacks, and psychotic behaviors, in addition to "psychogenic seizures." This definition of *non-epileptic seizures* is so broad that the term has either been used inconsistently, with authors assuming that readers understand what is meant in a particular context, or is qualified to be limited to a particular domain (e.g., "psychogenic" non-epileptic seizures).[13] Similarly, a myriad of classification systems have been proposed, with *non-epileptic seizures* variously defined or qualified. Thus, the term has come to have special yet inconsistent meanings, which unfortunately are not always clear to the reader.

Additionally, "non-epileptic seizures" are not commonly found in the psychiatric literature. In fact, outside of the group of investigators and clinicians with a special interest in this area, the term is virtually unknown. The term does not appear in *DSM-IV*. However, *DSM-IV* does refer to "seizures" in the list of conversion symptom examples as part of the "pseudoneurologic" symptom requirement for somatization disorder and as one type of conversion disorder: "with seizures or convulsions." As somatoform symptoms, such "seizures" are, by definition, "not fully explained by general medical conditions" (such as a metabolic disturbance or epilepsy). They are only seizures as modified by "somatoform" or "pseudoneurologic." Also, they are not "intentionally produced or feigned" (as in malingering or a factitious disorder). As a side note, although dissociative disorders are not included in the somatoform disorders grouping, *DSM-IV* includes dissociative complaints in the list of pseudoneurologic symptoms, which may fulfill requirements for somatization disorder. This represents a logical inconsistency in *DSM-IV*[14,15] and is also inconsistent with the *International Classification of Diseases*, Tenth Edition,[15] which uses a fused dissociative (conversion) disorder.[16]

Such inconsistent use of *non-epileptic seizures* cannot help but contribute to confusion in an already difficult area. If such inconsistent use is evident among academicians writing for their colleagues in peer-reviewed or editorially scrutinized venues, can use in clinical settings be expected to be any better? Nonetheless, the term has widely penetrated into clinical use and is minimally pejorative. It is the purpose of this chapter to propose a nosology and classification system that (1) is descriptively accurate, (2) is as free of inference and assumption as possible, (3) is logically consistent throughout, (4) is compatible with the classification systems most accepted in neurology and epileptology (International League Against Epilepsy classification)[17] and in psychiatry (*DSM-IV*),[12] (5) will facilitate differential diagnosis, and (6) is appropriate for communication with patients and families. The system is shown in outline form in Table 20.1 and algorithmically in the decision tree in Figure 20.1.

Decision Tree for the Differential Diagnosis of Seizure-Like Events

Following the algorithm of Figure 20.1, the process of differential diagnosis using the proposed nosology and classification can be determined by a series of "yes-no" questions in a decision-tree model. The following narrative describes the decision-making process in using the algorithm.

Explained by a General (Nonpsychiatric) Medical Condition or the Direct Effects of a Substance?

By design, seizure-like events represent a broad inclusive category of events intended to encompass a wide variety of paroxysmal events that are or could be misinterpreted as seizures. The question of whether the seizure-like events are explained by a general medical condition or are the direct effects of a substance is perhaps the most important and should first be applied to any paroxysmal event. Such a delineation is a basic dichotomization in psychiatry. Stated here in *DSM-IV* terminology, it corresponds to separating "organic" from "functional" conditions in previous classifications. The organic designation was abandoned as anachronistic, given progress in implicating "biological" (in many ways akin to organic) factors in traditionally designated functional disorders, such as depressive or bipolar mood disorders, schizophrenia and other psychotic disorders, panic disorder, and obsessive-compulsive disorder, to name a few.[18] In *DSM-IV*, the term *general medical condition* refers to all medical conditions that are not "psychiatric" or "mental." This is to emphasize that psychiatric conditions are still medical conditions. Thus, general medical conditions would include cardiovascular conditions that result in episodes of syncope, neurologic disorders with movements resembling seizures, and metabolic disturbances or epilepsy itself as an explanation for seizures. Various substances also fully explain seizures, some during intoxication (e.g., pentylenetetrazol), others during withdrawal (e.g., alcohol and other sedative-hypnotics).

TABLE 20.1
DSM-IV (Diagnostic and Statistical Manual of Mental Disorders, Fourth Edition)
Compatible Nosology and Classification of Seizure-Like Events

I. Explained by a general (nonpsychiatric) medical condition or the direct effect of a substance (intoxication or withdrawal)
   A. Paroxysmal nonseizure signs or symptoms of a general medical condition (e.g., syncope, transient ischemic attacks, tremors, dystonias, tics, migraine auras)
   B. Seizures (associated with abnormal paroxysmal discharge of cortical neurons)
      1. Symptomatic seizures (i.e., usually isolated seizures provoked by an identified precipitant [e.g., metabolic disturbances, high fever, blow to the head, electric shock, the direct effects of a substance])
      2. Epileptic seizures (chronic recurrent and unprovoked seizures, further differentiated according to the International League Against Epilepsy classification of epileptic seizures)
II. Not explained by a general medical condition or the direct effects of a substance
   A. Paroxysmal signs or symptoms explained by anxiety, mood, psychotic, or other mental disorder (e.g., panic attacks, profound psychomotor agitation or retardation, catatonia, hallucinations)
   B. Non-epileptic psychogenic seizures (seizures are simulated, either intentionally or unintentionally)
      1. Feigned seizures (i.e., intentionally produced)
         a. Malingered seizures (motivated by external incentives, such as avoiding military duty or work, obtaining financial compensation or drugs, evading criminal prosecution)
         b. Factitious seizures (apparent goal is to assume the patient role but is not otherwise motivated by objective external incentives or environmental advantages as in malingering)
      2. Somatoform seizures (not intentionally produced)
         a. Conversion seizures (presence of voluntary motor and/or sensory dysfunction or deficits)
            i. In conversion disorder (conversion symptoms only)
            ii. In somatization disorder (multiple somatic symptoms: pseudoneurologic somatoform symptoms and also at least four pain, two gastrointestinal, and one sexual or reproductive; for several years; begins before age 30 years)
            iii. In undifferentiated somatoform disorder (at least 6 months' duration; also other somatoform symptoms but criteria for somatization disorder not met)
            iv. In somatoform disorder not otherwise specified (less than 6 months' duration; also other somatoform symptoms)
         b. Dissociative seizures (dysfunction in consciousness, identity, or memory; in the absence of motor sensory components)
            i. In depersonalization disorder
            ii. In dissociative disorder not otherwise specified

Source: American Psychiatric Association. Diagnostic and Statistical Manual of Mental Disorders (4th ed). Washington, DC: American Psychiatric Association, 1994.

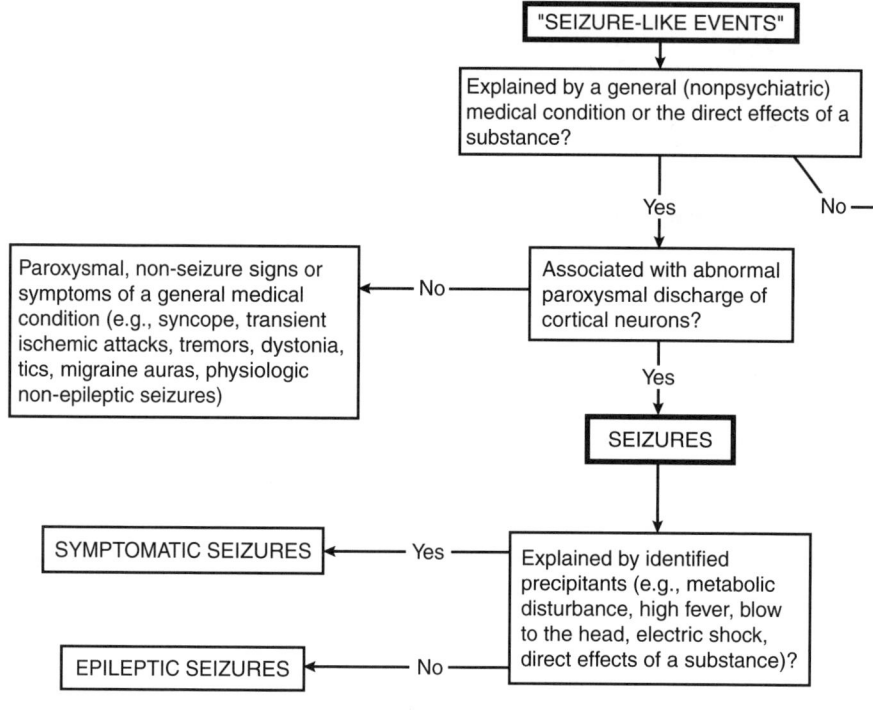

FIGURE 20.1. *DSM-IV (Diagnostic and Statistical Manual of Mental Disorders, Fourth Edition)* compatible nosology and classification of seizure-like events. (NOS = not otherwise specified.)

Nosology, Classification, and Differential Diagnosis of Non-Epileptic Seizures   259

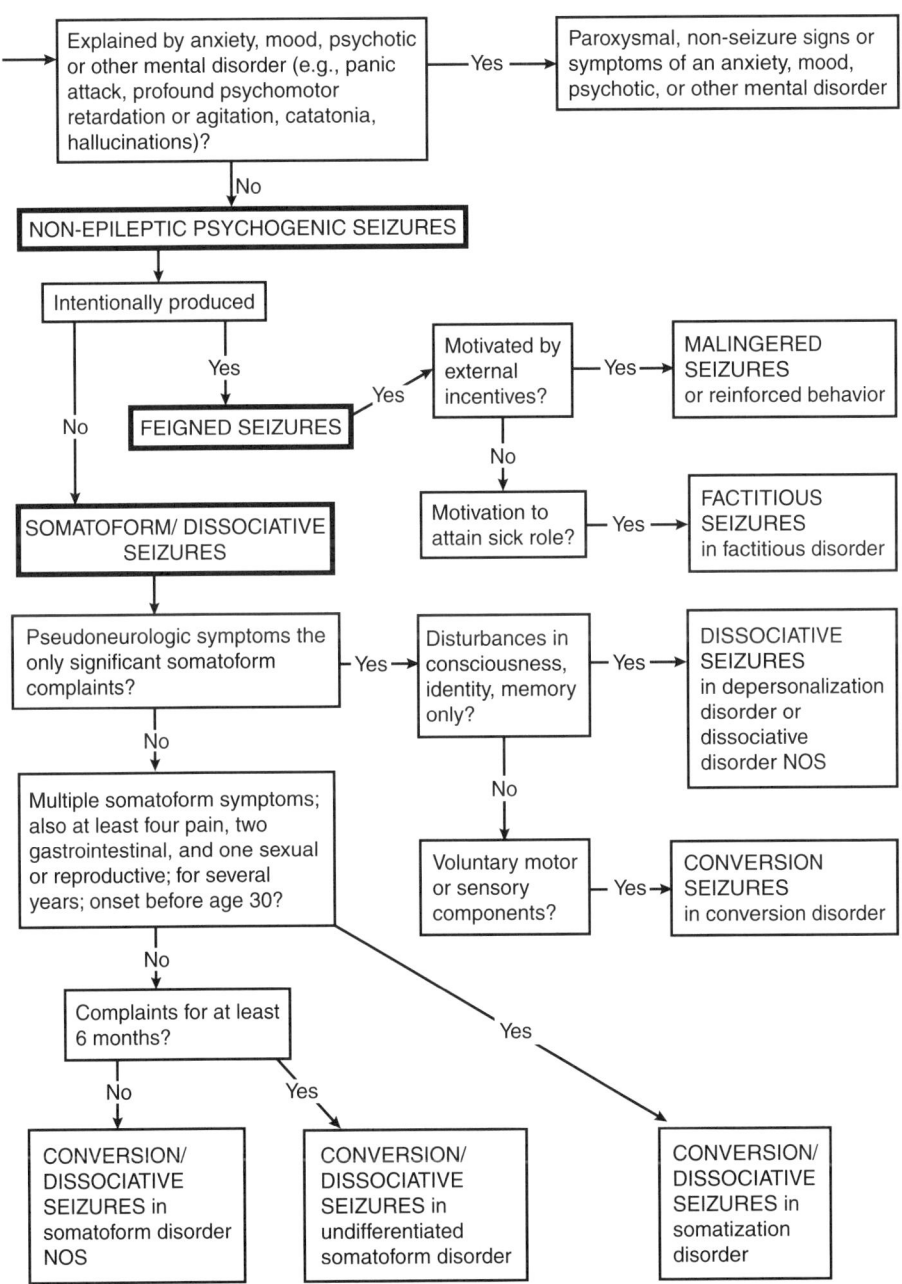

Yes

A yes answer signifies that the seizure-like event is fully explained as an effect of either an identified or presumed general medical condition or the direct effects of a substance as described previously.

No

A no answer signifies that the event is not fully explained on one of the previously mentioned bases and would lead to determination on the psychiatric arm of the algorithm. In this discussion, the "medically explained" arm is reviewed first.

Associated with Abnormal Paroxysmal Discharge of Cortical Neurons?

No

Not all medically explained events that are paroxysmal, and thereby may resemble seizures, meet the previously given definition of a seizure. Such events would be classified as "paroxysmal, nonseizure signs or symptoms of a general medical condition." Included here would be manifestations of a general medical condition such as vascular conditions that cause syncope or transient ischemic attacks. In syncope, brief loss of clear consciousness, sometimes accompanied by some spasmodic jerks, may resemble a seizure. In transient ischemic attacks, transient neurologic deficits may appear suddenly and then promptly resolve, resembling a seizure. Neurologic conditions, such as tremors, dystonias, and tics, may all be associated with sudden involuntary movements that may resemble seizures. Migraine auras may manifest with the sudden onset of sensory experiences (e.g., scintillating scotomas) or deficits that may be misinterpreted as seizures. However, all of these events, although paroxysmal, are not associated with the abnormal discharges of cortical neurons as in a seizure.

Yes

A yes answer designates that events are seizures. This leads to the question of cause, particularly as to whether they are non-epileptic or epileptic seizures.

Explained by Identified Precipitants?

Yes

A yes answer designates that the seizures are provoked by identified factors, such as metabolic disturbances (e.g., hypoxia or an electrolyte disturbance), high fever, or external causes such as a blow to the head or an electric shock or to the direct effects of a substance, whether it be intoxication or withdrawal.[6] With such a definition the occurrence of such seizures would parallel the precipitants and in most instances would be isolated events, limited to times during which the provoking precipitants were operative. These seizures, it can be argued, are symptomatic, whereby the events meet the definition of a seizure yet are not considered a result of epilepsy. This question is of major clinical importance in that for such symptomatic seizures there is generally no need for continued anti-epileptic drugs.

No

Exclusion of such factors leads to a determination of epileptic seizures. Epileptic seizures can be differentiated extensively according to current neurologic concepts,[16] but this is not the focus of this chapter, which is intended to expand on seizure-like events that do not have such physiologic explanations. Readers are directed to the International League Against Epilepsy classification for differentiation of epileptic seizures.[16]

Explained by an Anxiety, Mood, Psychotic, or Other Mental Disorder?

Backtracking to those events that are not explained by a general medical condition or the direct effects of a substance, the question of whether the event can be explained by an anxiety, mood, psychotic, or other mental disorder can be asked.

Yes

A yes designation signifies that the events are paroxysmal signs or symptoms of a mental disorder but that any resemblance to a seizure is incidental, that is, not consciously intended or motivated by factors out of awareness (i.e., "unconscious") to simulate a seizure. Examples of such events would include panic attacks, which may come on suddenly and be associated with some change in the level of awareness, resembling changes that occur with seizures. More rarely, profound psychomotor retardation or agitation also comes on suddenly and may be associated with apparent change in the level of awareness. Likewise, hallucinatory phenomena can come on suddenly and also may affect the level of awareness, thereby resembling a seizure. Paroxysms of false perceptions may resemble partial complex seizures, and disturbances in level of awareness may suggest absence seizures.

No

In the absence of such explanations, one is left with the probability that an event is a psychogenic seizure. That is, the events' resemblance to seizures is not incidental, as in the previously described events associated with anxiety, mood, or psychotic disorders. Rather, they actually simulate seizures either intentionally, as in malingering and factitious disorder, or unintentionally—that is, without conscious intent (unconsciously)—as in conversion or dissociative seizures. In each of these, there are some assumptions about psychological motivation or explanation, as are discussed later. Having determined that the event is a psychogenic seizure, the next task is to decide whether the event is produced intentionally, as alluded to above.

Intentionally Produced (Feigned)?

Yes

As used in *DSM-IV*, the term *intentionally* means conscious intent. Something can be unconsciously intentional but not fulfill the *DSM-IV* definition of intentional production. Determining whether conscious intent is present is difficult and not always clear-cut, if not impossible.[14] Some would argue that it should be abandoned. Yet, it remains a task intrinsic to Western legal systems, in which ascertaining intent is instrumental in determining the level of criminal responsibility (consider the differentiations of manslaughter versus second-degree murder). Even manslaughter is further subdivided as voluntary or involuntary.

Although imperfect, methods used in determining whether a seizure-like event is intentionally produced involve a "contextual analysis."[12] The presence of obvious objective goals, such as external incentives, avoiding military duty or work, obtaining financial compensation or drugs, or evading criminal prosecution, should make one especially suspicious of intentionality. The setting is also important to consider. In court or legal referrals, the military, or prison settings, intentionality is much more common.

If it is decided that a psychogenic seizure is intentionally produced, it is designated a *feigned seizure*. The next question pertains to the motivation for its conscious production.

Motivated by External Incentives?

This question involves whether the production is motivated by obvious external incentives as were listed previously.

Yes

If the answer is yes, the events are considered malingered seizures.

No

A no answer leads to the next question.

Motivation to Attain the Sick Role?

Yes

In the case of a yes answer, a diagnosis of factitious disorder would be considered, whereby the motivation is less obvious and involves the goal of assuming the "sick role." This is described elsewhere in *DSM-IV* as the "patient role," which is more accurate descriptively. In factitious disorders, there is some aspect about being a patient that is motivating for such individuals, perhaps in terms of the personal attention or perhaps in the procedures performed (which would be noxious to most people). In the case of a factitious seizure, the motivation could be the process of being evaluated and perhaps hospitalized, with the resultant care, concern, and attention that would be involved, as well as obtaining sometimes dramatic diagnostic procedures, such as electroencephalography, magnetic resonance imaging, computed tomography, and so forth. As strange as it may seem, procedures used for the evaluation of seizures in the past that might have included brain scans, angiography, and even the dangerous and often dreaded pneumoencephalography also were motivating. These motivations must be differentiated from others such as gaining admission to a hospital as a place to sleep and be given food and shelter, which would be considered malingering.

Another interesting although rare presentation is "factitious disorder by proxy,"[19] whereby a person, often a parent or caretaker, contrives to make it appear that another person, generally under his or her control or influence, such as a child, has some medical condition. In the case of seizures, the perpetrator might report symptoms that suggest a seizure, thereby obligating health care professionals to evaluate the victim, perform diagnostic procedures, and so forth.

Intentionally Produced?

No

In the absence of intentional production, psychogenic seizures are designated as somatoform or dissociative seizures either as symptoms of a dissociative or a conversion disorder itself or, depending on whether other somatoform symptoms are present, as components of another somatoform disorder. It is unfortunate that *DSM-IV* requires that a categorical distinction between dissociative and somatoform disorders must be made. As is explained below, perhaps a varietal differentiation would be more appropriate. In *DSM-IV*, dissociative disorders are not included as somatoform disorders in that, although they are medically unexplained symptoms that suggest a general medical condition, they do not involve *physical* symptoms. This distinction is arbitrary, however, because it appears that dissociative and conversion symptoms are closely related etiologically as well as phenomenologically.[14,15] They often coexist in the same patients. Even in

DSM-IV, dissociative symptoms are included as examples of pseudoneurologic symptoms in the criteria for somatization disorder.

Pseudoneurologic Symptoms the Only Significant Somatoform Complaints?

Yes

If the somatoform symptoms are limited to pseudoneurologic complaints, the somatoform seizure would be considered either a part of a dissociative or conversion disorder.

Disturbances in Consciousness, Identity, or Memory Only?

Yes

If the answer is yes, the event would be considered a dissociative seizure. Dissociative seizures may resemble complex partial seizures or even absence attacks. It has been argued by some that such events were actually associated with seizure activity, but this is not necessarily the case.[20,21]

No

If, on the other hand, only voluntary motor or sensory components are involved, the event would represent a conversion seizure. In some instances, of course, both voluntary motor or sensory and dissociative components may be involved. In such cases, a mixed conversion/dissociative seizure would be diagnosed. *DSM-IV* subtypes conversion disorder as "with motor symptom or deficit," "with sensory symptom or deficit," "with seizures or convulsions," or "with mixed presentation." If seizures are the only conversion symptoms, "conversion disorder with seizures or convulsions" would be diagnosed; if other conversion symptoms were seen as well, "with mixed presentation" would be the subtype.

Pseudoneurologic Symptoms the Only Significant Somatoform Complaints?

Backtracking to the question of whether no pseudoneurologic somatoform symptoms are present, the question of whether these symptoms are the only significant somatoform complaints should be asked.

No

According to *DSM-IV* definitions, if multiple nonpseudoneurologic somatoform symptoms are present, the next questions involve the following: Of which of the somatoform disorders are the somatoform seizures (whether dissociative or conversion) a component?

Multiple Somatoform Symptoms: In Addition to
Pseudoneurologic Symptoms, Also at Least Four Pain,
Two Nonpain Gastrointestinal, and One Nonpain
Sexual or Reproductive Symptoms, with an Onset before
Age 30 Years and a Duration of at Least Several Years?

Yes

If the criteria of multiple somatoform symptoms are met, somatization disorder is diagnosed. In such cases the conversion or dissociative seizures would be subsumed under this diagnosis because, as pseudoneurologic symptoms, they are a subset of the symptomatology of this disorder.[22] Conversion or dissociative disorder would not be diagnosed in addition.

No

If criteria for somatization disorder are not met but the symptoms have been present for at least 6 months, the conversion or dissociative seizures would be considered part of an undifferentiated somatoform disorder. If symptoms have been present for less than 6 months, somatoform disorder not otherwise specified would be diagnosed.

Advantages of the Proposed Nosology

It is argued that the nosology that has been outlined has major advantages over previously proposed systems, particularly in regard to differential diagnosis. It starts with making a fundamental dichotomization of seizure-like events as fully explained on the basis of a general medical condition or the direct substance effects versus those not so explained. On the medically/substance-explained side, it then differentiates between events that merely suggest seizures and the seizures themselves. The latter are dichotomized between those that are generally occasional events provoked by some identified (symptomatic) precipitant versus epileptic seizures, that is, those that occur spontaneously and recurrently. On the nonmedically/substance-explained side, the first group to be separated out have events that only incidentally (and generally not very convincingly) resemble seizures, leaving events that are designated psychogenic. Intentionally produced seizures, as are seen in malingering and factitious disorder, are then separated out leaving somatoform seizures, which are further subdivided as either dissociative or conversion seizures. It is argued that this nosology and classification can cover virtually any seizure-like event, placing the event unambiguously in the classification.

One argument against this system is that "psychogenic" and "somatoform" may be perceived as pejorative and thereby not optimally acceptable to patients. However, because these terms are "upstream" from the diagnosis, they are rather inevident to patients, who would be advised that they were manifesting a conversion or dissociative seizure. The term *somatoform* was, at least in part, adopted by psychiatry because of its neutrality. *Conversion* and *dissociative* can also be perceived as relatively neutral and nonjudgmental. Informing patients who are malingering or are manifesting a factitious disorder of the diagnosis may be more problematic. Such patients may simply withdraw from treatment. Still, unnecessary diagnostic and therapeutic procedures may have been avoided.

The authors welcome debate on this subject.

References

1. Carroll L. The Annotated Alice: Alice's Adventures in Wonderland and Through the Looking Glass. New York: Btamhall House, 1960;268–269.
2. Kendell RE. The Role of Diagnosis in Psychiatry. Oxford: Blackwell Scientific, 1975;vii–viii, 1–8.
3. Fenton GW. Epilepsy and hysteria. Br J Psychiatry 1986;149:28–37.
4. Trimble MR. Pseudoseizures. Neurol Clin 1986;4:531–548.
5. Gates JR, Mercer K. Nonepileptic events. Semin Neurol 1995;15:167–174.
6. Gates JR, Erdahl P. Classification of Non-Epileptic Events. In AJ Rowan, JR Gates (eds), Non-Epileptic Seizures. Boston: Butterworth–Heinemann, 1993;21–30.
7. Porter RJ. Epileptic and Non-Epileptic Seizures. In AJ Rowan, JR Gates (eds), Non-Epileptic Seizures. Boston: Butterworth–Heinemann, 1993;9–20.
8. Chabolla DR, Krahn LE, So EL, Rummans TA. Psychogenic nonepileptic seizures. Mayo Clin Proc 1996;71:493–500.
9. Martin RL, Yutzy SH. Somatoform Disorders. In RE Hales, JA Talbott, SC Yudofsky (eds), The American Psychiatric Press Textbook of Psychiatry (2nd ed). Washington, DC: American Psychiatric Press, 1994;591–622.
10. American Psychiatric Association. Diagnostic and Statistical Manual of Mental Disorders (3rd ed). Washington, DC: American Psychiatric Association, 1980.
11. American Psychiatric Association. Diagnostic and Statistical Manual of Mental Disorders (3rd ed, revised). Washington, DC: American Psychiatric Association, 1987.
12. American Psychiatric Association. Diagnostic and Statistical Manual of Mental Disorders (4th ed). Washington, DC: American Psychiatric Association, 1994.
13. Lesser RP, Krauss GL. Psychogenic Non-Epileptic Seizures Resembling Complex Partial Seizures. In AJ Rowan, JR Gates (eds), Non-Epileptic Seizures. Boston: Butterworth–Heinemann, 1993;39–45.
14. Martin RL. Conversion disorder, proposed autonomic arousal disorder, and pseudopsychosis. In TA Widiger, AF Frances, HA Pincus, et al. (eds), DSM-IV Sourcebook, vol 2. Washington, DC: American Psychiatric Association, 1996;893–914.

15. World Health Organization. The ICD-10 Classification of Mental and Behavioral Disorders Clinical Descriptions and Diagnostic Guidelines (10th rev). Geneva: World Health Organization, 1992.
16. Martin RL. Diagnostic issues for conversion disorder. Hosp Commun Psychiatry 1992;43:771–773.
17. Commission on Classification and Terminology of the International League Against Epilepsy. Proposal for revised clinical and electroencephalographic classification of epileptic seizures. Epilepsia 1981;22:489–501.
18. Tucker G, Popkin M, Caine E, et al. Reorganizing the "organic" disorders. Hosp Commun Psychiatry 1990;41:722–724.
19. Dreifuss FE. Munchausen Syndrome by Proxy. In AJ Rowan, JR Gates (eds), Non-Epileptic Seizures. Boston: Butterworth–Heinemann, 1993;203–207.
20. Devinsky O, Putnam F, Grafman J, et al. Dissociative states and epilepsy. Neurology 1989;39:835–840.
21. Ross C, Heber S, Anderson BA, et al. Differentiating multiple personality disorder and complex partial seizures. Gen Hosp Psychiatry 1989;11:54–58.
22. Martin RL, Yutzy SH. Somatoform Disorders. In A Tasman, J Kay, JA Lieberman (eds), Somatoform Disorders. Philadelphia: Saunders, 1997;1119–1155.

CHAPTER 21

Relationship of Remote and Recent Life Events to the Onset and Course of Non-Epileptic Seizures

Elizabeth S. Bowman

> *The hysterical fit of convulsions, far from being a simple phenomenon, is, on the contrary, a very variable and complex symptom. The convulsions have all sorts of meanings.*
> Pierre Janet, *The Major Symptoms of Hysteria*[1]

After a diagnosis of non-epileptic seizures (NES) has been made, clinicians and patients alike face an important question: "Why is *this* person having NES *now*?" The answer is important because the treatment should be tailored to the cause of the NES. Unfortunately, answering this question can be difficult because there is no single cause of NES and because each patient's life situation is unique.

Neurologists can address this problem with a general explanation that life stresses cause NES and that psychiatric evaluation is indicated. In addition to arriving at a concurrent psychiatric diagnosis (such as panic or major depression), mental health evaluators usually need a detailed understanding of the psychological function of NES (e.g., expression of anger, grief, etc.) if they are to successfully apply psychotherapeutic or behavioral treatments. The antecedent and concurrent life events of NES patients are often the key to the psychic reasons for the seizures and their treatment.

Interviewers who feel at a loss about what types of events might be important sometimes conduct an interview of blind general probing. This is as inefficient as driving from Chicago to Buenos Aires without a road map. You might (or might not) arrive at your destination, but the therapeutic journey is slow. Knowledge of the patterns of life events associated with NES is like a road map to guide interviews. The purpose of this chapter is to help clinicians understand what life events frequently contribute to NES so that they can organize their interviews efficiently (Appendix 21.1). This aim is accomplished by presenting an overview of the literature on precipitants of NES, as well as a discussion of the patterns of such life events found in one study of NES patients.

Literature Review

The literature on life events associated with NES consists mostly of case reports. Few systematic studies have been conducted, and little has been written about the patterns into which these events fall. The wide arrays of NES-associated events that have been identified fall into general categories: (1) childhood and adulthood trauma, (2) bereavement or losses, and (3) acute or situational stresses.

Childhood and Adulthood Trauma

Many reports comment on the association of childhood sexual abuse with conversion seizures. Between 1964 and 1996, 24 reports mentioned past or current sexual abuse or incest in adolescents or adults. Bowman[2] found that 11% of NES patients reported the initial onset of NES during ongoing childhood or adolescent sexual abuse. Goodwin et al.[3] and LaBarbera and Dozier[4] noted that termination or disclosure of incest precipitated NES in adolescents.

Five studies of series of NES patients have found that such individuals reported higher rates of physical and sexual child abuse than did general population subjects, with 24–58% reporting childhood sexual abuse and 15–71% reporting childhood physical abuse.[5-8] In comparison, North American general population rates are 5–13% for physical abuse[9,10] and 6–38% for sexual abuse.[11,12] Betts and Boden[13] found a significant association between a reported history of childhood sexual abuse and re-enactment and fainting types of NES.

The connection between conversion symptoms (including seizures) and trauma or adversity is not new. Janet[1] and Briquet[14] mentioned emotionally traumatic events, including the witnessing of trauma, as precipitants of a variety of conversion symptoms. Ljungberg[15] reported adverse childhood environments in 35% of his subjects with hysteria. Snyder et al.[6] found that 55% of their NES subjects had major childhood trauma.

Adulthood Trauma

Adulthood trauma can also precipitate NES. Bowman,[2] Caldwell and Stewart,[16] Kloster,[17] Nash,[18] and Shen et al.[19] noted rape as a precipitant of NES in males and females. Adulthood physical assaults[5,17] and a variety of accidents can also trigger the onset of NES. Accidents with even minor head injuries have long been noted to precede the onset of NES.[20] Lancman et al.[21] found that 16% of adult NES subjects had head injuries with loss of consciousness. The author found that 53% (24 of 45) of NES subjects reported a lifetime history of head injury with loss of consciousness, but these events were often remote and not always relevant to seizure onset (Bowman, unpublished data, 1996).

The literature suggests that NES begin or recur when childhood abuse is followed in adulthood by trauma or by events that are reminiscent of childhood trauma.[2,22,23] The author found that 11% of 27 subjects fell into this category.[2] Precipitating reminders of child abuse have included head traumas, surgery, accidents, changes in sexual activity,[2] rape,[2,18] and childbirth.[24] Domestic abuse was found in at least 42% of Bowman and Markand's[7] subjects and was reported by Fakhoury et al.[25] to precipitate NES as late as 50–60 years after childhood abuse. Even surgery may serve as a symbolic physical retraumatization, precipitating NES in victims of past abuse.[26]

Bereavement

In numerous reports, depression, bereavement, and a variety of losses have precipitated NES. The death of family members is mentioned most frequently.[17,21,27,28] Anniversaries of deaths or accidents have also been reported as precipitants, especially when grieving had been blocked or incomplete.[29,30] NES may also be associated with other losses, such as miscarriages, divorce, or children moving away.[28]

Acute or Situational Stresses

The third category of life events reported to precipitate NES is acute or situational stresses. One report mentions multiple life stresses in 11%,[2] and another notes acute situational stresses in 70%.[31] The most commonly mentioned stress is domestic problems or family conflicts, noted in 20%,[32] one-third,[21] and two-thirds[33] of NES subjects. Other acute stresses are illnesses and surgeries, lawsuits, and job pressures.[17,20,26,29,34]

Among children and adolescents, the most common life events mentioned are family conflict (in one-third[13]) and sexual abuse, especially incest.[3,4,20,35–39] In both cases, NES may be an indirect communication of personal distress about family life. Other precipitants of NES in youth are learning disabilities and school pressures,[40] parental loss,[41] and head injury.[35]

The literature indicates that the life events that trigger NES are not always discernible. One-fifth of subjects in Lancman et al.'s adult[21] and adolescent[35] series had no obvious abnormalities in social background. Guberman[29] noted that recent, obviously upsetting events were found in NES patients without long psychiatric histories. In patients with long psychiatric histories, however, precipitating events were less obvious (e.g., not getting a work promotion) but functioned as emotional traumas. Bjornes[42] summed up the implications concerning the precipitants of NES, noting that they constitute a psychological crisis that disturbs a balance between defenses and forbidden emotions or mental content. This general principle explains why NES are triggered by diverse events, ranging from the seemingly trivial to the catastrophic.

In the next section, results are presented from the only study that has systematically assessed remote and recent life events in relationship to NES in adults.

Research Data: Seizure-Associated Events in 58 Patients with Non-Epileptic Seizures

The Sample

As is more fully described in Bowman and Markand,[7] the author studied 58 adults (35 women and 23 men) at Indiana University's video-electroencephalography laboratory and epilepsy clinic between 1991 and 1995, with NES captured by video-electroencephalography. Subjects with below-normal IQ were excluded. Nine subjects had concomitant epilepsy. Because only adults were studied, the results from this sample should not be generalized to child or adolescent NES patients or to patients with subnormal intelligence.

Method of Study

The subjects gave informed consent to participate in a systematic assessment of psychiatric diagnosis (via structured interview) and life events previously reported as associated with NES (via an exploratory interview). Subjects completed self-report questionnaires about personal history and abuse or trauma. The author gathered information of life events associated with seizures in an extensive, unstructured interview that inquired about the onset and temporal course of seizures; the form of the seizures; childhood, home, and caretakers; education; military and vocational experiences; interpersonal and sexual relationships; family relationships in

TABLE 21.1
Frequent Immediate Precipitants of Non-Epileptic Seizures in Adults

	Frequencies in Samples		
	58 Adults	35 Women	23 Men
Accident, any type	11	9	2
Clustered life stresses	10	3	7
Role change	10	4	6
Personal illness or surgery	10	6	4
Bereavement or anniversary of loss	8	7	1
Relationship conflict	8	1	7
Sexual events*	8	7	1
Contact/impending contact with abuser or rapist	7	6	1
Spouse physical/sexual abuse	7	6	1
Job loss/pressures/conflicts	5	0	5

*Includes onset of menses, incestuous intercourse, first sexual activity, affairs, new romantic interest, homosexual advances.

childhood; current economic situation; disability-seeking; medical history; the details of any abuse in childhood or adulthood; and other childhood and adulthood losses and traumas. Subjects also described the way that conflicts and emotions such as anger or grief were handled by them and their family of origin and in their current family situation. Subjects also were asked why they thought they were having NES.

The interview placed the onset and recurrence of NES in the context of a timeline of life events, personal psychodynamics, and psychiatric illnesses. The timing and meaning of life events were compared to the onset and course of the seizures to look for patterns. This method yields data that are subjective, but the results resemble the outcome of a psychodynamically oriented psychiatric evaluation of the cause of NES.

Findings

The life histories of these subjects indicated that both remote and recent events were significant contributors to the onset, worsening, or recurrence of NES. The author found it useful to organize contributory life events into three categories, which are discussed in detail below: (1) immediate precipitants, (2) contextual contributors, and (3) remote contributors.

Immediate Precipitants

The author defined immediate precipitants as the most psychologically significant events that occurred in the minutes to weeks before the onset, recurrence, or exacerbation of NES. Subjects often experienced more than one category of event as an immediate precipitant. Table 21.1 shows the 10 most common categories of immediate precipitating events in the 58 subjects described previously.

Accidents were almost evenly divided between vehicular and other types, some of which were minor, but a number involved being struck in the head. Clustered life stresses generally involved stresses in several areas (job, marital, legal, familial, financial, etc.). Protracted divorce or custody battles contributed significantly to some of these clustered stresses. More than one-half of the role change stresses involved marital status changes (engagement, recent marriage, divorce). Seven of the eight relationship conflicts involved family. Contact or impending contact with abusers included stalking by abusive husbands and unexpected social contact with relatives who had been childhood abusers. For several women, protracted stalking encounters by abusive ex-spouses ended in beatings, death threats, or armed confrontations.

Less frequent immediate precipitants included contact with abused children, impending career success, acute depression, family illness, adulthood assault (not by spouse), rape, separation from abusive spouse, parental abandonment (precipitated childhood onset), parental separation, and pregnancy.

Some gender differences were apparent and may relate to the higher rates of childhood abuse and sexual abuse among female subjects. Women showed nonsignificant trends toward being more likely than men to have NES after abuse-related events ($p < .10$) or sexual events ($p = .05$, Z test). In men, NES were significantly more likely to have been precipitated by relationship conflicts ($p < .01$) or job stresses ($p < .02$).

Some immediate precipitants were easy to detect because of a close temporal relationship to seizure onset or recurrence or because they were obvious stressors (the death of a spouse, a recent rape, etc.). As case 1 illustrates, some precipitants are not obvious.

Case 1: A Less than Obvious Precipitant

A happily married woman in her 40s with a satisfying job had her first onset of NES without an obvious immediate precipitant. Exploration of her background revealed that early in childhood her sibship had been separated into different adoptive homes because of extreme child abuse. At approximately age 4 she was adopted by insecure parents who changed her first and last names and vigorously kept her from information about her family or contact with her siblings. Over the past several years she had been increasingly bothered by this loss and had sought to find her siblings. Seizures began shortly after she discovered that her adoptive mother had secretly blocked a recent attempt by her biological siblings to locate her. Perhaps her NES safely expressed an upsurge of simmering rage at her controlling mother and grief over her childhood losses. NES stopped when she located her lost siblings, who confirmed her memories of child abuse. This case illustrates how knowledge of a patient's early life can help to identify a seemingly minor recent event as stressful enough to precipitate NES.

Case 2: The Last Straw Precipitant

A married man in his 30s reported the first onset of NES within hours of being served with legal papers that demanded an increase in child support payments. Additional current life stresses were found, including financial problems and conflict with his stepchildren. Exploration of his past revealed a childhood marked by severe emotional rejection. He watched in helpless rage as his father beat his mother and molested his sisters. Lacking constructive outlets for anger, he acted out antisocially and abused substances until substance abuse treatment and a religious conversion ended access to these coping mechanisms. Subsequently, he became acutely depressed in the face of several years of protracted legal harassment, destruction of property, and life threats from his ex-wife. As in childhood, he felt enraged but helpless to respond. He admitted being afraid of his anger because of his history of destructive acting out. His NES consisted of amnesic episodes with shaking, crying, and moaning. He felt angry when awakening from them.

Cases 1 and 2 illustrate five key findings about the role of immediate precipitants and their relationship to life context and remote life events. First and most important, the significance of the immediate precipitant is often understandable only after learning more about the patient's past, especially personal relationships and earlier traumas. In case 2, for example, a history of helpless rage in the face of harassment and lack of family modeling of appropriate expressions of anger were critical to understanding the reaction to the new legal demands.

Second, although the immediate precipitant (e.g., the serving of legal papers in case 2) is often what the patient considers to be the cause of NES, it is usually not the ultimate dynamic or emotional cause (which in these two cases was suppressed anger). Third, immediate precipitants are often a real or symbolic last straw that breaks the ability of the person to cope with feelings they have barely kept in check. The precipitant may provide clues about the ultimate cause of the seizures (in case 2, anger about observing abuse while being helpless).

Fourth, a cluster of events may occur close together that serve as precipitants (such as a series of legal setbacks as in case 2). Fifth, the variety of immediate precipitating events is much greater than the number of basic underlying emotional causes of NES. This study found that immediate precipitants served three primary psychological functions: (1) arousal of the recollection of or the affect concerning past trauma, (2) the raising of chronic suppressed anger to an intolerable level, and (3) arousal of anxiety or sadness over past or impending losses.

In summary, immediate precipitants of NES may not be obvious. They generally cannot be understood without exploration of the patient's life history and current life context. Immediate precipitants generally function to stir up conflicted and unacceptable emotions to an intolerable pitch that results in release via NES.

TABLE 21.2
Frequent Life Contexts That Contribute to Non-Epileptic Seizures

1. Gradually increasing awareness of feelings or memories about child abuse experiences. Example: The patient's child is at the same age the patient was when the sexual abuse began.
2. A chronically frustrating but seemingly inescapable situation. Example: Chronic conflict with a boss in a job from which quitting or transfer is not an option.
3. Chronic marital tension or ongoing domestic abuse.
4. Irreconcilable family loyalty conflicts.

Contextual Contributors

Table 21.2 lists the contextual contributors to NES, found in three-fourths of our sample. Less common life context contributors include unresolved grief or multiple bereavements, middle-age job or life disappointments, loyalty conflict in enmeshed families, chronic legal battles, chronic physical illness or pain, anniversaries of traumas or losses, middle-age fears of illness or pain, and loss of previous outlet for feelings (e.g., cessation of substance abuse).

Contextual contributors are usually life situations rather than discrete life events. These psychodynamic and personal settings form the fertile ground on which a variety of immediate precipitants may fall, leading to the sprouting of NES. The limited ability of most NES patients to express emotions is, in a sense, the definitive context that contributes to their seizures, but it does not strictly qualify as a life event. In this study, 70% of subjects with marked emotional suppression were male and often came from backgrounds in which masculinity was equated with stoicism.

Contextual contributors and immediate precipitating events are not mutually exclusive. In case 2, for example, the precipitating event of a demand for more child support was part of the context of a protracted and frustrating legal battle. However, other parts of the patient's life (intrafamilial conflict, financial problems), although distinct from the immediate precipitant, contributed to his overall frustration.

Generally, when contextual factors are present, they appear more emotionally powerful than the immediate precipitant as a true cause for the NES. For instance, in case 1 the ongoing frustration with the controlling mother and the pressing desire for finding family roots were far more psychologically important than the final action of the mother in blocking access to the siblings. Indeed, the patient was angry because her mother had denied her requests for information about her family for several decades.

As the following case shows, some contextual contributors may be enough to precipitate NES without any final event.

Case 3: Trapped in a Context

> A young woman began having NES in her senior year of high school. Her history was devoid of significant losses, trauma, or overt conflicts with family or peers. She revealed that she believed her family expected her to attend college, but she felt emotionally unready and doubted her academic capabilities. She had not revealed this to them for fear that she would disappoint her parents. NES appeared to express her anxiety over feeling trapped between disappointing her parents or enduring the humiliation of anticipated academic failure. With encouragement, she revealed her feelings to her parents, who supported her decision to delay college. NES soon stopped.

Contextual contributors pose particular challenges for interviewers. Patients with NES often are either not conscious of contextual contributors or do not want to admit their existence. Thus, contexts must be ascertained indirectly by asking about a range of life situations (e.g., How do they like their job and boss? How are their children doing academically and socially? Have there been changes in whom they live with? How long have they been married, separated, or divorced? What is their satisfaction with their spouse? Are there current legal problems?). Sometimes, the context can be elicited by asking what has been on the patient's mind lately.

Remote Life Events

Some events contribute to the genesis of NES although they are temporally remote (arbitrarily defined as longer than 1 year previous to the onset of seizures). They are generally emotionally powerful events, commonly traumatic in nature. The emotional pain that these events generate can be so powerful that subjects repress or dissociate them from awareness or admit that they have actively avoided the feelings for years. These patients may have found it psychologically less painful to express affect about these events somatically in NES or other somatic symptoms than via direct conscious mechanisms.

Because of psychological and temporal remoteness, such contributing events may not be volunteered by patients and can easily be overlooked by interviewers. Subjects often have partial amnesia for these events. In our study of 45 subjects, we found that 73% had amnesia for significant blocks of childhood, and 82% reported amnesia for nonictal adulthood events.[7] However, some subjects voluntarily brought up these remote events as the likely cause of their NES.

Table 21.3 shows the seven most common remote contributing events found in our sample. The shared characteristic among these events is the resulting unresolved strong feelings. Remote contributors are usually childhood events, but unresolved feelings from adulthood traumas may also be important, especially when combined with a history of childhood trauma.

TABLE 21.3
Common Remote Events That Contribute to Non-Epileptic Seizures

1. Childhood sexual abuse
2. Childhood physical abuse
3. Chronic emotional rejection by parents
4. Childhood abandonment or other serious childhood trauma
5. Physical assaults or life-threatening events in adulthood
6. A chronically anger-engendering or violent family that punished the child's open expression of anger
7. Nonfamilial rape as an adolescent or adult

Two categories of remote events involved emotional rather than physical or sexual maltreatment: (1) chronic belittling rejection (found in one-third of subjects) and (2) an anger-inducing family (one-fifth of subjects). Both situations resulted in individuals who were filled with emotional pain without a safe way to express it. Information about anger-inducing families was elicited by asking how (in childhood and adulthood) the patient and each of his or her parents responded when angry. The anger-inducing families included those in whom all expression of anger was avoided, those with a battering father and a mother who tried to escape beatings by avoiding expressions of anger, and those in which the child was provoked but punished for responding with anger. These families produced adult patients who were cauldrons of unexpressed anger that they were unaware of or were terrified to express.

It is imperative to ask about these seven types of events but to anticipate false denials of them. Like Betts and Boden,[13] the author encountered initial denial of shame-inducing events, such as rape or sexual abuse. Disclosure was aided by building rapport, then asking about abuse near the end of the interview. A number of subjects denied trauma or abuse on the written checklist they completed before the interview but verbally disclosed these events in the interview. Some subjects had never been asked about or divulged rapes or childhood sexual abuse. However, a history of child abuse does not automatically mean that child abuse experiences are a cause of the NES. In 18% of our subjects who reported physical child abuse and 17% of those who reported childhood sexual abuse, we could find no plausible emotional connection between the abuse and the NES.

Temporally remote adolescent or adult rapes contributed to NES in one-fifth of subjects. Adulthood assaults or life-threatening events contributed to NES in two-fifths of subjects.

How can we know that events so remote are connected to the genesis of NES? First, strong emotional responses to questions about these events indicated that they were still causing considerable distress. Some subjects initially denied trauma with suddenly lowered heads, trembling chins, and tearful eyes.

Disclosure was aided by gently and softly remarking on the subject's pain and inviting more information but giving explicit permission to decline further discussion. Second, in a number of interviews, transient conversion symptoms (seizures, paralysis, tremors, numbness, deafness, muteness) and episodes of dissociative amnesia occurred when subjects began to discuss remote trauma or conflicts about anger. Third, a number of patients explicitly connected these remote events to NES or admitted that memories and feelings about remote traumas had been increasingly intrusive and distressing in recent years. Fourth, on follow-up, those who effectively dealt with their abuse or anger in therapy had marked reduction or cessation of NES.

Childhood abuse experiences are the most common remote event. Directly or indirectly, it appears that childhood sexual abuse contributed to NES in one-half and childhood physical abuse in one-third of the 58 adults.[7] Betts and Boden[13] and Arnold and Privitera[8] report similar findings. Female subjects reported significantly more childhood and adulthood physical and sexual abuse than male subjects—approximately twice the frequency in most categories of trauma.[43] In addition to frank childhood abuse, other childhood traumas (being orphaned, abandoned, or chronically exposed to domestic violence) occurred in 40% of patients but appeared unrelated to the NES in one-third of this group.

Remote traumas and emotional conflicts set the stage for NES when the emotions they engendered are not dealt with. This is particularly likely to happen when dissociation severs the affect or part of the memory of the event from conscious access. Like old volcanoes, these simmering emotions lie partially dormant until painful life contexts and immediate precipitants jolt them to life. How these categories of life events combine is the subject of the final section of this chapter.

Patterns of Life Events Associated with Seizures

The variety of life events associated with NES is vast. Thus, finding recurrent patterns of remote and recent events that contribute to NES is essential for conducting efficient interviews. Our subjects had four general patterns of events, or life pathways, to NES.

The most common event pathway is the reactivation of emotions about child abuse by a variety of adulthood precipitants. This pattern occurred in one-half of consecutive NES subjects and was significantly more frequent in women (22 of 35, 63%) than in men (4 of 23, 17%). In this group, adulthood precipitants included trauma (e.g., spouse abuse) or more mundane events that symbolized earlier trauma or threatened to bring a re-experience of traumatic feelings (e.g., an incest victim awakening in genital pain after gynecologic surgery or an abused schoolteacher encountering abused children for the first time in adulthood). Events that would have been mere stresses for other people became emotional traumas because of unresolved feelings about child abuse. Adulthood sexual demands (not normally considered a stress) served as a seizure precipitant for some women with a history of childhood sexual abuse.

The second pattern is chronic repression of anger followed by a series of adulthood frustrations. This occurred in one-fourth of the subjects and was more common in men (8 of 23, 35%) than in women (2 of 35, 6%). This pattern was accompanied by a family history of dysfunctional handling of anger, personal denial of feeling or expressing anger, or distorted beliefs about anger (e.g., anger can only be expressed in violence and therefore it is unsafe even to feel it). Commonly, midlife family or job disappointments contributed to the gradual rise of repressed anger to a point at which NES were the only acceptable outlet. Interviewers should look first for these two patterns because they accounted for NES in three-fifths of consecutive adult subjects with NES.[7]

The third pattern, evident in approximately 10% of NES patients, is a relationship of NES to trauma solely in late adolescence or adulthood. In such cases the precipitants are more obvious because the trauma is generally quite severe. NES in these subjects may represent an expression of dissociated terror occurring during severe accidents, rapes, or assaults.

The fourth pattern is NES in response to nontraumatic adulthood stresses that are unrelated to chronic anger. This pattern is evident in fewer than 10% of the subjects. It is noted in individuals with low-normal IQs or in persons with very immature coping abilities who are limited in their general ability to express a variety of emotions verbally or to manage them cognitively. NES in these subjects may represent an outlet for a variety of emotions. Because persons with below-normal IQs were excluded from this study, these data probably underestimate the frequency of this pattern of precipitating life events. Among cognitively intact subjects in this group, precipitating stresses were more severe (i.e., chronic physical pain or multiple losses in close succession).

In conclusion, although a wide variety of life events contribute to NES, these events generally fall into a handful of narrative patterns that represent a combination of emotionally powerful remote events, ongoing stressful life contexts, and recent "final straw" events that precipitate the actual onset of the NES. In general, life events contribute to NES by creating overwhelming feelings of terror, anger, or loss that are kept out of awareness or whose direct expression is viewed by the patient as forbidden.

References

1. Janet PF. The Major Symptoms of Hysteria. New York: Macmillan, 1907;22.

2. Bowman ES. Etiology and clinical course of pseudoseizures. Relationship to trauma, depression, and dissociation. Psychosomatics 1993;34:333.
3. Goodwin J, Simms M, Bergman R. Hysterical seizures: a sequel to incest. Am J Orthopsychiatry 1979;49:698.
4. LaBarbera JD, Dozier JR. Psychologic responses of incestuous daughters: emerging patterns. South Med J 1981;74:1478.
5. Alper K, Devinsky O, Perrine K, et al. Nonepileptic seizures and childhood sexual and physical abuse. Neurology 1993;43:1950.
6. Synder SL, Rosebaum DH, Rowan AJ. SCID diagnosis of panic disorder in psychogenic seizure patients. J Neuropsychiatry Clin Neurosci 1994; 6:261.
7. Bowman ES, Markand ON. Psychodynamics and psychiatric diagnoses of pseudoseizure subjects. Am J Psychiatry 1996;153:57.
8. Arnold LM, Privitera MD. Psychopathology and trauma in epileptic and psychogenic seizure patients. Psychosomatics 1996;37:438.
9. Finkelhor D. Child Sexual Abuse—New Theory and Research. New York: Free Press, 1984.
10. Russell DEH. The incidence and prevalence of intrafamilial and extrafamilial sexual abuse of female children. Child Abuse Neglect 1983;7:133.
11. Stein MB, Walker FR, Anderson G, et al. Childhood physical and sexual abuse in patients with anxiety disorders and in a community sample. Am J Psychiatry 1996; 153:275.
12. Mullen PE, Romans-Clarkson SE, Walton VA, et al. Impact of sexual and physical abuse on women's mental health. Lancet 1988;1:841.
13. Betts T, Boden S. Diagnosis, management and prognosis of a group of 128 patients in non-epileptic attack disorder. Part II. Previous childhood sexual abuse in the etiology of these disorders. Seizure 1992;1:27.
14. Mai FM, Merskey H. Briquet's "Treatise on Hysteria." Arch Gen Psychiatry 1980;37:1401.
15. Ljungberg L. Hysteria. A clinical, prognostic and genetic study. Acta Psychiatr Scand 1957;32(Suppl 112):1.
16. Caldwell TA, Stewart RS. Hysterical seizures and hypnotherapy. Am J Clin Hypn 1981;23:294.
17. Kloster R. Pseudo-Epileptic vs. Epileptic Seizures: A Comparison. In L Gram, SI Johannessen, PO Osterman, M Sillanpaa (eds), Pseudoepileptic Seizures. Petersfield, UK: Wrightson Biomedical, 1993;3–16.
18. Nash JL. Pseudoseizures: etiologic and psychotherapeutic considerations. South Med J 1993;86:1248.
19. Shen W, Bowman ES, Markand ON. Presenting the diagnosis of pseudoseizure. Neurology 1990;40:756.
20. Liske E, Forster FM. Pseudoseizures: a problem in the diagnosis and management of epileptic patients. Neurology 1964;13:41.
21. Lancman ME, Brotherman TA, Asconape JJ, Penry JK. Psychogenic seizures in adults: a longitudinal analysis. Seizure 1993;2:281.

22. Blumer D, Montouris G, Herman B. Psychiatric morbidity in seizure patients on a neurodiagnostic monitoring unit. J Neuropsychiatry 1995;7:445.
23. Torem MS. Non-Epileptic Seizures as a Dissociative Disorder. In AJ Rowan, JR Gates (eds), Non-Epileptic Seizures. Boston: Butterworth–Heinemann, 1993;173–179.
24. Miller HR. Psychogenic seizures treated by hypnosis. Am J Clin Hypn 1983;25:248.
25. Fakhoury T, Abou-Khalil B, Newman K. Psychogenic seizures in old age: a case report. Epilepsia 1993;34:1049.
26. Ward PE, McCarthy DJ, Nyman GW. Podiatric implications of psychogenic seizures. J Foot Surg 1998;27:222.
27. Standage KF. The etiology of hysterical seizures. Can Psychiat Assoc J 1975;20:67–73.
28. Gardner DL, Goldberg RL. Psychogenic seizures and loss. Int J Psychiatry Med 1982–83;12:121.
29. Guberman A. Psychogenic pseudoseizures in non-epileptic patients. Can J Psychiatry 1982;27:401.
30. Ramchandani D, Schindler BA. Distinguishing features of pseudocomplex partial seizures. Bull Menninger Clin 1992;56:479.
31. Pakalinis A, Drake ME, Phillips B. Neuropsychiatric aspects of psychogenic status epilepticus. Neurology 1991;41:1104.
32. Lempert T, Schmidt D. Natural history and outcome of psychogenic seizures: a clinical study in 50 patients. J Neurol 1990;237:35.
33. Buchanan N, Snars J. Pseudoseizures (non epileptic attack disorder)—clinical management and outcome in 50 patients. Seizure 1993;2:141.
34. Parry T, Hirsch N. Psychogenic seizures after general anaesthesia. Anaesthesia 1992;47:534.
35. Lancman ME, Asconape JJ, Graves S, Gibson PA. Psychogenic seizures in children: long-term analysis of 43 cases. J Child Neurol 1994;9:404.
36. McAnarney E. The older abused child. Pediatrics 1975;55:298.
37. LaBarbera JD, Dozier E. Hysterical seizures: the role of sexual exploitation. Psychosomatics 1980;21:897.
38. Gross M. Incestuous rape: a cause for hysterical seizures in our adolescent girls. Am J Orthopsychiatry 1979;49:704.
39. Goodwin J. Pseudoseizures and incest. Am J Psychiatry 1979;136:1231.
40. Silver LB. Conversion disorder with pseudoseizures in adolescence: a stress reaction to unrecognized and untreated learning disabilities. J Am Acad Child Psychiatry 1982;21:508.
41. Glenn TJ, Simonds JF. Hypnotherapy of a psychogenic seizure disorder in an adolescent. Am J Clin Hypn 1977;19:245.
42. Bjornes H. Aetiological Models as a Basis for Individualized Treatment of Pseudo-Epileptic Seizures. In L Gram, SI Johannessen, PO Osterman, M Sillanpaa (eds), Pseudo-Epileptic Seizures. Petersfield, UK: Wrightson Biomedical, 1993.
43. Bowman ES, Maybury BG. Psychiatric diagnoses and abuse histories of males with nonepileptic seizures. Epilepsia 1996;37(Suppl 5):17.

Appendix 21.1. Paradigm for Interviewing Patients with Non-Epileptic Seizures

The steps below constitute a useful way to approach interviewing about life events associated with non-epileptic seizures (NES). With practice, such an assessment can usually be accomplished in a 90-minute exploratory interview, and a reasonable working model for the cause of NES can be formulated.

1. Ask about remote trauma or early emotional pain.
2. Ask about cumulative losses: death, health, job, finances, moves, and relationships (from divorce to "empty nest" syndrome).
3. Assess the patient's usual way of coping with feelings (the family can sometimes tell you this information most accurately). Look specifically at anger, depression or grief, and anxiety.
4. Look for current life contexts (listed in Table 21.2) that often contribute to stress or conflict. Families may be helpful sources of such information.
5. Look for discrete events (see Table 21.1) that might be immediate precipitants of the NES, and look for symbolism that might tie events to remote conflicts.
6. Look for three general patterns: (1) old trauma and recent reminders, (2) solely adulthood trauma, and (3) a gradual buildup of adverse life events or frustrations in a person with marginal emotional coping ability.

Be humble! A few patients will baffle you!

CHAPTER 22

Non-Epileptic Seizures as a Paradigm for Research on Historical Theories of Conversion

Kenneth R. Alper

This chapter summarizes clinical research on non-epileptic seizures (NES) at the New York University Comprehensive Epilepsy Center (NYU CEC). The high rate of presentation of patients with NES to CECs, as well as the relatively high comorbidity of epilepsy and NES,[1] makes the CEC an excellent environment in which to study patients with conversion disorder presenting as NES. A major advantage is the medical diagnostic accuracy conferred by video-electroencephalographic (VEEG) monitoring under the supervision of qualified epileptologists. We report here about research on patients with conversion disorder presenting as NES as it relates to some of the major historical theories on conversion, namely, those of Jean Martin Charcot and his two students, Sigmund Freud and Pierre Janet.

The study of NES has the potential for a richly productive research paradigm for psychoanalytic theory. The distinction between the subconscious versus conscious self-experience is a fundamental theoretical tenet of dynamic psychiatry and was originally stated by Sigmund Freud in 1893 in the context of his clinical observations on patients with "hysterical fits."[2] *DSM-IV (Diagnostic and Statistical Manual of Mental Disorders, Fourth Edition)* claims an "atheoretical" orientation. Yet, its definition of conversion is basically the same entity that Freud originally proposed. It still invokes the concept of a distinction between unconscious and conscious self-experience and the production of symptoms by subconscious intent to achieve the primary gain of neutralizing painful affect.

The advent of the neo-Freudian or ego psychology school has intensified interest in borderline levels of personality organization and their relation to dissociative states. Dissociation can be viewed as the disruption of the conscious experience or internal representation of the self. It is seen as a defensive response to trauma, functioning to mitigate an intolerable experience of the self interacting with the external world by interrupting or altering the self experience. Pierre Janet's emphasis on dissociation and the relationship of personality to the capacity for its development remains, to date, an influential contribution to dynamic psychiatry as evidenced by the classification of conversion in the *ICD-10 (International Classification of Diseases*, Tenth Edition) system in a merged dissociative (conversion) disorder category, as well as the significant body of clinical research on dissociation and its relationship to personality.[3]

In contrast to the historical tendency toward divergence between psychiatry and neurology, the recent past has seen the development of the fields of neuropsychiatry and behavioral neurology. Consistent with this trend is a reconsideration of Charcot's theory that some hysterical patients had a biological diathesis that conferred vulnerability for the development of conversion. Charcot held a view that agreed with his pupil, Freud, as to the psychological nature of symptom production in conversion but differed from Freud in viewing the tendency toward conversion as biologically determined, in other words, as "something a patient had, rather than did."[4]

At the NYU CEC, the diagnosis of NES is found in roughly 15–20% of admissions, which is within a similar range to the prevalence reported in most other CECs.[1] The diagnosis of conversion NES (C-NES) is made on the basis of an absence of epileptiform activity during the patient's typical events on 24-hour VEEG monitoring and a positive response to placebo in provoking or terminating typical episodes. Patients in whom NES is suspected are seen by the CEC neuropsychiatrist (KA) for a structured psychiatric assessment that includes the Structured Clinical Interview for *DSM-III-R* (Revised; SCID),[5] the self-rated version of the SCID-II,[6] the Dissociative experiences scale (DES),[7] the Beck anxiety inventory,[8] the Beck Depression Inventory,[9] the Hamilton Anxiety Scale,[10] and the Hamilton Depression Scale.[11] Abuse histories are obtained using the methodology described previously.[12] The definition of C-NES and its distinction from non-conversion NES (NC-NES) are also provided elsewhere.[13]

Hypotheses Regarding Conversion

Using the above methodology, we have had the opportunity to investigate some of the major hypotheses of Freud, Janet, and Charcot regarding conversion in patients with NES. In the remainder of this chapter, clinical findings are presented that relate to the following hypotheses:

1. Childhood trauma is a pathogenetic factor in conversion disorder.
2. As a defensive operation, conversion serves a primary gain function—that is, to mitigate or neutralize unpleasant conscious experience.
3. The clinical features of a conversion event tend to symbolically represent an underlying intrapsychic stressor.
4. There is an increased tendency toward dissociation in conversion disorder.
5. Neurologically evident brain dysfunction confers risk for conversion symptoms.

Childhood Trauma Is a Pathogenetic Factor in Conversion Disorder

Freud, Janet, and Charcot agreed on a pathogenetic contribution of childhood trauma to the subsequent development of conversion disorder. Charcot included both physical and emotional trauma as risk factors for conversion, as evidenced by his concept of "hysterotraumatism."[14,15] Janet emphasized the role of trauma in the genesis of dissociative pathology in vulnerable individuals.[3,4] Freud viewed conversion as an intrapsychic conflict expressed as a bodily symptom and, particularly in his earlier work, emphasized the role of childhood abuse in the formation of sexual conflict.[14]

As described elsewhere,[12] we routinely assess abuse histories at the NYU CEC. In the most recent gender-matched series of 132 patients with C-NES and 169 control subjects with complex partial epilepsy (CPE), childhood abuse was reported by 38% of patients with C-NES and 20% in CPE ($p = .007$). The C-NES patients also had a greater degree of severity in the type of sexual abuse in terms of incestuousness and sexual invasiveness.[12] A relationship of abuse severity to the tendency toward C-NES was not seen in patients reporting only physical abuse.

The greater qualitative severity of sexual, but not nonsexual, physical abuse in this study supports Freud's emphasis on sexual trauma in childhood as a pathogenetic factor in the later development of conversion. However, the data do not support Freud's attribution of exclusively sexual content to the production of conversion symptoms.[14] Although relatively more C-NES than CPE patients reported a history of abuse in childhood, a majority did not. This supports the existence of important determinants of conversion in addition to childhood sexual trauma.

Further evidence consistent with a distinctive pathogenetic contribution of childhood abuse to the development of conversion is the distinction of NC-NES from C-NES.[13] Seventy-one patients with C-NES and 21 patients with NC-NES were compared. NC-NES consisted of nonconversion psychiatric presentations, including panic disorder, psychotic disorders, or tic disorders. In this sample, a history of abuse in childhood was seen in 32% of those with C-NES and only 9% of the non-gender-matched

NC-NES subjects ($p = .03$). The female gender predominance commonly reported in C-NES[1] was not seen in the NC-NES sample. These findings are consistent with a specific relationship of abuse in childhood to the later development of conversion.

A methodological note should be made regarding the acquisition of abuse histories. The clinical dilemma concerning the reliability of memories of childhood abuse is represented in Freud's abandonment of the seduction theory and in the contemporary forensic controversy regarding recovered memories.[16,17] No doubt, individual patients may have elaborated or even fabricated such a history, whereas others may have omitted disclosing one. A specific step taken to improve the reliability of research data is the use of relatively conservative criteria to define childhood sexual abuse.[12] Generally, a positive correlation exists between reliability and the degree of conservatism in a clinical definition, and abuse is not likely to be an exception in this regard. In obtaining an abuse history, an effort is made not to lead patients or to communicate an excessive sense of salience about this issue. In such regard, inquiry about abuse is placed toward the middle of the interview, when professional rapport has been established during exploration of more neutral and less intimate topics. Questions regarding childhood abuse follow a sequence of inquiries that begin with ones that are unambiguously neurologic in nature. Patients are first asked about head trauma, then about physical trauma or assault as an adult, and only then about childhood abuse.

As a Defensive Operation, Conversion Serves a Primary Gain Function to Attenuate or Neutralize Unpleasant Conscious Experience

Freud's concept of primary gain remains consistent with the contemporary *DSM-IV* definition of conversion disorder, which retains a criterion for associated psychological factors.[18-20] Clinical data relating to this issue include the results of a questionnaire completed by 155 patients with CPE and 73 with C-NES.[21] The questionnaires probed patient beliefs that psychological stress served as a precipitant of their events. Seventy-one percent of the CPE patients perceived an association between the experience of psychological stress and more frequent events. This figure is very close to the 72% reported in another series of CPE patients.[22] However, only 46% of patients with C-NES acknowledged a relationship of psychological stress to their events, a highly significant difference ($p < .0005$).

One interpretation of these results is that C-NES patients may not be aware of the relationship of their events to stress precisely because of the primary gain involved. That is, the patient remains unaware because the conversion symptom serves to alleviate the subjective experience of psychological stress, allowing the patient to avoid the conscious experience of an unendurable affect without consciously mastering or resolving underlying stressful issues.

Clinical Features of a Conversion Event Tend to Symbolically Represent an Underlying Intrapsychic Stressor

The idea of symbolic content is stated by Freud: "The motor phenomena of hysterical attacks can be interpreted partly as universal forms of reaction appropriate to the affect accompanying memory . . . partly as a direct expression of these memories."[23] VEEG affords the opportunity to systematically analyze and classify ictal phenomenology.[24] One hundred fifty C-NES patients were studied. Conversion events were classified according to the epilepsy-like syndrome most strongly resembled. Events were therefore classified as resembling a generalized tonic-clonic seizure (GTCS), a complex partial seizure, a simple partial seizure, or a syncopal episode. In addition, potentially symbolic ictal phenomena, such as violent behavior (thrashing, kicking, punching, screaming), pelvic thrusting, crying, spitting, and side-to-side head movement, were noted.

Some interesting associations between ictal symptomatology and abuse history were found in these individuals with C-NES. Patients with differing types of trauma appeared to manifest different behaviors during events. Patients with NES resembling GTCS reported more frequent histories of childhood sexual abuse with greater degrees of sexual invasiveness and coerciveness than did the other phenomenologic types, findings similar to those reported previously by Betts and Boden.[25] The syncopal-NES type of event appeared to be associated with physical abuse.

These findings are generally compatible with a formulation of the symbolic representation of trauma in conversion symptoms. A GTCS-like event might be expected to more closely resemble movements suggestive of sexual intercourse than would syncopal events or NES that resemble most partial epileptic events. The movements of subjects whose episodes resembled syncopal events could be plausibly regarded as symbolically reenacting their movements while being victimized by violence or reenacting a behavioral adaptation to evade further physical assault.

There Is an Increased Tendency toward Dissociation in Conversion Disorder

DSM-IV provides separate categories for dissociative disorders and subsumes conversion under the somatoform disorders[18–20] that could be interpreted to imply that dissociation and conversion are distinct processes. This implication is not universally accepted, as evidenced by the classification of conversion disorder as a dissociative (conversion) disorder in the *ICD-10* system.

At the heart of the theoretical distinction of conversion from dissociation is Freud's formulation of repression as the essential defensive operation in conversion. Freud emphasized a model of conversion in which a wish or self-image that was incompatible with the idealized self-representation of the superego is actively excluded from conscious awareness. The self-experience remains intact and continuous, whereas the repressed contents remain sequestered from awareness. This contrasts with dissociation, which Janet viewed as contributing to conversion by causing "a retraction of personal consciousness," which then permits the behavioral acting out of dissociated memories and personality functions.[26] In repression, the model stresses the active exclusion of a particular stressor from an otherwise intact self-experience. In dissociation, the formulation emphasizes the failure of controlling and monitoring functions of the self in the context of a weakening of the executive functions of the personality.

Janet's ideas regarding dissociation and its relationship to conversion have an interesting resonance with current theoretical interest in ego psychology and dissociative phenomena. There is a general correspondence between Janet's concept of failure to regulate behavior due to the dissociation of the observing from the controlling self and the concept of ego weakness giving rise to impulsive acting out. With trauma, there is an increased liability for dissociation, as well as for the development of states characterized by ego weakness such as borderline personality disorder.[3] Janet believed that a loss of "nervous energy" resulted in the failure of normally integrated functions mediating between intentional action and conscious experience.[27] There is a resonance between this idea and the current concept that borderline personality disorder involves recurrent chronic exposure to stress in development, giving rise to states of impaired ego functions that result in the dissociation of the monitoring and controlling functions of the self. At the NYU CEC we administered the DES[7] to 132 patients with C-NES and 169 with CPE.[28] The control groups were matched for age, gender, and educational status. We hypothesized that the overall DES score would be higher in C-NES. However, only a trend was seen in this direction, with a mean DES score of 15.1 in C-NES and 12.7 in CPE ($p = .079$). These scores are elevated above those reported in normal populations but below the cutoff of 20 suggested for the dissociative disorders.[7]

We also hypothesized that the DES has a heterogeneous underlying item content. Principal component analysis with varimax rotation yielded five factors that accounted for nearly 54% of the variance. Three of these factors appeared to be interpretable and reasonably robust statistically and were in general agreement with other factor analytic studies of the DES. The factor that accounted for the greatest share of variance appeared to constellate items relating directly to derealization and depersonalization. This factor was elevated in C-NES ($p = .005$), but the difference was marginal when the C-NES subjects who reported a history of childhood abuse were withheld from the comparison ($p = .064$). This result is consistent with childhood trauma as an important mediating factor in the relationship of dissociation to conversion but suggests that dissociation is more strongly related to childhood trauma than to the tendency toward conversion symptoms. The relatively nonspecific nature of the relationship of dissociation to conversion found in this study tends to support the current *DSM-IV* distinction of conversion disorder from the dissociative disorders.

Another factor, termed *absorption-imaginative involvement*, appeared to contain some features seen in post-traumatic stress disorder, such as vivid memories and difficulties with attention and concentration. This factor may be related to childhood trauma. It was elevated in abused subjects irrespective of their neurologic diagnosis ($p = .001$) and was not different in C-NES versus CPE when subjects reporting abuse were withheld from the analysis ($p = .203$). Again, a history of abuse in childhood, and not conversion per se, appeared to be the more consistent correlate of dissociation.

A third factor, termed simply *amnesic*, appeared to constellate items of the DES that could be attributed to poor memory, such as not remembering important people or events or misplacing objects. This factor showed no significant relationship to a history of abuse in childhood. Scores on this factor showed a trend toward being greater in C-NES than CPE patients ($p = .056$), suggesting that the items might be caused by memory impairment due to a neurologic condition. The amnesic factor appears to have partially confounded the C-NES versus CPE distinction using total DES scores because these were greater in CPE patients, whereas scores on the other factors were generally higher in those with C-NES.

Neurologically Evident Brain Dysfunction Confers Risk for Conversion Symptoms

Charcot believed in the existence of a neurologically determined diathesis toward conversion, even when a specific lesion could not be explicitly demonstrated.[26] Charcot's general formulation is supported by a substantial literature on the occurrence of conversion symptoms in neurologic or other medical conditions. A study using operationally defined criteria for Charcot's syndrome of hysteria found it to be associated with diffuse brain injury due to trauma, anoxia, or hypoglycemia.[29] The exacerbation of NES by anti-epileptic drug toxicity is another example of an apparent association between conditions that diffusely affect the brain and conversion.[30]

An observation that might bear on Charcot's concept of conversion is the comorbidity of NES and epilepsy. The rate at the NYU CEC has been 20%,[12] which is the range generally reported for CECs.[1] This rate is obviously much greater than the expected association on the basis of chance alone and implies a causal relationship between epilepsy and the subsequent development of NES. Several mechanisms could account for this relationship, including symptom modeling, a specific effect of epilepsy, or a general risk associated with multiple neurologic conditions including epilepsy. The available evidence suggests that epilepsy does not confer greater risk for conversion symptoms than for other neurologic symptoms but that the epileptic patient with conversion is relatively more likely to manifest NES due to symptom modeling.[1]

References

1. Alper K. Nonepileptic seizures. Neurol Clin 1994;12:153.
2. Freud S. On the Physical Mechanism of Hysterical Phenomena: Preliminary Communication. In J Strachey, A Freud (eds), The Standard Edition of the Complete Psychological Works of Sigmund Freud, vol 2. London: Hogarth, 1965;3–17.
3. Spiegel D, Cardena E. Disintegrated experience: the dissociative disorders revisited. J Abnorm Psychol 1991;100:366.
4. Slavney PR. Perspectives on Hysteria. Baltimore: Johns Hopkins University, 1990.
5. Spitzer RL, Williams JB, Gibbon M, First MB. Structured Clinical Interview for DSM-III R (patient ed). With Psychotic Screen—SCID-P, version 1.0. Washington, DC: American Psychiatric Press, 1990.
6. Spitzer RL, Williams JB, Gibbon M, First MB. Structured Clinical Interview for DSM-III-R. Personality Disorders (SCID-II, questionnaire). Washington, DC: American Psychiatric Press, 1990.
7. Bernstein EM, Putnam EW. Development, reliability, and validity of a dissociation scale. J Nerv Ment Dis 1986;174:727.
8. Beck AT, Brown G, Epstein N, Steer RA. An inventory for measuring clinical anxiety: psychometric properties. J Consult Clin Psychol 1988;56:893.
9. Beck AT, Ward CH, Mendelson M, et al. An inventory for measuring depression. Arch Gen Psychiatry 1961;4:561.
10. Hamilton M. The assessment of anxiety states by rating. Br J Med Psychol 1959;32:50.
11. Hamilton M. Rating depressive patients. J Clin Psychiatry 1980;41:21.
12. Alper K, Devinsky O, Perrine K, et al. Nonepileptic seizures and childhood sexual and physical abuse. Neurology 1993;43:1950.
13. Alper K, Devinsky O, Perrine K, et al. Psychiatric classification of nonconversion nonepileptic seizures. Arch Neurol 1995;52:199.
14. Mace CJ. Hysterical conversion I: a history. Br J Psychiatry 1992;161:369.
15. Toone B. Disorders of Hysterical Conversion. In CM Bass, RH Cawley (eds), Somatization: Physical Symptoms and Psychological Illness. Oxford: Blackwell Scientific, 1990;207–234.
16. Loftus EF. The reality of repressed memories. Am Psychol 1993;48:518.
17. Gutheil TG. True or false memories of sexual abuse? A forensic psychiatric view. Psychiatr Ann 1993;23:527.
18. Martin RL. Diagnostic issues for conversion disorder. Hosp Comm Psychiatry 1992;43:771.
19. Martin RL. DSM-IV: changes for the somatoform disorders. Psychiatr Ann 1995;25:29.

20. Martin RL. Conversion Disorder, Proposed Autonomic Disorder, and Pseudocysesis. In TA Widiger, AJ Frances, HA Pincus, et al. (eds), DSM-IV Source Book, vol 2. Washington, DC: American Psychiatric Association, 1996;893.
21. Luciano D, Perrine K, Clayton B, Devinsky O. Stress as a seizure precipitant and its relationship to ictal focus. Epilepsia 1992;33(Suppl 3):130.
22. Fenton GW. Epilepsy and hysteria. Br J Psychiatry 1986;149:28.
23. Freud S. Some General Remarks on Hysterical Attacks (1908). In J Strachey, A Freud (eds), The Standard Edition of the Complete Psychological Works of Sigmund Freud, vol 9. London: Hogarth, 1959;229–234.
24. Luciano D, Barkan M, Devinsky O, et al. Abuse history and ictal semiology of nonepileptic psychogenic seizures. Epilepsia 1995;36(Suppl 4):161.
25. Betts T, Boden S. Diagnosis, management and prognosis of a group of 128 patients with nonepileptic attack disorder. Part 2. Previous childhood sexual abuse in the aetiology of these disorders. Seizure 1992;1:27.
26. Nemiah J. Somatoform Disorder. In HS Kaplan, BJ Sadock (eds), Comprehensive Textbook of Psychiatry. Baltimore: Williams & Wilkins, 1985;924–942.
27. Nemiah J. Dissociative Disorders (Hysterical Neurosis, Dissociative Type). In HS Kaplan, BJ Sadock (eds), Comprehensive Textbook of Psychiatry. Baltimore: Williams & Wilkins, 1985;942–957.
28. Alper K, Devinsky O, Perrine K, et al. Dissociation in epilepsy and conversion non-epileptic seizures. Epilepsia 1997;38:991–997.
29. Eames P. Hysteria following brain injury. J Neurol Neurosurg Psychiatry 1992;55:1046.
30. Niedemeyer E, Blumer D, Holscher E, et al. Classical hysterical seizures facilitated by anticonvulsant toxicity. Psychiatr Clin 1970;3:71.

CHAPTER 23

Use of Hypnosis to Differentiate Epileptic from Non-Epileptic Events

John J. Barry and Orit Atzmon

In 1861, Hughlings Jackson introduced our present understanding of seizures as originating from abnormal structures that produce "excessive and disorderly discharge of nerve tissue."[1,2] Epilepsy results from chance paroxysmal discharge. Non-epileptic events (NEE) are episodic behavioral changes that resemble epileptic events (EE) but are without abnormal brain electrical discharges as measured by the electroencephalogram (EEG).

NEE can be divided into two categories, those that are physiologic and those that arise from psychological causes, often termed *pseudoseizures*. In the former category, syncopal episodes of cardiac and noncardiac origin, as well as sleep, metabolic, and other neurologic disorders, must be ruled out.[2] Frontal lobe epileptic events are particularly difficult to discriminate from NEE because EEG changes often are not present.[3] Investigators have used a variety of diagnostic methods to discriminate between NEE and EE. Because NEE of psychological origin and EE can occur in the same individual (in 8–40%), the task is formidable.[4]

NEE are responsible for between 5% and 20% of the patients evaluated for epilepsy and between 10–40% of patients referred to comprehensive epilepsy centers.[5-8] It is estimated that 200,000–400,000 patients who experience NEE have been evaluated medically. The importance of a correct diagnosis cannot be overemphasized. The inappropriate use of anti-epileptic drugs alone or in combination can have significant side effects, from respiratory arrest in patients with pseudostatus[9] to potential teratogenicity of anti-epileptic drugs in patients with NEE.

Once physiologic causes in the patient with NEE have been ruled out, psychological investigations become of paramount importance. NEE from psychological etiologies can be further divided into those events that occur with unconscious versus conscious awareness. The latter group are examples of factitious disorder or malingering.

Non-Epileptic Events as a Somatoform Disorder

Those patients whose "seizures" occur without conscious awareness of the event or its cause represent the majority of patients with NEE. Most of these patients meet criteria for a somatoform disorder, often of a conversion type, that is, unexplained neurologic-appearing deficits that are judged to be secondary to psychological causes.[10] Blumer[11] has coined the term *paroxysmal somatoform disorder* to emphasize the association of other somatic complaints, especially chronic pain, in these patients. A more severe form of this disorder, called *somatization disorder* or *Briquet's syndrome*, was described by Perly and Guze[12] and requires multiple unexplained medical symptoms, often including pseudoneurologic complaints.

Katon et al.[13] have emphasized the association of depression and somatization. They conceptualized that these patients have a language dysfunction. Because of sociocultural and childhood experiences, affective and cognitive components of their depression are ignored, and distress is expressed in somatic ways.

The role of trauma in the etiology of NEE has been commented on by Bowman in two reviews. The first study included 27 patients with NEE and found that 88% had some form of trauma, most with a positive history of sexual abuse.[14] In the second, 45 patients with NEE were evaluated; 89% were diagnosed with dissociative disorders, and another 49% met criteria for post-traumatic stress disorder.[10]

Charcot popularized the term *hysteroepilepsy* for seizures of psychological origin. He was also responsible for a provocative test to both elicit and terminate these events.[4] The link between dissociation and trauma was originally clarified by Janet.[15] Having learned the technique from Charcot, he used hypnosis as a tool to uncover a wide variety of dissociative phenomena.

Peterson et al.[16] used hypnosis and a recall technique to help discriminate between patients with EE and those with NEE. They reasoned that epileptic patients would be amnesic for events that occurred during a seizure, whereas patients with NEE would retain good recall. These postulates were borne out when they hypnotized 45 patients. The 20 epileptics had amnesia for the details of their seizures. In contrast, the 25 NEE patients remembered the environmental particulars that occurred during their psychogenic events.

Schwartz et al.[17] used hypnosis to induce NEE. In a trance state they simulated previous "seizure"-instigating situations. In the 16 patients evaluated with histories of epileptic events, none had their seizures induced. Ten patients with NEE experienced events without EEG changes. Interestingly, two of this group had a history of positive EEGs in the past, therefore representing examples of patients with both EE and NEE.

Diagnostic Techniques Including Suggestion

In addition to unique clinical and historical characteristics, a variety of diagnostic tests have been used to discriminate between patients with EE and those with NEE. These include the Minnesota Multiphasic Personality Inventory,[18-20] the Millon Clinical Multiaxial Inventory,[21] the Wechsler Adult Intelligence Scale,[22] the Dissociative Experiences Scale,[23] auditory evoked potential,[24] elevations, and prolactin increases after an event.[25]

All of these methods have been reported to have varying degrees of sensitivity and specificity. The most valid diagnostic method is the occurrence of a patient's typical events during video-EEG monitoring.[26,27] Even this technique is not without error, however. Scalp EEG can be normal in patients with EE, especially in patients with simple partial seizures.[28] Frontal lobe complex partial seizures, especially of medial and orbital frontal regions, often occur in the presence of a normal EEG.[29] These patients often present with "hysterical" features. Their events characteristically occur nocturnally and are of short ictal duration with stereotyped movements.

In patients who present with histories of sexual abuse, an affective disorder, and prolonged epileptic events (usually beyond 90 seconds), a diagnosis of NEE must be strongly entertained.[3] The use of suggestion to secure a diagnosis is an extremely helpful tool. A psychogenic seizure can be induced and terminated by several different techniques. One must adhere to several caveats, however.

It is important to recall that up to 8–40% of patients evaluated in an inpatient setting have both NEE and EE.[4] It is therefore imperative to make sure that an individual event is a typical one. In patients with several different types of events, some may be NEE and may be able to be precipitated by suggestion. Others emanate from a true epileptic focus and generally are nonresponsive to these techniques.

TABLE 23.1
Hypnotic Induction Profile

Measure of hypnotizability
Combines a measure of the patient's innate ability to be hypnotized, as measured by the eye-roll sign, with a measure of hypnotic expression, the induction score
Scores range from 0 to 10
Hypnotic potential without hypnotizability = decrement profile

---

Three primary types of suggestion induction techniques have been described. All are used while the patient is being monitored with continuous video-EEG. The placebo intravenous infusion method uses saline as a seizure precipitating agent.[30] In a similar fashion, the alcohol patch method attempts to induce a psychogenic seizure by placing the device on the patient's neck, with the individual being told that it contains an agent that may promote an event.[31] Both methods require less than full disclosure at the specific agent used and may result in compromising the patient's trust. Instead of promoting an atmosphere of cooperation, a therapeutic barrier[4] may result.

Hypnotic Induction Profile with Seizure Initiation

The Hypnotic Induction Profile (HIP) was developed by Spiegel and Spiegel in the 1970s.[32] It is a measure of a patient's hypnotizability and dissociability traits, which are frequently seen in individuals with NEE. It correlates well with other hypnotizability scales[33] and is described in Table 23.1.

After an HIP score is obtained, the use of hypnosis for seizure induction ensues (Table 23.2). With the patient hypnotized, a split-screen technique is used. The subjects imagine a safe secure scene on one side of the screen and then shifts their attention to the other side. The patient is then asked to imagine viewing himself or herself having a typical event. The subject is asked to recall a recent "seizure" and to describe it in full. As with Peterson's previous study, full recall, except with frontal lobe complex partial seizures, is usually pathognomonic of an NEE. Patients are then asked to experience the event being witnessed, and seizure induction follows. Patients can shift from one screen to the other, starting and stopping events, thereby increasing the diagnostic validity of the test. Because the entire procedure is explained to the patients, full disclosure takes place. Furthermore, the patient is taught the technique and can use it to control events in the future.[34–36]

TABLE 23.2
Hypnosis and Seizure Induction

Patient is hypnotized and taught relaxation
Split-screen technique is used
Patient is asked to recall his or her last seizure, and the extent of memory for that event is determined
An attempt at seizure induction ensues
Patient is taught the technique and can often self-induce and terminate non-epileptic events

Comparison Reliability of Diagnostic Tests

Walczak et al.[37] used the placebo infusion method in 68 patients and found that 82% of subjects with NEE had typical psychogenic events induced by the procedure. In 8% of the NEE group, atypical events were produced. In two (10%) epileptic patients, the placebo infusion method resulted in the induction of true epileptic seizures. Lancman et al.[31] used the alcohol patch method in 93 cases of patients with NEE and found a diagnostic sensitivity of 77.4% and a specificity of 100%.

In a current study by the authors, preliminary results indicate that the sensitivity of hypnosis with seizure induction to discriminate between NEE and EE is similar to the other suggestion techniques noted previously. Overall HIP scores appear lower for epileptic patients than for the NEE group or those patients with both EE and NEE.

Patients who demonstrate the ability to be hypnotized during the hypnotic induction but who go on to show little further ability to be hypnotized are given a decrement profile on the HIP. To date, most of the patients with NEE in the aforementioned study who failed to experience induction of their typical events via hypnosis had decrement scores on the HIP; additionally, they were considered to have a possible diagnosis of factitious disorder or malingering because of significant drug abuse histories, apparent antisocial personality disorders, and/or florid secondary gain issues. It also has been noted by Spiegel and Spiegel[32] that a decrement profile is often associated with significant psychopathology. The use of the HIP to diagnose these patients is hypothetical and must be further clarified, but it might help to identify this very difficult-to-diagnose population.

Hypnosis with seizure induction is also being compared by the authors in another study, with other diagnostic tests reported to be useful for discriminating between NEE and EE. Only hypnosis with seizure induction and a diagnosis on the SCID-E[38] (Structured Clinical Interview for the *Diagnostic and Statistical Manual of Mental Disorders,* Third Edition [Revised], Epilepsy Version) of major depressive disorder, past or present, has thus far proved significantly discriminatory. Both studies suggest the validity of the use of hypnosis as a diagnostic tool.

Overview

Five subgroups of patients with NEE have been proposed.[39] These categories include those patients who misinterpret abnormal physical sensations as seizures, often after neurologic consultation. Another group has documented seizure activity in addition to NEE. Hypnosis may be very useful for these groups, teaching relaxation techniques and showing patients how to use hypnosis to turn their events on and off.

Two other cohorts present a different set of problems. Those patients who are psychotic need psychotropic drugs and are not good hypnosis candidates.[32] Individuals who are of borderline intellectual ability may present with NEE. These patients generally manifest behavioral dysfunction to express distress generated from psychosocial difficulties. A search for an environmental cause is usually curative, coupled with behavioral interventions.[39]

By far the largest and most challenging group consists of patients who express emotional conflict via somatic channels and present with symptoms of NEE. The vast majority of these patients have experienced some form of abuse, either physical, psychological, or both.[14] These experiences have biological and psychological consequences.

Trauma can cause organic changes, resulting in individuals becoming hypersensitive to their surroundings. Neurotransmitters may be permanently affected, with the development of decreased serotonin levels and abnormal down-regulation of norepinephrine. Corticosteroids and endogenous opioids also may be affected. In addition, heightened sensitization of the amygdala and right hemispheric activity have been noted.[40] These changes may explain the frequent occurrence of depression and personality dysfunction in patients who have experienced trauma. The usefulness of antidepressants in patients with NEE may stem from these physiologic changes.

Psychologically, throughout life the human organism strives to develop an environment that is predictable and safe. Those individuals who have experienced a severe break in attachment, via trauma, may never develop this concept of the world[41] and, as noted previously, this is a frequent occurrence in patients with NEE. Dissociation becomes the primary defense mechanism that protects the patient from past, present, and future distress. Hypnosis is an excellent tool in measuring dissociability and is, therefore, an ideal technique to diagnose the presence of NEE.

Hypnosis has other unique features. It dramatically helps the patient accept the diagnosis of NEE by giving the individual a means to potentially decrease these events. It is critical to remember that NEE represents a safeguard against severe emotional tumult, and it cannot be taken away without a replacement for this treasured defensive tool. Hypnosis offers not only a technique to modulate these events but, more important, increases the therapeutic alliance with the patient, an absolute necessity for eventual cure. In the authors' experience, it provides a useful conduit to longer-term therapy by allowing the patient a method to control events while an atmosphere of trust develops. Eventually, as the therapy progresses, "seizures" often abate and are replaced by increased verbal ability to define an underlying conflict. With this increased awareness, the patient may become depressed or may have a previously apparent depression worsen. Psychopharmacologic intervention often becomes imperative.

Although the technique just described is no panacea, it can be a useful instrument to discriminate between NEE and EE. In an age of managed care, developing a diagnosis and treatment plan often must be accomplished in the shortest possible period of time. Hypnosis can facilitate this goal by giving the patient a tool to decrease events. It also helps the individual accept the results of the evaluation. Finally, hypnosis assists in the introduction of individual, and possibly group, psychotherapy.

References

1. Glaser OH. Historical Perspectives and Future Directions. In E Wyllie (ed), The Treatment of Epilepsy: Principles and Practice. Philadelphia: Lea & Febiger, 1993;3–10.
2. Rowan AJ. An Introduction to Current Practice in the Diagnosis of Nonepileptic Seizures. In AJ Rowan, JR Gates (eds), Non-Epileptic Seizures. Boston: Butterworth–Heinemann, 1993;1–9.
3. Saygi S, Katz A, Marks DA, Spencer S. Frontal lobe partial seizures and psychogenic seizures: comparison of clinical and ictal characteristics. Neurology 1992;42:1274–1277.
4. Gates JR, Luciano D, Devinsky O. The Classification and Treatment of Nonepileptic Events. In O Devinsky, WH Theodore (eds), Epilepsy and Behavior. New York: Wiley-Liss, 1991;251–263.
5. Lempert T, Schmidt D. Natural history and outcome of psychogenic seizures: a clinical study of 50 patients. J Neurol 1990;237:35–38.
6. Lesser RP. Psychogenic seizures. Neurology 1996;46:1499–1507.
7. Volvow MR, Durham NC. Pseudoseizures: an overview. South Med J 1986;79:600–607.
8. Krumholtz A, Niedermeyer E, Alkaitis D, Morel R. Psychogenic seizures: a five year follow-up study. Neurology 1980;30:392.
9. Howell SJL, Owen L, Chadwick DW. Pseudostatus epilepticus. QJM 1989;71:507–519.
10. Bowman ES, Markand ON. Psychodynamics and psychiatric diagnoses of pseudoseizure subjects. Am J Psychiatry 1996;153:1:57–63.

11. Blumer D. The Paroxysmal Somatoform Disorder: A Series of Patients with Nonepileptic Seizures. In AJ Rowan, JR Gates (eds), Non-Epileptic Seizures. Boston: Butterworth–Heinemann, 1993;165–173.
12. Katon W, Lin E, Von Korff M, et al. Somatization: a spectrum of severity. Am J Psychiatry 1991;148:34–40.
13. Katon W, Kleinman A, Rosen O. Depression and somatization: a review. Parts 1 and 2. Am J Med 1982;72:127–135,241–247.
14. Bowman ES. Etiology and clinical course of pseudoseizures; relationship to trauma, depression, and dissociation. Psychosomatics 1993;34:333–342.
15. van der Kolk BA, van der Hart O. Pierre Janet and the breakdown of adaptation in psychological trauma. Am J Psychiatry 1989;146:1530–1540.
16. Peterson DB, Sumner JW, Jones GA. Role of hypnosis in differentiation of epileptic from convulsive-like seizures. Am J Psychiatry 1950;107:428–432.
17. Schwartz BE, Bickford RG, Rasmussen WC. Hypnotic phenomena, including hypnotically activated seizures, studied with electroencephalogram. J Nerv Ment Dis 1955;122:564–574.
18. Wilkus RJ, Dodrill CB, Thompson PM. Intensive EEG monitoring and psychological studies of patients with pseudoepileptic seizures. Neurology 1984;25:100–107.
19. Henrichs TF, Tucker DM, Farha J, Novelly RA. MMPI indices in the identification of patients evidencing pseudoseizures. Epilepsia 1988;29:184–187.
20. Vanderzant CW, Giordani B, Berent S, et al. Personality of patients with pseudoseizures. Neurology 1986;36:664–668.
21. Thompson PM, Batzel LW, Wilkus RJ. Millon clinical multiaxial inventory assessments of patients manifesting either psychogenic or epileptic seizures. J Epilepsy 1992;5:226–230.
22. Mason S, Risse GL, Gates JR, Relick N. The relationship between subjective memory complaints and objective test performance in patients with psychogenic seizures. Epilepsia 1992;33:134.
23. Alper K. Use of the dissociative experiences scale in differentiating epileptic from non-epileptic patients. Presentation at Non-Epileptic Seizures, A Consensus Conference on the Diagnosis and Treatment, Washington, DC, April 1996.
24. Drake ME, Huber ST, Pakalnis A, Phillips BB. Neuropsychological and event-related potential correlates of nonepileptic seizures. J Neuropsychiatry 1993;5:102–104.
25. Pritchard PB. The effect of seizures on hormones. Epilepsia 1991;32:S46.
26. Meierkord H, Will B, Fish D, Shorvon S. The clinical features and prognosis of pseudoseizures diagnosed using video-EEG telemetry. Neurology 1991;41:1643–1646.
27. Pierelli F, Chatrian GE, Erdly WW, Swanson PD. Long-term EEG-video-monitoring: detection of partial epileptic seizures and psychogenic episodes of 24-hour EEG record review. Epilepsia 1989;30:513–523.
28. Cascino GD. Ictal Extracranial EEG. In E Wyllie (ed), The Treatment of Epilepsy: Principles and Practice. Philadelphia: Lea & Febiger,1993;261–267.

29. Williamson PD, Spencer DD, Spencer SS, et al. Complex partial seizures of frontal lobe origin. Ann Neurol 1985;18:497–504.
30. Cohen R, Suter C. Hysterical seizures: suggestion as a provocative EEG test. Ann Neurol 1982;11:391–395.
31. Lancman ME, Asconape JJ, Craven WJ, et al. Predictive value of induction of psychogenic seizures by suggestion. Ann Neurol 1994;35:359–361.
32. Spiegel H, Spiegel D. Trance and Treatment: Clinical Uses of Hypnosis. New York: Basic Books, 1978.
33. Frischholz EJ, Spiegel D, Spiegel H. The hypnotic induction profile and absorption. Am J Clin Hypn 1987;30:2:87–94.
34. Bush E, Barry J, Spiegel D, et al. The successful treatment of pseudoseizures with hypnosis. Epilepsia 1992;33:135.
35. Gravitz MA. Hypnotherapeutic management of epileptic behavior. Am J Clin Hypn 1979;21:282–284.
36. Miller HR. Psychogenic seizures treated by hypnosis. Am J Clin Hypn 1983;25:248–252.
37. Walczak TS, Williams DT, Berten W. Utility and reliability of placebo infusion in the evaluation of patients with seizures. Neurology 1994;44:394–399.
38. Victoroff JI, Spitzer RL, Williams JB, et al. Structured Clinical Interview for DSM III-R Epilepsy Version. Los Angeles: UCLA School of Medicine, Department of Neurology, 1989.
39. Gates JR, Erdahl P. Classification of Nonepileptic Events. In AJ Rowan, JR Gates (eds), Non-Epileptic Seizures. Boston: Butterworth–Heinemann, 1993;21–31.
40. van der Kolk BA. The Body Keeps the Score: Approaches to the Psychobiology of Posttraumatic Stress Disorder. In BA van der Kolk, AC McFarlane, L Weisaeth (eds), Traumatic Stress: The Overwhelming Experience of Mind, Body, and Society. New York: Guilford, 1996;214–241.
41. van der Kolk BA, van der Hart O, Marmar CH. Dissociation and Information Processing in Posttraumatic Stress Disorder. In BA van der Kolk, AC McFarlane, L Weisaeth (eds), Traumatic Stress: The Overwhelming Experience of Mind, Body, and Society. New York: Guilford, 1996;303–327.

CHAPTER 24

On the Psychobiology of Non-Epileptic Seizures

Dietrich Blumer

The predicament is familiar. On completing intensive neurodiagnostic procedures, the patient is informed that he or she has non-epileptic seizures (NES). There is no need for anti-epileptic medication, and it may be much better not to have epilepsy. The patient asks for the name of the disorder and is told, in so many words, that it is psychogenic seizures. The predicament of experiencing uncontrollable fits of passing out and convulsing as the result of a mental problem is both embarrassing and difficult for the patient to grasp.

NES frequently are the somatic result of unbearable past events and a currently conflicted life situation. The patient, who has valiantly brushed aside the impact of painful memories, finds it difficult to verbalize conflicts in psychotherapy and hesitates to comply with such treatment. On the other hand, NES also exist that are not related to painful life events.

A better understanding of the psychobiology of NES may render the condition less embarrassing and more treatable. The disorder that presents with NES as the main symptom was termed *hysteria* in premodern medicine; in modern psychiatry, it is listed among the somatoform disorders. Preferable terminology would reflect specifically the psychobiology of the disorder, if it can be identified.

This chapter is based on the findings of the evaluation and treatment of patients with NES at the Epi-Care Center over the past 10 years. The topic is complex and the formulations admittedly tentative.

Findings

In a series of 34 consecutive patients with NES, a very high prevalence of somatoform symptoms and of pain in particular (in 82% of the patients) was noted.[1] In almost one-half of the patients, severe pain was a prodrome to the attack, often in a crescendo pattern, increasing to the point of becoming unbearable as the attack became manifest. A history of prolonged physical or sexual abuse, or both, was frequently obtained. On the other hand, all but 8 of the 34 patients had at least some evidence of cerebral impairment, by significant history, magnetic resonance imaging, electroencephalography, or neuropsychological testing. The psychiatric history showed a high prevalence of mostly unipolar depressive episodes, suicide attempts, and psychiatric hospitalizations. A basic depressive state can be recognized in patients with NES, less by the presence of overt depressed mood than by an anergic state and the complaint of persistent, bodily experienced pain. Before the manifestation of their illness, they typically had maintained an adjustment as hard-working citizens.

In a more recent series, the presence of pain, as well as the history of psychologically traumatic events in patients with epileptic seizures (ES) and NES, was studied.[2] In this series of 68 patients, all of whom underwent long-term video-electroencephalographic monitoring, 32 had ES, 17 had NES, and 11 had both ES and NES (8 had other or undetermined events). Prodromal pain, occurring in 75%, was noted almost exclusively among the NES patients. Pain after the attack was present more evenly among the two groups, whereas significant pain in between the attacks was found twice as often among the patients with NES (82%). The prodromal pain occurred again, often in the previously described crescendo pattern, and can be considered virtually pathognomonic for NES. The history of trauma and abuse was more prevalent among the patients with NES.

Apart from the two series, we have observed four patients over the past several years who since childhood reacted to either sudden fear or pain with an NES-like startle response but who had no history of either brain damage or painful psychological trauma. They may be recognized as individuals with an innate low threshold for NES or startle response.

Psychobiology of Non-Epileptic Seizures

Where there is much atypical pain, there is much hidden suffering and often a history of psychological trauma and abuse. It is plausible that the past experience of severe and protracted trauma, the impact of which was brushed aside, may return in a flashback and be reenacted in the attack.

Kretschmer[3] had a view of hysterical events surprisingly similar to that of Freud, but Kretschmer further postulated that the hysterical reaction made use of "reflex, instinctive or otherwise biologically preformed mechanisms," particularly in the form of either a *motility storm* consisting of regression in a state of terror with hyperkinesis, screaming, trembling, and convulsing, or of *sham death* with stupor, immobilization, hiding, or a hypnoid state. These are the same primitive reactions that can be observed when healthy individuals experience mortal fear on being faced with a sudden life-threatening catastrophe, such as an earthquake or a bombardment.

The archaic or primitive reactions are paroxysmal in nature but may be prolonged. In post-traumatic hysteria or NES, the original trauma appears to be relived, with screams absent, eyes shut, inability to run, and intense pain typically present.

What could be the neurologic basis of the biologically preformed mechanisms of the hysterical reaction or of NES, respectively? Matsumoto and Hallett[4] have discussed the startle syndromes, and under the heading of hyperexplexia (which includes any movement disorder in which there is a physiologic demonstration of exaggerated startle reflexes) they list post-traumatic startle disorders together with those secondary to brain damage (particularly involving the brain stem and thalamus) and idiopathic cases. Similarly, many patients can be observed whose NES appear secondary to past emotional trauma, a smaller group with NES after brain damage, and a few individuals who, in the absence of preceding mental or cerebral trauma, have reacted since childhood to either sudden physical pain or a sudden fear with an NES-like startle response.

Startle responses in animals may result in powerful motor innervation. Human startle responses, as studied in the laboratory with the help of an unexpected loud noise, are rather subtle. The eyes close, and a grimace occurs with a predominantly flexor motor innervation and assumption of a defensive posture; this is followed by more varied and complex components.[5] The response is less stereotyped than an ES. The acoustic startle circuit has been well established by animal experiments[6] as a pathway involving four neuronal zones: from the ventral cochlear nucleus to the ventral nucleus of the lateral lemniscus, to the motor effector area for the startle response in the pontomedullary reticular formation (nucleus reticularis pontis caudalis), and via reticulospinal pathways to the alpha motor neurons. Furthermore, and of particular importance if one considers that fear must be involved in the startle response, the existence of a ventral amygdalofugal tract that projects from the central amygdaloid nucleus to the motor effector area of the startle response in the brain stem has been established. The same pathways are present in humans.

Exaggerated startle reflexes have been documented both in war veterans and in women with sexual assault–related post-traumatic stress disorder.[7-9] In both groups, startle would increase after the exposure to trauma but would tend to normalize with the passage of time. Three of our patients with long-standing NES were studied for abnormal startle reflexes in Mark Hallett's laboratory at the National Institutes of Health with no significant findings. The challenge to document the plausible kinship of NES to exaggerated startle reflexes remains.

The startle (or surprise) response or reflex obviously occurs not merely on sudden unexpected sensory input as practiced in the laboratory experiment but notably on frightening and terrifying events and has the value of a basic instinct to secure survival. Szondi[10] viewed this archaic paroxysmal instinct as the basis of a universal human need to protect from danger; this need becomes engaged in hysteria as the individual responds to an unbearable threat by various forms of motility storm or immobilization.

The extraordinary prevalence of patients with NES who have memories of terrifying life events suggests that the startle mechanism may become engaged in a chronically recurrent pattern in these individuals.

Terminology

In a search for the neural basis of the NES, the hypothesis of its kinship to the startle syndromes has been offered. Once this kinship is found acceptable, one can choose the term *complex startle seizures* for NES and *complex startle disorder* for the illness. The syndrome associated with complex startle seizures (NES) commonly includes anergia, pain, and other somatoform symptoms but still needs to be better established. The novel term would seem preferable to the term *paroxysmal somatoform disorder*, which was earlier proposed[1] in keeping with a modern psychiatric terminology that focuses on the description of syndromes.

Hysteria was named according to the basic mechanism that was believed to be involved (the wandering womb). The ancient name was only recently discarded. The term *startle disorder* would recognize the primary neural mechanism in NES and has no offensive connotation. Patients with seizures who are told they do not have epilepsy could relate to a designation of their illness that emphasizes the role of a universal human reflex in the response to exceptionally painful life events. The same understanding would be helpful to professional observers, who tend to react with dismay to a paroxysm that they do not recognize as a neurologic disorder.

The startle disorder, although commonly post-traumatic, may also occur secondary to brain damage. Impairment of cerebral functions, perhaps most importantly epilepsy, appears to facilitate NES. Finally, there is a small group of individuals with idiopathic startle disorder whose condition could be termed *simple startle disorder*.

Treatment

The treatment for NES at the Epi-Care Center consists of prescribing an antidepressant combined with an antianxiety drug or the beta-adrenergic blocker propranolol (often at a high dose), or both, and if possible with psychotherapy. In a few patients, antidepressants alone have been surprisingly effective for NES.

Propranolol has been useful for post-traumatic stress disorder[11] and, at exceptionally high doses, for individuals who had been exposed to prolonged extreme abuse in childhood and developed a dissociative identity disorder in later life.[12] It has not been unusual for us to find patients with dissociative identity disorder among those diagnosed as having NES, and we can confirm the effectiveness of their treatment with high doses of propranolol combined with psychotherapy. Patients with NES and individuals with dissociative identity disorder notably have in common the unbearable headaches that precede a seizure or a dissociative event, respectively.

NES usually are more prolonged than ES and on occasion may present resembling status epilepticus. Misdiagnosis and heroic treatment of such "NES status" with anti-epileptic drugs can be fatal.[13] At the Epi-Care Center, we have been able to terminate NES status by the intramuscular injection of a strong analgesic; prolonged experience of severe pain appeared to have prolonged the attack. In our present opinion, the pharmacologic treatment for NES is definitely helpful but needs further corroboration and improvement.

Conclusion

A theory of NES needs to consider its common post-traumatic nature, the near omnipresent experience of pain with frequent crescendo before the attacks, and the dynamic psychobiological nature of the events. The premodern findings on what was then termed *hysteria*, with its paroxysmal and more persistent presentation, should not be ignored. The role of brain damage and the relationship to epilepsy also need to be considered. Finally, the theory should have a bearing on how the disorder can be treated or perhaps prevented.

In its conventional use, the term *startle response* refers to the effect of a sudden, unpleasant sensory input. The assumption that the same innate response apparatus is set in motion on sudden danger or fright is not farfetched. Trauma causes pain, and unbearable pain is often dealt with by repression or dissociation. Yet the concealed painful memories remain present as dynamic factors and are triggered in flashbacks at a later time. Thus, an exogenous paroxysmal response (hysterical attack) is provoked and may be mistaken for an endogenous epileptic paroxysm. The vulnerability to suffer a complex startle attack (NES) appears to be enhanced in individuals with epilepsy, as well as after certain forms of brain damage, and the phenomenon of startle epilepsy has been documented.

It appears that not only psychotherapy but pharmacologic interventions promise help for NES. A combination of the two types of interventions may be most effective. By preventing wars, we are more successful in saving soldiers from trauma. Finding a means to prevent domestic abuse with women and children as the victims remains a problem.

References

1. Blumer D. The Paroxysmal Somatoform Disorder: A Series of Patients with Non-Epileptic Seizures. In AJ Rowan, JR Gates (eds), Non-Epileptic Seizures. Boston: Butterworth–Heinemann, 1993;165–172.
2. Blumer D, Phillips B, Montouris G, et al. Pain associated with epileptic and non-epileptic seizures. Epilepsia 1995;36(Suppl 4):158.
3. Kretschmer E. Hysteria. New York: Nervous and Mental Disease Publishing Co, 1926.
4. Matsumoto J, Hallett M. Startle Syndromes. In CD Marsden, S Fahn (eds), Movement Disorders. Oxford: Butterworth–Heinemann, 1994:418–433.
5. Landis C, Hunt WA. The Startle Pattern. New York: Farrar and Rinehart, 1939.
6. Davis M, Gendelman DS, Tischler MD, Gendelman PM. A primary acoustic startle circuit: lesion and stimulation studies. J Neurosci 1982;2:791.
7. Morgan CA III, Grillon C, Lubin H, Southwick SM. Startle reflex abnormalities in women with sexual assault-related posttraumatic stress disorder. Am J Psychiatry 1997;154:1076.
8. Grillon C, Morgan CA III, Davis M, Charney DS. Baseline startle amplitude and prepulse inhibition in Vietnam veterans with posttraumatic stress disorder. Psychiatry Res 1996;64:169.
9. Morgan CA III, Grillon C, Southwick SM, et al. Exaggerated acoustic startle reflex in Gulf War veterans with posttraumatic stress disorder. Am J Psychiatry 1996;153:64.
10. Szondi L. Triebpathologie. Bern, Switzerland: Hans Huber, 1952.
11. Silver JM, Sandberg DP, Hales RE, et al. New approaches in the pharmacotherapy of posttraumatic stress disorder. J Clin Psychiatry 1990;51(Suppl 10):33.
12. Braun B. Unusual medication regimens in the treatment of dissociative disorder patients. Part 1: Noradrenergic agents. Dissociation 1990;3:144.
13. Pakalnis A, Drake ME Jr, Phillips B. Neuropsychiatric aspects of psychogenic status epilepticus. Neurology 1991;41:1104.

CHAPTER 25

Treatment of the Adult Patient with Non-Epileptic Seizures

Venkat Ramani

The neuropsychiatrists of the early nineteenth century were quite familiar with the clinical problem of feigned epilepsy. *Hysteroepilepsy*, a term coined by Charcot, was a subject of intense interest for neurologists during the second half of the 1800s. The term *pseudoseizures* was introduced by Liske and Forster in 1964. The modern era in the study of non-epileptic seizures (NES) began in the mid-1970s with the availability of electrophysiologic intensive monitoring techniques in comprehensive epilepsy centers. The diagnostic approach to NES became progressively more refined over the next two decades. Today, simultaneous video-electroencephalographic (EEG) monitoring technology is firmly established as the gold standard for the diagnosis of NES, especially in complex cases in which NES may coexist with genuine epilepsy. Despite these advances in the diagnostic aspects of NES, treatment of this disorder has not received systematic attention. Charcot used ovarian compression for the treatment of hysteria, and Gowers prescribed iron tonic to correct the presumed underlying anemia. The psychiatric profession until now has largely ignored a systematic approach to the treatment of the NES patient, presumably because of the inherent diagnostic ambiguities and the general pessimism among mental health professionals regarding the therapeutic results with somatoform disorders.

A comprehensive review of the treatment strategies in NES can be found in the first edition of this book and in several sections of this, the second edition. This chapter will highlight the treatment strategies and consensus from Part IV of this volume.

Based on two decades of experience, there is now a general consensus among epileptologists that NES is a treatable condition. Most investigators have emphasized a multidisciplinary team approach. A number of unanswered questions remain, however. The criteria for treatment success have not been established, and the various treatment techniques have not been standardized. One long-term follow-up study, which found that NES may substantially improve after diagnostic clarification even without formal psychotherapy, raises important questions about the place of long-term psychiatric treatment in today's cost-conscious managed care environment. It is very encouraging to note the current progress in quantitative assessment of psychopathology and neuropsychological deficits in NES patients. It is hoped that advances in these areas can provide a rational basis for identifying clinical subgroups among NES patients based on which specific treatment strategies can be developed for each group. In the following section, the views expressed by a panel of experts on treatment of NES are summarized.

Dr. Elizabeth Bowman

According to Dr. Elizabeth Bowman, the study of NES has moved a long way since the days when all such patients were classified as hysterics. Research on the classification of the underlying causes of NES is far ahead of research on treatment. This is appropriate because treatment properly rests on accurate diagnostic classification and a search for the etiology of seizures. It is only in the past 5–10 years that any order has begun to emerge from the diagnostic chaos, thus allowing us to study treatment and its outcome. The literature shows that most authors agree that NES has no single cause. Accordingly, no single treatment has dominated. Over the years, proposed treatments have ranged from ovarian manipulation to exorcism, hypnosis, and psychoanalytically oriented psychotherapies. Outcome has not correlated well with treatment approaches or even with receiving treatment. Is there any way to bring order to such a confusing situation? Dr. Bowman believes that treatment is best approached by viewing NES as the presenting symptom of several clusters of problems and then tailoring treatment to the underlying problem. These problems have been repeatedly identified in the literature, as discussed below.

Major depression or grief and bereavement associated with losses may underlie NES in some cases. Patients in this cluster seem to respond best to a combination of antidepressant medication and psychotherapy. Panic attacks are often misdiagnosed as seizures. In this group, treatment with antianxiety medications alone is not uniformly helpful. Therapeutic exploration of the underlying trauma that might be contributing to the panic or dissociative flashbacks may be indicated in these patients. The role of childhood abuse and trauma in the etiology of conversion disorders has been well emphasized in the literature. In this group, a combination of hypnosis and individual psychotherapy may be effective in abreacting and achieving control over dissociative seizure symptoms. It is important to realize that some patients in this dissociative group report auditory hallucinations, which may result in misdiagnosis of the condition as atypical psychosis. Dr. Bowman recommends the following systematic approach to the treatment of NES:

1. Assess for depression. If major depression is present, start treatment with antidepressant drugs and plan to treat for at least 6 months. Assess if psychotherapy is also needed. Indications for psychotherapy (in addition to medications) include depression related to incomplete bereavement and depression related to ongoing conflicts or stress.
2. Assess for panic disorder. If panic is a regular feature of the clinical episodes, begin an antipanic drug. Try initial low doses of selective serotonin reuptake inhibitors (SSRIs) such as fluoxetine and sertraline first. Use benzodiazepines only temporarily or if an adequate dose of SSRI is ineffective. Cognitive therapy to reduce and prevent panic attacks is essential to prevent relapse when antipanic medications are withdrawn.
3. Assess for a history of trauma (adulthood trauma and child abuse). If it seems etiologically related to the seizures, psychotherapy to process the trauma is essential. This generally involves verbal processing of the trauma, abreaction of the related emotions, and cognitive restructuring to reduce the impact.
4. Assess for dissociative disorders (amnesia, fugue, depersonalization, derealization, and identity alterations). These are usually related to a history of psychological trauma. If NES are related to such trauma that resultant dissociated ego states of personality exist, psychotherapy should be started to facilitate the expression of the dissociated affect and the reduction of amnesic barriers. Hypnosis may be helpful in bridging amnesia between ego states and in helping the person access affect about the trauma.
5. Assess for other life events or conflicts that may be causing NES. Identify complicated bereavement, family or marital conflict, or unexpressed anger/frustration and direct therapy to address these issues.
6. Finally, if the cause for NES is not clear, hypnosis (see Dr. Barry's discussion) may be helpful in teaching the patient how to control the expression of seizures.

Dr. Kent Mercer

Dr. Kent Mercer reports that the comprehensive inpatient treatment approach is used at the Minnesota Epilepsy Group for the management of

NES. This approach does not differentiate assessment/diagnosis from treatment. The inpatient milieu is sensitive to the possibility of NES. A supportive, nonjudgmental attitude is maintained. All events are treated as bona fide seizures until proved otherwise by video-EEG evidence. The diagnosis of NES is made based on definitive video-EEG recording of multiple events without ictal EEG correlate. A comprehensive inpatient evaluation is conducted by a multidisciplinary treatment team consisting of the epileptologist, a clinical neuropsychologist, a social worker, dedicated nursing staff, EEG technologists, and a consulting psychiatrist. Careful psychosocial assessment examines the relative strengths and weaknesses of the patient and the environmental support systems; treatment guidelines are based on this evaluation. Comprehensive psychosocial history focuses on past trauma, recent stressors, and current support systems. A great deal of attention is paid to the presentation of the diagnosis of NES to the patient and the family members. This is done in a carefully orchestrated manner by the multidisciplinary treatment team in order to facilitate insight and to set the stage for continued psychotherapy. The patient's understanding of the nature of his or her condition and its psychological causes is considered important for successful treatment outcome.

Dr. Mercer has reported the results of the Minnesota Epilepsy Group experience with 29 adult NES patients who were followed for an average of 27 months after the diagnosis. Patients did not receive any systematic outpatient psychiatric follow-up treatment. The outcome was evaluated by a telephone survey using a 15-item questionnaire. At follow-up, 11 patients were free of seizures, whereas 18 continued to experience NES. The author emphasizes the importance of early diagnosis of NES as well as psychoeducational efforts designed to improve patient understanding of the NES diagnosis and treatment recommendations.

Dr. Kenneth Alper

Dr. Kenneth Alper emphasizes the presentation of the diagnosis of NES to the patient as the crucial first step in treatment. After accurate video-EEG diagnosis of NES, the diagnosis is presented to the patient by the multidisciplinary team. An aggressive search for a primary *DSM-IV (Diagnostic and Statistical Manual of Mental Disorders*, Fourth Edition) axis I disorder is made and, if present, is treated vigorously. In some cases, axis II conditions or personality disorders may be important in treatment considerations. In all cases the symptom is seen as a coping mechanism, and the treatment is directed at helping the patient to learn more appropriate coping ways to deal with stress. Depression may emerge during the course of treatment (as in the treatment of addictions), as the patient gives up maladaptive old ways while trying to learn more appropriate new coping strategies.

Dr. Alper emphasizes the following points in the treatment of NES:

1. Treatment begins with the presentation of the diagnosis of NES.
2. Treat the underlying axis I pathology appropriately.
3. There is an analogy between NES and addictions in that both conditions involve compulsive behaviors whose motivation is not consciously recognized by the patient, and the behavior serves the primary gain of avoiding stress/conflict.
4. A commitment to change on the part of the patient is more important for a favorable treatment outcome than the physician's ability to come up with causal explanations for the seizures.

Dr. Dietrich Blumer

Dr. Dietrich Blumer emphasizes a number of important factors in therapy for NES. He stresses the importance of a trusting relationship between the patient and the therapist and the problems patients often have in this area because of prior abuse or trauma. He also stresses the potential negative influence of a dysfunctional family milieu in therapy. A subgroup of patients whose seizures are triggered by pain, fatigue, stress, and fear may do well with supportive therapy. Ideally, psychotherapy is indicated in most cases of NES, but Dr. Blumer calls attention to the limitations to proper psychotherapy by the constraints of time and financial issues in today's health care environment. A judicious use of psychoactive drugs is important in the therapy of NES. Overtreatment with drugs may result in toxic encephalopathies, secondary emergence of regressive behavioral patterns, and increased frequency of NES.

Dr. John Barry

Like the other authors, Dr. John Barry emphasizes the importance of how the diagnosis of NES is initially presented to the patient and family. He stresses the importance of recognizing axis I disorders. He also calls attention to the cultural underpinnings of the conversion symptomatology. He emphasizes the value of hypnosis in certain subsets of NES patients. Patients who misinterpret their abnormal physical sensations as seizures and those who augment their seizure symptoms may be good candidates for relaxation therapy and hypnosis. Psychotic patients who require drug therapy and patients with borderline intelligence may be good candidates for environmental therapy, but hypnotherapy may not be appropriate.

The most challenging group consists of patients who express emotional conflicts through somatic channels or NES. The vast majority of these patients have a history of physical, emotional, or sexual trauma. In this group, hypnosis can be very effective. It dramatically helps the patient to accept the diagnosis of NES by giving the individual a means to potentially decrease these events. It provides the patient a sense of self-control. Hypnosis also facilitates therapeutic alliance, which is the basis for long-term psychotherapy. Dr. Barry cautions about the limitations of telephone surveys in treatment outcome research because of the tendency of NES patients to minimize their symptoms in order to please the physician. In his concluding remarks, Dr. Barry calls attention to the problem of inadequate financial reimbursement for psychotherapy and the need to develop cost-effective group therapeutic strategies for NES in today's cost-conscious managed health care environment.

Summary

There is a good deal of agreement among the authors regarding the nature of NES, its treatment, and its outcome. They are unanimous in their opinion that NES is treatable. NES is a heterogeneous condition with diverse etiologies, and treatment should, therefore, be individualized. Accurate video-EEG diagnostic confirmation is important before treatment. The diagnosis of NES should be presented to the patient and the family in a supportive, nonjudgmental fashion by a multidisciplinary treatment team. Treatment should be individualized with an appropriate combination of drug, cognitive, behavior, psychodynamic, and family therapies as well as hypnosis. Depression, panic disorder, and personality disorders should be addressed in therapy when appropriate. A history of physical, emotional, and sexual trauma is frequently present in NES patients that render them vulnerable to dissociative and conversion disorders. These issues should be dealt with in psychotherapy for successful treatment outcome in NES.

Index

Note: Page numbers followed by *f* indicate figures; page numbers followed by *t* indicate tables.

Abdominal epilepsy, 59
Absence seizures, 21
Absence status, 63
Acute stress disorder, 12
Adolescents, non-epileptic seizures in, perceptions of, 227–235, 247–248
  by adolescents, 229–232
  interviews for, 228–229
  by parents, 232–234
  qualitative methodologies for, 228
Alcoholic blackout, 65
Alternating hemiplegia of childhood, 97
Alternating hemiplegia of infancy, 64
Amnesia, 24, 58t
  after temporal lobe seizure, 64
Amok, 11
Anxiety disorders, 11–12, 151–156, 154t
  decision tree for, 257t, 259f, 261–262
  neuropsychological testing in, 120–121
Aprosexia, 126
Arousal
  disorders of, 73–75
    model of, 74
    treatment of, 74
  pure tonic seizures and, 77
  recurrent, seizures and, 78
Arrhythmias, 24, 53
Asthma, anoxic convulsions in, 53, 56
Asystole, syncope and, 53
Ataque de nervious, 11
Ataxia, paroxysmal, 60

Atropine, in breath-holding spells, 100
Auditory reflex epilepsy, 43
Automatisms
  in frontal lobe seizures, 40
  in temporal lobe seizures, 41
Autonomic seizures, pure tonic seizures with, 77–78
Avoidance behavior, during psychogenic non-epileptic seizures, 20

Behavior patterns, reinforcement of, 13
Benign myoclonus, 96
Benign paroxysmal vertigo, 98–99
Breath-holding spells, 64–65, 99–100
Briquet's syndrome, 254
Bulimia, nocturnal, 73
Button game, in pediatric evaluation, 214–215, 216f

California Verbal Learning Test, 134
Cataplexy, 65
Child/person in rain technique, in pediatric evaluation, 217, 218f
Children
  alternating hemiplegia in, 64, 97
  benign myoclonus in, 96
  benign paroxysmal vertigo in, 98–99
  breath-holding spells in, 64–65, 99–100
  cardiac arrhythmias in, 100
  conversion reaction in, 101
  night terrors in, 100

317

Children (continued)
    non-epileptic seizures in, 95–106,
        197–205. See also specific
        disorders.
        age-based differences in, 198
        case studies of, 102–106
        categories of, 96, 96f
        demographic factors in, 199–200,
            199t, 204
        developmental history and, 200
        medical history and, 201, 205
        misdiagnosis of, 95
        neurologic history and, 201–202, 205
        onset of, 202, 202f, 203f
        physiologic, 96–101, 103f
        prevalence of, 102
        psychiatric disorders and, 202–203
        psychiatric history and, 201, 204
        psychogenic, 101–102, 185–194. See
            also Psychogenic non-epileptic seizures, pediatric.
        psychosocial stressors and,
            200–201
        risk factors for, 197–202
        school performance and, 200, 204
        stressors and, 200–201, 204
    shuddering attacks in, 64
    spasmus nutans in, 97
Choreoathetosis, paroxysmal, 60
Classification, 256–266, 257t,
        258f–259f. See also Seizure-like events, decision tree for.
Cognition, 125, 139–149
    evaluation of, 142–144, 144t. See also
        Neuropsychological testing.
    in adult non-epileptic seizures,
        126–134, 128t, 130t, 131f,
        132f, 132t
    in pediatric non-epileptic seizures,
        191–193, 191t, 192t, 193t
    patient reports on, 142, 142t
    psychiatric disorders and, 125–126
    Wechsler Adult Intelligence Scale
        for, 140
Cognitive reflex epilepsy, 42–43

Complex partial seizures
    frontal lobe, 40
    temporal lobe, 41
Confusion, 58t
Conversion disorder, 8–9, 185, 246. See
        also Psychogenic non-epileptic seizures, pediatric.
    features of, 187–188, 188t
    historical theories of, 285–292
        brain dysfunction and, 291–292
        childhood trauma and, 287–288
        dissociation and, 289–291
        primary gain function and, 288
        symbolic content and, 289
    neuropsychological testing in,
        117–118
    sexual abuse in, 188–189, 188t
    stressors in, 188–189, 188t, 190–191,
        190t, 191t
Crying, during psychogenic non-epileptic seizures, 20

Decerebrate attacks, 7, 65
Depersonalization disorder, 11
Depression, 151–156, 154t
    neuropsychological testing in,
        119–121
    somatization and, 296
Diencephalic seizures, pure tonic
        seizures with, 77–78
Diencephalic syndromes, 62–63
Dissociative disorders, 10–11, 286,
        289–291
    vs. parasomnias, 81, 82
Dissociative disorders not otherwise
        specified, 11
Dissociative fugue, 10
Dreams, seizures as, 76
Drop attacks, 65
Dyskinesias, paroxysmal, 60–61
Dystonia, paroxysmal, 60

Electroencephalography, 35
    in nocturnal seizures, 78–79
Enuresis, 23, 62

Epilepsy, terminological use of, 254–255
Epileptic seizures. *See also specific types.*
　misdiagnosis of, 36–38, 37t, 52
　vs. non-epileptic seizures, 20–21, 33–45, 34t, 37t, 39t
　non-epileptic seizures and, 4–5, 45–46
　quality of life and, 160–161
Episodic nocturnal wanderings, 76–77

Factitious disorder, 12–13
Finger-tapping speed test, 117
Focal epileptic seizures, 21
Frontal lobe seizures, 20–21, 38, 39t, 40
Fugue states, 10–11, 24, 63–64

Gastroesophageal reflux, in children, 97–98
Gelastic seizures, 44–45

Hallucinations, 58t, 62–63
Hallucinosis, peduncular, 63
Halstead-Reitan index, 125, 126
Hamartoma, hypothalamic, 39t, 44–45
Hemiplegia, alternating
　of childhood, 97
　of infancy, 64
House-tree-person technique, in pediatric evaluation, 215–216, 217f
Hyperexplexia, 61
　neonatal, 98
Hypnogenic paroxysmal dystonia, 77
Hypnotic induction profile, 298, 298t, 299t
Hypnotism, 242
Hypochondriasis, 10
Hypoglycemia, 65
Hypothalamic hamartoma, 44–45
Hysteria, 3–4
　Minnesota Multiphasic Personality Inventory tests for, 131f, 132t, 133, 146, 147f
Hysterical epilepsy, 5–6

Infant. *See also* Children.
　alternating hemiplegia in, 64, 97
　benign paroxysmal vertigo in, 98–99
　breath-holding spells in, 99–100
　gastroesophageal reflux in, 97–98
　hyperexplexia in, 98
　masturbation in, 98
　shuddering attacks in, 98
　spasmus nutans in, 97

Jumping, 61–62
Juvenile myoclonic epilepsy, 44

Kleine-Levin syndrome, 63

Latah, 11
Light-sensitive epilepsy, 42
Likert scale analogue, in pediatric evaluation, 213, 215f
Locomotor centers, in rapid eye movement behavior disorder, 75–76
Long-QT syndrome, in children, 100

Malingering, 12–13, 24–25
　decision tree for, 257t, 259f, 262–263
　neuropsychological testing in, 117–118
Masturbation, infantile, 98
Migraine headache, 7, 22, 54t, 56–57
Minnesota Multiphasic Personality Inventory, 26–27, 124–125, 126, 129–130, 131f, 132f, 132t, 133
　cognition study and, 145–146, 147f
　literature review on, 123, 172t, 173t–178t, 174–179, 176t
　quality of life study and, 161–162, 163, 164–165, 165t
Mood disorders, 12, 126, 151–156, 154t. *See also specific disorders.*
　decision tree for, 257t, 259f, 261–262
Movement disorders, 7, 22, 54t, 56t, 60–62
Multiple sclerosis, tonic attacks in, 60

Munchausen syndrome by proxy, 101, 237–241
  clinical characteristics of, 238–240
  management of, 240–241
Myoclonic jerks, 39t, 44
Myoclonus, 61–62
  benign, 96
  non-epileptic, 54t
Myorhythmia, 61

Narcolepsy, 23
Neonate. *See* Infant.
Neuropsychological testing, 26–27, 115–122, 125. *See also* Minnesota Multiphasic Personality Inventory.
  case studies of, 117–121
  components of, 116–117
  contextual evaluation of, 9
  empirical study of, 126–134, 128t, 130t, 131f, 132t
  future of, 10
  limitations of, 117, 148
  literature review of, 170–171
  original studies of, 171–174, 172t, 173t
  in psychiatric disorders, 125–126, 129–130, 130t, 148
Night terrors, 23, 62, 73–75, 100
Nightmares, seizures as, 76
Nocturnal dystonia, paroxysmal, 61
Nocturnal myoclonus, 62, 80
Nocturnal seizures, 76–78
  diagnosis of, 78–80
Non-epileptic paroxysmal neurologic events, 51–66, 54t–55t, 56t, 57t, 58t
Non-epileptic seizures, 6f, 32t
  clinical presentation of, 33–35, 34t
  convulsive, 35
  diagnosis of, 31–46, 112
    electroencephalogram in, 35–36
    patient history in, 33
    prolactin measurement in, 36
  epidemiology of, 4–5, 111
  vs. epileptic seizures, 33–45, 34t, 37t, 39t
  epileptic seizures and, 45–46
  historical perspective on, 3–4, 33
  incidence of, 4–5, 111
  life event precipitants of, 269–271
    case studies of, 274–277
    contextual, 276–277, 276t
    immediate, 273–276
    investigation of, 272–279, 273t
    literature review on, 270–272
    recurrent patterns of, 279–280
    remote, 277–279, 278t
    stressful, 271–272
    traumatic, 270
  physiologic, 6–7, 7f, 21–25. *See also specific disorders.*
  placebo activation of, 45
  psychobiology of, 305–310
    pain and, 306
    primitive reactions and, 307–308
  psychogenic, 8–13, 8f. *See also* Psychogenic non-epileptic seizures.
  terminology for, 5–6, 254–255
  treatment of, 46, 308–309, 311–316
Nosology, 256–266, 257t, 258f–259f. *See also* Seizure-like events, decision tree for.

Oral fluency test, 116

Panic disorder, 11–12
  vs. parasomnias, 82
Parasomnias, 62, 71–83, 72f, 551
  categories of, 72–73
  primary, 73–76
  vs. psychiatric disorders, 80–82
  vs. psychogenic non-epileptic seizures, 22–23
  secondary, 76–80
Paroxysmal toxic disorders, 6–7
Paroxysmal vertigo, benign, 98–99
Peduncular hallucinosis, 63

Pelvic movements, in psychogenic non-epileptic seizures, 19
Periodic limb movement disorder, 80
Personality, 123–125. *See also* Minnesota Multiphasic Personality Inventory.
Petit mal seizures, vs. psychogenic non-epileptic seizures, 21
Photosensitive epilepsy, 42
Physiologic non-epileptic seizures, 6–7, 7f, 21–25. *See also specific disorders.*
Piplokto, 11
Post-traumatic stress disorder, 12
  neuropsychological testing in, 119–120
  vs. parasomnias, 81, 82
Posturing
  dystonic, in psychogenic non-epileptic seizures, 19
  tonic, in supplementary motor area seizures, 39
Pregnancy, dystonic attacks during, 60
Projective tests, in pediatric evaluation, 214–220, 216f
Prolactin, serum, 26, 36
Propranolol, in non-epileptic seizures, 309
Proprioceptive reflex epilepsy, 43
Pseudoseizure, 5
Pseudotemporal lobe epilepsy, 66
Psychogenic amnesia, 24
Psychogenic non-epileptic seizures, 8–13, 8f
  avoidance behavior during, 20
  cessation of, 18
  clinical signs of, 18–20
  crying during, 20
  diagnosis of, 15–29
    clinical signs in, 18–20
    differential, 20–25
    neuropsychological testing in, 26–27. *See also* Neuropsychological testing.
  patient history in, 16–18

  prolactin measurement in, 26
  video-electroencephalography monitoring in, 25–26
  differential diagnosis of, 20–25
  dystonic posturing in, 19
  emotional reaction to, 17
  emotional trigger of, 18
  epilepsy and, 17
  vs. epileptic seizures, 20–21, 34–45, 34t, 37t, 39t
  frequency of, 16
  hospitalizations and, 17
  injury in, 18
  motor activity in, 19
  observation of, 16–17
  onset of, 18
  pediatric, 101–102, 185–194
    A-B-C triplet change model for, 209, 210t
    cognitive function and, 191–193, 191t, 192t, 193t
    comorbid psychiatric disorders in, 189, 192, 192t
    demographic features of, 187, 187t, 189–190, 190t
    investigation of, 189–193, 190t, 191t, 192t, 193t
    literature review on, 185–189, 186t, 187t, 188t, 189t
    psychological assessment of, 207–225, 246–247
      button game for, 214–215, 216f
      child/person in rain technique for, 217, 218f
      follow-up for, 221
      goals of, 210–211
      house-tree-person technique for, 215–216, 217f
      initial meeting for, 212
      Likert scale analogue for, 213, 215f
      projective tests for, 214–220, 216f
      resistance in, 212, 220, 221
      rosebush technique for, 218, 219f
      squiggle game for, 218–219

Psychogenic non-epileptic seizures
    (*continued*)
  symptom externalization for,
      212–213, 213f, 214f
  sexual abuse in, 188–189, 188t
  stressors in, 188–189, 188t,
      190–191, 190t, 191t, 245–246
  symptoms management program
      for, 208–210, 210t
  treatment of, 208–210, 210t
    psychological, 220–221,
        222–225, 222t, 223t, 224t
  pelvic movements in, 19
  vs. physiologic non-epileptic seizures,
      21–25
  progression of, 18–19
  psychiatric disorders and, 18
  sexual abuse and, 17, 188–189, 188t
  suggestion and, 20, 45
  treatment of, 27–29
    anti-epileptic drugs in, 16
    multidisciplinary team for, 28, 46
    response to, 16
Psychosis, 12, 126
  decision tree for, 257t, 259f, 261–262
Pure tonic seizures, with arousal, 77

Quality of life, 159–161
Quality of Life in Epilepsy 89 study,
    163–168, 166t

Rapid eye movement behavior disorder,
    23–24, 62, 75–76
Reading reflex epilepsy, 42
Reflex epilepsy, 39t, 42–44
Rey Auditory Verbal Learning Test,
    116–117
Rhythmic movement disorder, 80
Romano-Ward syndrome, 53
Rosebush technique, in pediatric evaluation, 218, 219f

Sandifer's syndrome, 97–98
Schizophrenia, 12, 126
  decision tree for, 257t, 259f,
      261–262

Seizure-like events, 254
  decision tree for, 256–265, 258f–259f
    feigned events and, 257t, 259f,
        262–263
    medical condition and, 256, 257t,
        258f, 260–261
    mental disorder and, 257t, 259f,
        261–262
    psychogenic disorder and, 257t,
        259f, 262–265
    somatoform disorders and, 257t,
        259f, 263–265
    substance and, 256, 257t, 258f,
        260–261
Self-induced seizures, 43–44
Sexual abuse, 17, 188–189, 188t
Shuddering, 64, 98
Sleep, injury during, 75
Sleep disorders, 55t, 62, 71–83, 72f
  categories of, 72–73
  primary, 73–76
  vs. psychiatric disorders, 80–82
  vs. psychogenic non-epileptic
      seizures, 22–23
  secondary, 76–80
Sleep drunkenness, 62, 74
Sleep terrors, 23, 62, 73–75, 100
Sleepwalking, 23, 73–75, 76–77
Somatization disorder, 9, 254
Somatoform disorders, 8–10, 254, 255.
    See also Conversion
    disorder.
  decision tree for, 257t, 259f, 263–265
  non-epileptic events as, 296–297
  undifferentiated, 9–10
Somatosensory reflex epilepsy, 43
Spasmus nutans, 97
Speaking reflex epilepsy, 42
Squiggle game, in pediatric evaluation,
    218–219
Startle, 43, 54t, 61, 307–308, 309
Stokes-Adams attacks, 24
Stress disorder
  acute, 12
  post-traumatic, 12, 81, 82
Stretching, syncope and, 53

Subcortical seizures, pure tonic seizures with, 77–78
Suggestion induction techniques, 20, 45, 296–301, 298t, 299t
Supplementary motor area seizures, 20–21, 38, 39t, 40
Svengali syndrome, 241–244
Syncope, 6, 22, 53, 54t, 56
Syndrome de la calotte pedonculaire de l'Hermitte, 63
Syphilis, tertiary, 65

Temporal lobe seizures, 39t, 40–42
   amnesia after, 64
Thinking reflex epilepsy, 42–43
Transient global amnesia, 24, 64
Transient ischemic attack, 7, 24

Tremor, valproic acid and, 60

Valproic acid, tremor with, 60
Vascular headache, 59
Vasovagal attack, 64–65
Ventricular tachycardia, 24, 53
Vertigo, paroxysmal, benign, 98–99
Video-electroencephalography monitoring, 25–26, 35–36
Visual hallucinations, in temporal lobe seizures, 41
Visual illusions, in temporal lobe seizures, 41
Visual self-induced seizures, 43–44

Writing reflex epilepsy, 42